Contributions to Statistics

The series **Contributions to Statistics** features edited and conference volumes in theoretical and applied statistics. Composed of refereed selected contributions, the volumes present the latest developments in all the exciting areas of contemporary statistical research.

Preface

'Developments in Statistical Modelling' is a collection of 40 papers to be presented at the 38th International Workshop on Statistical Modelling (IWSM), which is held from 14th to 19th of July 2024 in Durham City, UK. The IWSM is the annual workshop of the Statistical Modelling Society, with the purpose of promoting important developments, extensions, and applications in statistical modelling and bringing together statisticians working on related problems from various disciplines. The contributions to this volume hence reflect this spirit.

The IWSM series has its roots in some rather informal meetings in the late 80s arising out of the GLIM community, which then got formalized in subsequent years to become a regular series of workshops. It has since travelled a few times to the UK: 1994 to Exeter, 2010 to Glasgow, 2018 to Bristol, and now in 2024 to Durham. Along this way, the initially informal network matured, with the launch of a journal, 'Statistical Modelling: An International Journal', in 2000, and the foundation of the Statistical Modelling Society in 2003.

We are honoured and delighted to be able to host this workshop at Durham, which, we believe, is a lovely location to host a conference in summer. The cathedral and the river wear equip the historic city centre with some unique flair. All relevant locations in the city can be reached by foot, and there is a stunning countryside—with the Pennines in the West and the Coast in the East—that delegates will have opportunity to explore. At this occasion, some rather distinctive mathematical history of Durham may also be mentioned: The Benedictine monk and historian Bede introduced in 725 a novel technique for finger counting; that is to count, with 10 fingers only, numbers up to 9999. The tradition of the name 'Bede' is still living forth: Durham is host to the Tier 2 supercomputer Bede, a facility of the N8 Centre of Excellence in Computationally Intensive Research (CIR).

The papers published in this volume were submitted in early 2024 for presentation at the conference, for either oral or poster presentation, and underwent a careful refereeing process involving the 18 members of the Scientific Committee plus a few other referees drawn from the Organizing Committee of the conference. Papers which were eligible for this volume (and consented to publication) underwent a second round of review. It is noted that this process did not distinguish between oral and poster submissions. As such, 29 of the 40 papers contained in this volume are presented orally at the conference, and 11 as posters. Notably, about half of the papers contained in this volume are presented by PhD students. It is noted that papers which are presented at the conference but which do not appear in this volume are provided in the conference online PDF proceedings volume which is available at https://maths.dur.ac.uk/iwsm2024/.

The papers presented in this volume cover developments in a wide range of disciplines including generalized linear models, mixture models, regularization techniques, hidden Markov models, smoothing methods, censoring and imputation techniques, Gaussian processes, spatial statistics, shape modelling, goodness-of-fit problems, network analysis, among others. A wide range of applications is considered within these papers, where a particular abundance of contributions in the field of biostatistics is notable. The contributions are equally frequentist and Bayesian—but this is anyway a categorization which this community has synergetically overcome.

We would like to draw particular attention to the keynote contribution 'Statistical Modelling for Big and Little Data' by Robin Henderson, which looks at contemporary data problems from the wider viewpoint of data science, encompassing statistics and machine learning, highlighting that both small and large data sets come with their own challenges, and can be equally simple—or hard!—to model and analyse.

We are looking forward to an enjoying and stimulating conference, and we hope that this volume will contribute to initiating and sustaining discussions about problems in statistical modelling, potentially triggering new developments and ideas. We are already now looking forward to the next edition of the workshop in Limerick in 2025 where perhaps some of these will be presented.

Acknowledgements. The Editors wish to thank the Durham Research Methods Centre (DRMC) for their financial support of the conference.

May 2024

Jochen Einbeck
Hyeyoung Maeng
Emmanuel Ogundimu
Konstantinos Perrakis

Contents

REML for Two-Dimensional P-Splines

Martin P. Boer(✉)

Wageningen University and Research, Wageningen, The Netherlands
martin.boer@wur.nl

Abstract. We propose a new method based on residual (or restricted) maximum likelihood (REML) for P-splines. Existing methods use a transformation of P-splines to a mixed model; in the new model it is shown that a more direct method can be used keeping the sparse structure of P-splines. The method is illustrated with a two-dimensional example using the R-package `LMMsolver` on CRAN. We will show that for this example `LMMsolver` is several orders of magnitude faster than other methods, which use a transformation of P-splines to mixed models where the sparse structure of P-splines is lost.

Keywords: Mixed models · Precision Matrices · Sparse Matrix Algebra

1 Introduction

Using B-splines for penalized regression, also known as P-splines [3], can offer computational efficiency due to the local character of B-splines. This results in sparse linear equations that can be solved easily. However, the primary challenge lies in determining the optimal penalty parameter. One effective approach to tackle this issue is through mixed models and restricted maximum likelihood (REML) [8]. Various methods have been suggested to convert the original penalized B-spline model into a mixed model. The drawback of most existing transformations to mixed models lies in their inability to preserve the local character of B-splines, consequently diminishing computational efficiency.

In [1] a new method was proposed, using a sparse transformation to mixed models. This method is computationally more efficient than other approaches. In this paper we will show that REML can be used directly for P-splines, without a transformation to a mixed model.

2 Sparse Mixed Models for P-Splines

We will first briefly discuss the sparse mixed model formulation proposed by Boer [1]. For the moment we will assume the one-dimensional case, to keep notation simple, and extend to two-dimensional case later on. First we introduce some notation. Let $\mathbf{y} = (y_1, y_2, \ldots, y_n)'$ be the response variable, depending on the

J. Einbeck et al. (Eds.): IWSM 2024, CONTRIB.STAT., pp. 1–6, 2024.
https://doi.org/10.1007/978-3-031-65723-8_1

variable $\mathbf{x} = (x_1, x_2, \ldots, x_n)'$, defined in the interval $[x_{\min}, x_{\max}]$. Let $\mathbf{B}$ be a $n \times q$ matrix, with (i,j)th entry $B_{j,p}(x_i)$, where $B_{j,p}$ are p-th degree B-splines functions for $j = 1, \ldots, q$. The constants $\xi_{i,j,p}$ are defined by

$$x^i = \sum_{j=1}^{q} \xi_{i,j,p} B_{j,p}(x), \quad x \in [x_{\min}, x_{\max}].$$

Analytic expressions for $\xi_{i,j,p}$ are given in [6]. The matrix $\mathbf{G}$ is a $q \times k$ matrix with (i,j)th entry $\xi_{i,j,p}$. The $q \times (q-k)$ matrix $\mathbf{D}$ has k-th order difference penalties. The matrix $\mathbf{X}$ is defined by $\mathbf{X} = \mathbf{BG} = [\mathbf{1}|\mathbf{x}^1|\ldots|\mathbf{x}^{k-1}]$, where $\mathbf{DG} = \mathbf{0}$. Let $\mathbf{B}_*$ be a $k \times q$ matrix, with (i,j)th entry $B_{j,p}(x_{*,i})$, where the k reference points $x_{*,i}$ can be chosen arbitrarily, with condition $|\mathbf{B}_*\mathbf{G}| \neq 0$, see [1] for further details.

The sparse mixed model formulation for P-splines is defined by [1]

$$\mathbf{y} = \mathbf{X}\boldsymbol{\beta} + \mathbf{Z}\mathbf{u} + \mathbf{e}, \quad \mathbf{u} \sim N(\mathbf{0}, \boldsymbol{\Sigma}), \quad \mathbf{e} \sim N(\mathbf{0}, \mathbf{R}), \tag{1}$$

with $\mathbf{X} = \mathbf{BG}$, $\mathbf{Z} = \mathbf{B}$, $\mathbf{R}^{-1} = \theta_0 \mathbf{I}_n$ and $\boldsymbol{\Sigma}^{-1} = \theta_1 (\mathbf{D}'\mathbf{D} + \mathbf{B}_*'\mathbf{B}_*)$. The restricted log-likelihood of Eq. (1) is given by

$$2 \log \mathcal{L} = \log|\mathbf{R}^{-1}| + \log|\boldsymbol{\Sigma}^{-1}| - \log|\mathbf{C}| - \hat{\mathbf{e}}'\mathbf{R}^{-1}\hat{\mathbf{e}} - \hat{\mathbf{u}}'\boldsymbol{\Sigma}^{-1}\hat{\mathbf{u}}, \tag{2}$$

where $\hat{\mathbf{e}} = \mathbf{y} - \mathbf{X}\hat{\boldsymbol{\beta}} - \mathbf{Z}\hat{\mathbf{u}}$. The mixed model equations are given by

$$\begin{pmatrix} \mathbf{X}'\mathbf{R}^{-1}\mathbf{X} & \mathbf{X}'\mathbf{R}^{-1}\mathbf{Z} \\ \mathbf{Z}'\mathbf{R}^{-1}\mathbf{X} & \mathbf{Z}'\mathbf{R}^{-1}\mathbf{Z} + \boldsymbol{\Sigma}^{-1} \end{pmatrix} \begin{pmatrix} \hat{\boldsymbol{\beta}} \\ \hat{\mathbf{u}} \end{pmatrix} = \begin{pmatrix} \mathbf{X}'\mathbf{R}^{-1}\mathbf{y} \\ \mathbf{Z}'\mathbf{R}^{-1}\mathbf{y} \end{pmatrix}, \tag{3}$$

with on the left hand side the mixed model coefficient matrix $\mathbf{C}$. The matrices $\mathbf{R}^{-1}$, $\boldsymbol{\Sigma}^{-1}$, and $\mathbf{C}$ are sparse for the mixed model P-splines model, and therefore $\log \mathcal{L}$ and the partial derivatives with respect to precision parameters θ_m can be calculated in a computationally efficient way.

Extension to two-dimension P-splines is relative straightforward. For details and extension to higher dimensions see [1]. First we define the covariates $\mathbf{x}_1$ and $\mathbf{x}_2$, with corresponding $n \times q_i$ matrices $\mathbf{B}_i$ $(i = 1, 2)$. The $n \times q$ matrix $\mathbf{B}$ is defined by $\mathbf{B} = \mathbf{B}_1 \otimes_r \mathbf{B}_2$, where $\otimes_r$ denotes the row-wise Kronecker product, and with $q = q_1 \cdot q_2$. Matrix $\mathbf{G} = \mathbf{G}_1 \otimes \mathbf{G}_2$ has dimension $k \times q$, with $k = k_1 \cdot k_2$. The matrix $\mathbf{B}_* = \mathbf{B}_{*,1} \otimes \mathbf{B}_{*,2}$ has dimension $k \times q$. Finally, for $\boldsymbol{\Sigma}$ we have

$$\boldsymbol{\Sigma}^{-1} = \theta_1 \mathbf{D}_1'\mathbf{D}_1 \otimes \mathbf{I}_{q_2} + \theta_2 \mathbf{I}_{q_1} \otimes \mathbf{D}_2'\mathbf{D}_2 + (\theta_1 + \theta_2)\mathbf{B}_*'\mathbf{B}_*, \tag{4}$$

where $\mathbf{D}_1$ and $\mathbf{D}_2$ are difference penalty matrices.

3 Back Transformation from Mixed Models to P-Splines

In this section we will show how the restricted log-likelihood can be written in terms of P-splines, without transformation to mixed models. We define the following invertible linear transformation [1]:

$$\begin{pmatrix} \boldsymbol{\eta} \\ \mathbf{a} \end{pmatrix} = \begin{pmatrix} \mathbf{0}_k & \mathbf{B}_* \\ \mathbf{G} & \mathbf{I}_q \end{pmatrix} \begin{pmatrix} \boldsymbol{\beta} \\ \mathbf{u} \end{pmatrix}, \tag{5}$$

with determinant

$$\left|\begin{pmatrix} \mathbf{0}_k & \mathbf{B}_* \\ \mathbf{G} & \mathbf{I}_q \end{pmatrix}\right| = (-1)^k |\mathbf{B}_*\mathbf{G}| \neq 0. \tag{6}$$

The vector $\mathbf{a}$ is of length q and $\boldsymbol{\eta}$ is a vector of length k. The matrix coefficient matrix $\mathbf{C}$ can be decomposed as

$$\mathbf{C} = \begin{pmatrix} \mathbf{0}_k & \mathbf{G}' \\ \mathbf{B}_*' & \mathbf{I}_q \end{pmatrix} \begin{pmatrix} (\theta_1+\theta_2)\mathbf{I}_k & \mathbf{0} \\ \mathbf{0} & \mathbf{B}'\mathbf{R}^{-1}\mathbf{B}+\mathbf{P} \end{pmatrix} \begin{pmatrix} \mathbf{0}_k & \mathbf{B}_* \\ \mathbf{G} & \mathbf{I}_q \end{pmatrix}. \tag{7}$$

where

$$\mathbf{P} = \theta_1 \mathbf{D}_1'\mathbf{D}_1 \otimes \mathbf{I}_{q2} + \theta_2 \mathbf{I}_{q_1} \otimes \mathbf{D}_2'\mathbf{D}_2. \tag{8}$$

Using Eqs. (3), (5), and (7) it can be derived that the estimates for $\hat{\boldsymbol{\eta}}$ and $\hat{\mathbf{a}}$ are given by

$$\begin{pmatrix} (\theta_1+\theta_2)\mathbf{I}_k & \mathbf{0} \\ \mathbf{0} & \mathbf{B}'\mathbf{R}^{-1}\mathbf{B}+\mathbf{P} \end{pmatrix} \begin{pmatrix} \hat{\boldsymbol{\eta}} \\ \hat{\mathbf{a}} \end{pmatrix} = \begin{pmatrix} \mathbf{0} \\ \mathbf{B}'\mathbf{R}^{-1}\mathbf{y} \end{pmatrix}$$

From this it follows that $\hat{\boldsymbol{\eta}} = \mathbf{0}$ and

$$(\mathbf{B}'\mathbf{R}^{-1}\mathbf{B}+\mathbf{P})\hat{\mathbf{a}} = \mathbf{B}'\mathbf{R}^{-1}\mathbf{y}. \tag{9}$$

Using Eqs. (5) and (9) we obtain

$$2\log\mathcal{L} = \log|\mathbf{R}^{-1}| + \log|\boldsymbol{\Sigma}^{-1}| - \log|\mathbf{C}| - \hat{\mathbf{e}}'\mathbf{R}^{-1}\hat{\mathbf{e}} - \hat{\mathbf{a}}'\mathbf{P}\hat{\mathbf{a}}, \tag{10}$$

where $\hat{\mathbf{e}} = \mathbf{y} - \mathbf{B}\hat{\mathbf{a}}$.

From Eq. (7) it follows that $\log|\mathbf{C}|$ can be decomposed as

$$\log|\mathbf{C}| = \log|\mathbf{B}'\mathbf{R}^{-1}\mathbf{B}+\mathbf{P}| + 2\log|\mathbf{B}_*\mathbf{G}| + k\log(\theta_1+\theta_2). \tag{11}$$

Using some linear algebra it can be shown that $\log|\boldsymbol{\Sigma}^{-1}|$ can be decomposed as

$$\log|\boldsymbol{\Sigma}^{-1}| = \log|\mathbf{P}|_+ - \log|\mathbf{G}'\mathbf{G}| + 2\log|\mathbf{B}_*\mathbf{G}| + k\log(\theta_1+\theta_2). \tag{12}$$

where the pseudo determinant $|\mathbf{P}|_+$ is defined as the product of the $q-k$ non-zero eigenvalues of $\mathbf{P}$. The pseudo determinant $|\mathbf{P}|_+$ can be obtained in an efficient way, by using the spectral decomposition of $\mathbf{D}_i'\mathbf{D}_i = \mathbf{U}_i\boldsymbol{\Lambda}_i\mathbf{U}_i^{-1}$, where $\boldsymbol{\Lambda}_i$ is a diagonal matrix with the eigenvalues of $\mathbf{D}_i'\mathbf{D}_i$ $(i = 1, 2)$. The two-dimensional penalty matrix $\mathbf{P}$ defined by Eq. (8) can be written as [2]

$$\begin{aligned}\mathbf{P} &= (\theta_1\mathbf{U}_1\boldsymbol{\Lambda}_1\mathbf{U}_1^{-1}) \otimes (\mathbf{U}_2\mathbf{I}_{q_2}\mathbf{U}_2^{-1}) + (\theta_2\mathbf{U}_1\mathbf{I}_{q_1}\mathbf{U}_1^{-1}) \otimes (\mathbf{U}_2\boldsymbol{\Lambda}_2\mathbf{U}_2^{-1}) \\ &= (\mathbf{U}_1 \otimes \mathbf{U}_2)(\theta_1\boldsymbol{\Lambda}_1 \otimes \mathbf{I}_{q_2} + \theta_2\mathbf{I}_{q_1} \otimes \boldsymbol{\Lambda}_2)(\mathbf{U}_1 \otimes \mathbf{U}_2)^{-1}.\end{aligned}$$

From this we obtain that $|\mathbf{P}|_+$ can be calculated as the product of the non-zeros of a diagonal matrix

$$|\mathbf{P}|_+ = |\theta_1\boldsymbol{\Lambda}_1 \otimes \mathbf{I}_{q_2} + \theta_2\mathbf{I}_{q_1} \otimes \boldsymbol{\Lambda}_2|_+. \tag{13}$$

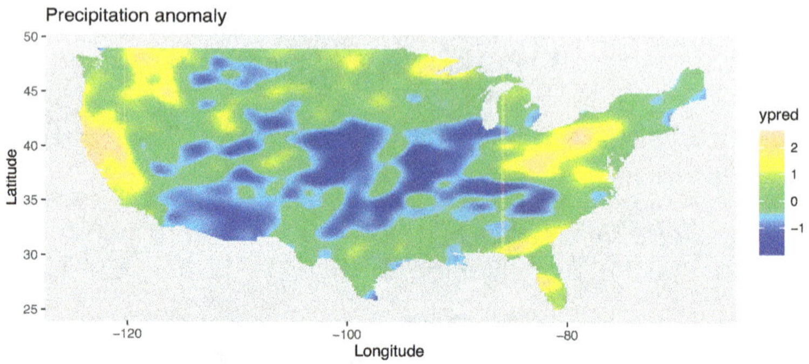

Fig. 1. Fitted surface for monthly precipitation anomalies in USA for April 1948, using `LMMsolver` with 40 segments in both directions. Computation time is less than one second, and 250 times faster than the `SOP` package, which gives the same fit.

Substituting Eqs. (11) and (12) into Eq. (10) gives the following expression for the REML log-likelihood

$$2\log\mathcal{L} = \log|\mathbf{R}^{-1}| + \log|\mathbf{P}|_{+} - \log|\mathbf{G}'\mathbf{G}| - \log|\mathbf{C}_{*}| - \hat{\mathbf{e}}'\mathbf{R}^{-1}\hat{\mathbf{e}} - \hat{\mathbf{a}}'\mathbf{P}\hat{\mathbf{a}}, \quad (14)$$

where $\mathbf{C}_{*} = \mathbf{B}'\mathbf{R}^{-1}\mathbf{B}+\mathbf{P}$. An efficient way to obtain $\log|\mathbf{C}_{*}|$ and to solve Eq. (9) is by using a sparse Cholesky decomposition of $\mathbf{C}_{*}$.

The expressions for the REML log-likelihood for P-splines and for standard mixed models have a similar structure, as can be seen from the comparison between Eqs. (2) and (14). There are two main differences. First, the precision matrix $\mathbf{\Sigma}^{-1}$ in Eq. (2) is positive definite, $\mathbf{P}$ in Eq. (14) is singular. However, $\log|\mathbf{P}|_{+}$ can be calculated using Eq. (13) in an efficient way. A second difference is an extra constant $-\log|\mathbf{G}'\mathbf{G}|$ in the REML P-splines formulation in Eq. (14), which can be easily calculated or just ignored.

An important element needed to calculate Eq. (14) and the partial derivatives with respect to precision parameters θ_m in an efficient way is avoiding the calculation of the inverses of the precision matrices, which are not sparse. One way to do this is to calculate the so-called sparse inverse. In `LMMsolver` [1] Automated Differentiation of the Cholesky algorithm [11] was implemented. Backward differentiation was used, which calculates the partial derivatives of the likelihood efficiently [11]. A detailed example for one-dimensional P-splines is given by Eilers and Boer [4]. The automated differentiation was implemented in `LMMsolver` using supernodal Cholesky factorization [7]. The implementation was written in `C++` using the `Rcpp` package.

4 An Application and Comparison of Computation Times

We will use two-dimensional P-splines for the `USprecip` data set from the `spam` R package [5]. There are n = 5,906 observations, with longitude-latitude positions of monitoring stations, and standardized precipitation for April 1948, see [1] and

Learning Bayesian Networks from Ordinal Data - The Bayesian Way

Marco Grzegorczyk(✉)

Bernoulli Institute, FSE, Groningen University, Groningen, The Netherlands
m.a.grzegorczyk@rug.nl
https://www.math.rug.nl/stat/People/Marco

Abstract. We propose a new Bayesian method for Bayesian network structure learning from ordinal data. Our Bayesian method is similar to a recently proposed non-Bayesian method, referred to as the ordinal structural expectation maximization (OSEM) method. Both methods assume that the ordinal variables originate from Gaussian variables, which can only be observed in discretized form, and that the dependencies in the unobserved latent Gaussian space can be described in terms of Gaussian Bayesian networks. In our simulation studies the new Bayesian method yields significantly higher network reconstruction accuracies than the OSEM method.

Keywords: Bayesian networks · ordinal data · latent Gaussian space · Markov Chain Monte Carlo (MCMC)

1 Introduction

Bayesian networks (BNs) make use of directed acyclic graphs (DAGs) to describe the conditional dependencies among random variables $X_1, \ldots, X_n$. The large majority of BN models assumes that the n random variables have either a joint multivariate Gaussian distribution (see, e.g., [1,2]) or that each of the n variables has a nominal (categorical) distribution (see, e.g., [3]). BNs for variables with ordinal (categorical) distributions have been scarcely explored in the literature. Recently, Luo et al. [4] proposed the so called OSEM ('ordinal structural expectation maximization') method for BN learning from ordinal data. Luo et al. assume that there is a Gaussian Bayesian network (DAG) among continuous variables but that the continuous variables cannot be observed directly. The continuous variables can only be observed in discretized form; i.e. each Gaussian variable is in one-to-one correspondence with an ordinal (categorical) variable, obtained through discretization of the corresponding Gaussian variable. Figure 1 provides a graphical illustration of the relationships between the unobserved latent Gaussian variables and the observable ordinal variables. BN structure learning then aims at learning the DAG among the non-observable latent Gaussian variables from the observable discretized (ordinal) variables.

We propose a Bayesian variant of OSEM, and we refer to it as the BoB method ('**B**ayesian way of modelling **o**rdinal data in form of latent **B**ayesian

J. Einbeck et al. (Eds.): IWSM 2024, CONTRIB.STAT., pp. 7–13, 2024.
https://doi.org/10.1007/978-3-031-65723-8_2

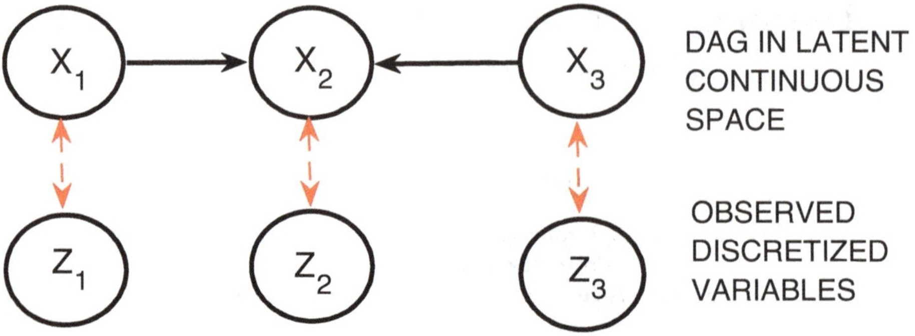

Fig. 1. Graphical illustration of the underlying relationships for $n = 3$ random variables. We assume that each X_i can only be observed in discretized form Z_i ($i = 1, 2, 3$). The goal is to learn the DAG in the latent Gaussian space, $X_1 \rightarrow X_2 \leftarrow X_3$, from the observed discretized variables Z_1, Z_2, and Z_3.

networks'). Unlike the OSEM method that searches for one single best DAG and has to rely on numerical approximations of expected sufficient statistics [4], the BoB method uses Markov Chain Monte Carlo (MCMC) simulations to posterior sample DAGs as well as the values of the latent Gaussian variables. Henceforth, the BoB method allows for Bayesian model averaging across the DAGs and takes the uncertainty about the values of the unobserved latent Gaussian variables into account. Another advantage of our new BoB method is the following one: Unlike the OSEM method, the BoB method can easily be applied to data sets that feature a mixture of both: ordinal variables and continuous variables.

Conceptually, our BoB method combines the 'Bayesian metric for Gaussian networks having score equivalence' (BGe score) from Geiger and Heckerman [1,2], MCMC techniques for BN structure learning [5,6], the 'extended rank likelihood' from Hoff [7], and the parameter sampling algorithm for Gaussian Bayesian networks from Grzegorczyk [8].

2 Mathematical Details

2.1 Bayesian Networks

In Bayesian networks directed acyclic graphs (DAGs) are used to model the conditional dependencies among random variables $X_1, \dots, X_n$. Any DAG $\mathcal{G}$ implies for each individual variable X_i a parent node set $\boldsymbol{\pi}_i$ and the assumption is that the joint distribution can be factorized into a product of n univariate conditional distributions, where each variable X_i just depends on his parent nodes (variables) in $\boldsymbol{\pi}_i$, symbolically:

$$p(X_1, \dots, X_n|\mathcal{G}) = \prod_{i=1}^{n} p(X_i|\boldsymbol{\pi}_i) \tag{1}$$

We define the random vector $\mathbf{X} := (X_1, \ldots, X_n)^\mathsf{T}$, and we assume that we have a data set $\mathcal{D}$ that consists of N observations of $\mathbf{X}$.

For the posterior probability of the DAG $\mathcal{G}$ we have:

$$p(\mathcal{G}|\mathcal{D}) = \frac{p(\mathcal{D}|\mathcal{G})p(\mathcal{G})}{p(\mathcal{D})} \propto p(\mathcal{D}|\mathcal{G})p(\mathcal{G}) \tag{2}$$

where $p(\mathcal{D}|\mathcal{G})$ and $p(\mathcal{G})$ are the marginal likelihood and the prior of $\mathcal{G}$, and

$$p(\mathcal{D}) := \sum_{\mathcal{G}} p(\mathcal{D}|\mathcal{G})p(\mathcal{G})$$

is a normalization constant.

Given a complete data set $\mathcal{D}$, standard Markov Chain Monte Carlo (MCMC) algorithms for BN structure learning (see, e.g., [5,6]) can be used to sample DAGs $\mathcal{G}$ from the posterior distribution, defined in Eq. (2).

2.2 Gaussian Bayesian Networks (BGe Score)

The 'Bayesian metric for Gaussian networks having score equivalence' (BGe score) from Geiger and Heckerman [1,2] assumes the vector $\mathbf{X}$ to have a multivariate Gaussian distribution and imposes a normal-Wishart prior on the mean vector $\boldsymbol{\mu}$ and precision matrix $\boldsymbol{\Sigma}^{-1}$, symbolically:

$$\mathbf{X} \sim \mathcal{N}_n(\boldsymbol{\mu}, \boldsymbol{\Sigma}) \quad \text{with} \quad \boldsymbol{\mu} \sim \mathcal{N}_n(\boldsymbol{\mu}_0, \lambda^{-1}\boldsymbol{\Sigma}) \quad \text{and} \quad \boldsymbol{\Sigma}^{-1} \sim \mathcal{W}(w, \mathbf{T})$$

where $\boldsymbol{\mu}_0 \in \mathbb{R}^n$, $\lambda > 0$, $w > n+1$ and $\mathbf{T} \in \mathbb{R}^{n,n}$ are fixed hyperparameters. Geiger and Heckerman show that the normal-Wishart prior yields that the marginal likelihood $p(\mathcal{D}|\mathcal{G})$ can be factorized like in Eq. (1). That is, $p(\mathcal{D}|\mathcal{G})$ factorizes into n local factors referring to the conditional distributions $p(X_i|\boldsymbol{\pi}_i)$, and each of those n factors can be computed analytically.

2.3 New Bayesian Network Model ('BoB Method')

We assume that we can partition the n random variables into two disjoint subsets $\mathcal{S}_1$ and $\mathcal{S}_2$ with $\mathcal{S}_1 \cup \mathcal{S}_2 = \{X_1, \ldots, X_n\}$, and that we can observe the continuous values of the variables in $\mathcal{S}_1$, while we can observe the values of the variables in $\mathcal{S}_2$ only in discretized form. That is, instead of $X_i \in \mathcal{S}_2$, we observe an ordinal variable Z_i with the following relationship between the N continuous values $x_{1,i}, \ldots, x_{N,i}$ of X_i and the corresponding N ordinal values $z_{1,i}, \ldots, z_{N,i}$ of Z_i:

$$z_{k,i} < z_{l,i} \quad \Rightarrow \quad x_{k,i} < x_{l,i} \qquad \forall k, l \in \{1, \ldots, N\} \tag{3}$$

The observed ordinal values of Z_i imply conditions for the latent continuous values of X_i. For any latent value $x_{k,i}$ of X_i we have the constraint:

$$l_{k,i} < x_{k,i} < u_{k,i} \tag{4}$$

where the lower bound $l_{k,i}$ is the maximal value $x_{l,i}$ with $z_{l,i} < z_{k,i}$, and the upper bound $u_{k,i}$ is the minimal value $x_{l,i}$ with $z_{l,i} > z_{k,i}$.[1] The bounds $l_{k,i}$ and $u_{k,i}$ ensure that Eq. (3) is fulfilled.

The extended rank likelihood from Hoff [7] is the joint probability of observing for the random variables from $\mathcal{S}_1$ the actually observed values $\mathcal{D}_1$ and of observing for the random variables from $\mathcal{S}_2$ any values $\mathcal{D}_2$ that satisfy the imposed constraints, cf. Eqs. (3–4); symbolically we write: $\mathcal{D}_2 \in \mathcal{C}$ to indicate that the latent values $\mathcal{D}_2$ fulfill the necessary constraints.

2.4 MCMC Inference

We use Markov Chain Monte Carlo (MCMC) simulations to generate posterior samples for the BoB method. Our MCMC algorithm consists of three consecutive sampling steps (1–3):

(1) Given valid values $\mathcal{D}_2 \in \mathcal{C}$ for the latent Gaussian variables, we merge $\mathcal{D}_1$ and $\mathcal{D}_2$ to a complete data set $\mathcal{D}$. Given complete data $\mathcal{D}$ and the BGe score [1,2] the marginal likelihood $P(\mathcal{D}|\mathcal{G})$ can be computed analytically and standard MCMC techniques for BN structure learning (see, e.g., [5,6]) can be applied to sample DAGs from the posterior distribution $p(\mathcal{G}|\mathcal{D})$; cf. Eq. (2).

(2) Given complete data $\mathcal{D}$ and the current DAG $\mathcal{G}$, we can use the Gaussian Bayesian network parameter sampling algorithm from Grzegorczyk [8] to posterior sample a mean vector $\boldsymbol{\mu}$ and a covariance matrix $\boldsymbol{\Sigma}$. The algorithm ensures that the covariance matrix $\boldsymbol{\Sigma}$ is coherent with the current DAG $\mathcal{G}$; i.e. that $\mathcal{G}$ and $\boldsymbol{\Sigma}$ imply the same conditional dependence relations among the random variables $X_1, \ldots, X_n$ yielding the factorization:

$$p(X_1, \ldots, X_n|\mathcal{G}) = \prod_{i=1}^{n} p(X_i|\boldsymbol{\pi}_i)$$

In a Gaussian BN with $\mathbf{X} \sim \mathcal{N}_n(\boldsymbol{\mu}, \boldsymbol{\Sigma})$ each conditional distribution $X_i|\boldsymbol{\pi}_i$ is a univariate (conditional) Gaussian distribution of the form:

$$X_i|\boldsymbol{\pi}_i \sim \mathcal{N}\left(\boldsymbol{\mu}_i + \sum_{X_k \in \boldsymbol{\pi}_i} b_{i,k}(X_k - \boldsymbol{\mu}_k),\ \sigma_i^2\right) \qquad (i = 1, \ldots, n)$$

where $\boldsymbol{\mu} = (\boldsymbol{\mu}_1, \ldots, \boldsymbol{\mu}_n)^{\mathsf{T}}$, the parameters $b_{i,k}$ can be thought of as regression coefficients, and the σ_i^2 parameters are the conditional variances.

(3) Given a covariance matrix $\boldsymbol{\Sigma}$ that is coherent with $\mathcal{G}$, the observed Gaussian values $\mathcal{D}_1$, and the constraint $\mathcal{D}_2 \in \mathcal{C}$, the unobserved latent values $\mathcal{D}_2$ can be posterior sampled from truncated conditional Gaussian distributions, as outlined in detail in the next subsection.

[1] If $z_{k,i}$ is the lowest possible discrete value, there is no lower bound and we set $l_{k,i} := -\infty$. Correspondingly, we set $u_{k,i} := \infty$ if $z_{k,i}$ is the largest possible discrete value, so that no upper bound is required.

2.5 Sampling the Latent (Unobserved) Gaussian Values

Each random variable $X_i \in \mathcal{S}_2$ can only be observed in discretized form. That is, instead of the continuous values $x_{1,i}, \ldots, x_{N,i}$ of X_i, only the corresponding ordinal values $z_{1,i}, \ldots, z_{N,i}$ of Z_i can be observed. For each unobserved latent value $x_{k,i}$ we have the constraint $l_{k,i} < x_{k,i} < u_{k,i}$ from Eq. (4). As the random vector $\mathbf{X} = (X_1, \ldots, X_n)^\mathsf{T}$ has an n-dimensional Gaussian distribution

$$\mathbf{X} \sim \mathcal{N}_n(\boldsymbol{\mu}, \boldsymbol{\Sigma})$$

the conditional distribution of X_i given the values $\mathbf{x}_{k,-i}$ of the $n-1$ other random variables $\mathbf{X}_{-i} := (X_1, \ldots, X_{i-1}, X_{i+1}, \ldots, X_n)^\mathsf{T}$ is a conditional Gaussian distribution. For the k-th observation this Gaussian distribution is subject to the truncation constraint $l_{k,i} < x_{k,i} < u_{k,i}$ from Eq. (4). We have

$$X_i | \left(\mathbf{X}_{-i} = \mathbf{x}_{k,-i},\; X_i \in [l_{k,i}, u_{k,i}]\right) \sim \mathcal{N}_{[l_{k,i}, u_{k,i}]}(\theta_{k,i}, \sigma_i^2) \quad \text{, where}$$

$$\begin{aligned} \theta_{k,i} &:= \boldsymbol{\mu}_i + \boldsymbol{\Sigma}_{i,-i} \cdot \boldsymbol{\Sigma}_{-i,-i}(\mathbf{x}_{k,-i} - \boldsymbol{\mu}_{-i}) \\ \sigma_i^2 &:= \boldsymbol{\Sigma}_{i,i} - \boldsymbol{\Sigma}_{i,-i} \cdot \boldsymbol{\Sigma}_{-i,-i} \cdot \boldsymbol{\Sigma}_{-i,i} \end{aligned}$$

and the subscript '$-i$' indicates all rows/columns except for the i-th and the truncation $X_i \in [l_{k,i}, u_{k,i}]$ is made explicit as a subscript of the Gaussian distribution symbol $\mathcal{N}(.,.)$.

For re-sampling the latent data, $\mathcal{D}_2$, in the third sampling step (3) from the previous subsection, we need to loop through the N values $x_{i,1}, \ldots, x_{i,N}$ of each of the random variables that has only been observed in discretized form, $X_i \in \mathcal{D}_2$. Hence, in total, $N \cdot |\mathcal{D}_2|$ unobserved latent values $x_{i,k}$ have to be sampled from such truncated Gaussian distributions to get a new realization of the unobserved latent data $\mathcal{D}_2 \in \mathcal{C}$, fulfilling the constraints from Eqs. (3–4).

2.6 Simulation Details

To take into account that the parameters $\boldsymbol{\mu}$ and $\boldsymbol{\Sigma}$ of the joint Gaussian distribution of the latent variables are not fully identifiable [4,7], we modify the BGe score [1,2] by enforcing the mean to be equal to zero, $\boldsymbol{\mu} = \mathbf{0}$, and we follow Hoff [7] and re-scale the sampled covariance matrix $\boldsymbol{\Sigma}$ to a correlation matrix, before resampling the unobserved latent values, as explained in the previous subsection.

For the graph prior in Eq. (2) we use

$$P(\mathcal{G}) \propto \prod_{i=1}^{n} \binom{n-1}{|\boldsymbol{\pi}_i|}^{-1}$$

where $|\boldsymbol{\pi}_i|$ is the cardinality of the parent set $\boldsymbol{\pi}_i$. In each MCMC iteration we perform a structure MCMC move [5,6], but we only re-sample the latent data $\mathcal{D}_2$ with probability $q = 0.05$. We run all MCMC simulations with $3000k$ iterations and withdraw the first half of the samples to account for a burn in phase. We apply the OSEM method as described in Luo et al. [4].

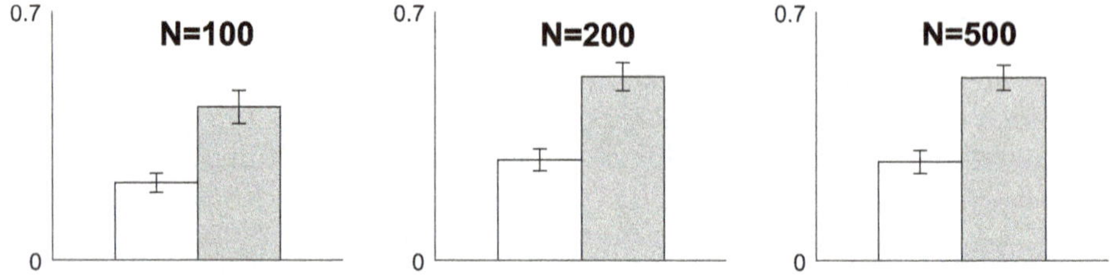

Fig. 2. AUC network reconstruction scores for fully discretized ECOLI70 data: OSEM (white) vs. BoB (gray). For three sample sizes N the average AUCs are across 10 discretized data sets and the error bars indicate 95% confidence intervals.

3 Empirical Results

ECOLI70 is a benchmark Gaussian Bayesian network with $n = 46$ nodes and 70 edges. We generate ten ECOLI70 data sets for each of three sample sizes $N \in \{100, 200, 500\}$; i.e. 30 data sets on total. In each data set we z-score standardize and discretize *all* variables, as described in [4]. Full discretization refers to $\mathcal{S}_1 = \emptyset$. We use areas under precision-recall curves (AUC$\in [0, 1]$) to quantify the network reconstruction accuracy. Figure 2 shows the average AUCs of OSEM and BoB. The AUC differences are in favour of BoB and statistically significant. The BoB method can also learn BNs from mixed data with ordinal and continuous variables; i.e. from data with $\mathcal{S}_1 \neq \emptyset$. To demonstrate this, we distinguish six fractions $p \in \{0, 0.2, 0.4, 0.6, 0.8, 1\}$ of discretized variables. For each data set we randomly select a fraction p of the $n = 46$ variables and discretize only the selected variables. $p = 0$ refers to the latent Gaussian data without any discretization, while $p = 1$ refers to the fully discretized data with $\mathcal{S}_1 = \emptyset$. Since OSEM cannot be applied to mixed data, we here compare the BoB method with traditional Gaussian Bayesian networks (GBNs) using the BGe score with $\boldsymbol{\mu} = \mathbf{0}$. This ensures that the two methods (BOB and GBNs) are identical for $p = 0$. For the GBNs with $p > 0$ we z-score standardize the ordinal variables

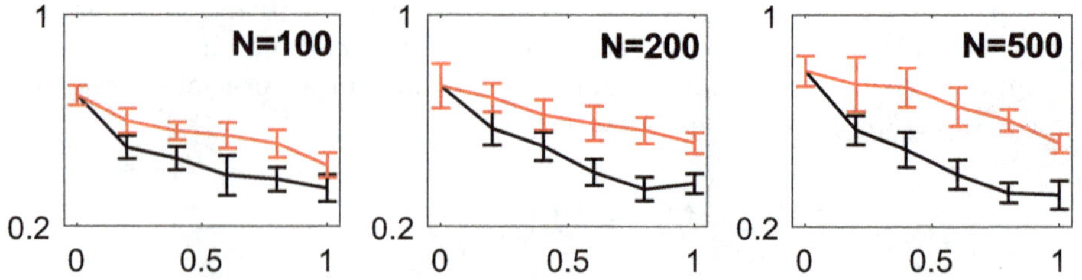

Fig. 3. AUC network reconstruction accuracy scores for mixed ECOLI70 data: GBNs (black) vs. BoB (red). For three sample sizes N the average AUC scores have been plotted against six fractions p of discretized variables. Averages are across ten data instantiations and error bars indicate 95% confidence intervals.

and treat them as if they were continuous variables. Figure 3 monitors the AUC scores across for different fractions p of discretized variables. Again, the AUC network reconstruction scores are significantly in favour of the new BoB method.

4 Conclusion

We have proposed a Bayesian approach for modelling the dependencies among ordinal variables via latent Gaussian Bayesian networks. The new BoB method can be seen as the Bayesian counterpart of the OSEM method, recently proposed by Luo et al. [4]. Both methods assume that the ordinal variables originate from latent Gaussian variables that have only been observed in discretized form. In our simulation study the new BoB method led to significantly better network reconstruction results than the OSEM method. In addition, we have shown that the BoB method can also be applied to learn BNs from mixed data and then performs better than traditional Gaussian Bayesian networks. We note that an extended paper of this short IWSM conference paper has been submitted [9] and that our work was inspired by Dobra et al. [10] and Mohammadi et al. [11] who proposed a similar Bayesian framework for 'Gaussian graphical models'.

References

1. Geiger, D., Heckerman, D.: Parameter priors for directed acyclic graphical models and the characterization of several probability distributions. Ann. Stat. **30**, 1412–1440 (2002)
2. Kuipers, J., Moffa, G., Heckerman, D.: Addendum on the scoring of Gaussian directed acyclic graphical models. Ann. Stat. **42**(4), 1689–1691 (2014)
3. Heckerman, D., Geiger, D., Chickering, D.: Learning Bayesian networks: the combination of knowledge and statistical data. Mach. Learn. **20**, 197–243 (1995)
4. Luo, X.G., Moffa, G., Kuipers, J.: Learning Bayesian networks from ordinal data. J. Mach. Learn. Res. **22**, 1–44 (2021)
5. Madigan, D., York, J.: Bayesian graphical models for discrete data. Int. Stat. Rev. **63**, 215–232 (1995)
6. Giudici, P., Castelo, R.: Improving Markov chain Monte Carlo model search for data mining. Mach. Learn. **50**, 127–158 (2003)
7. Hoff, P.D.: Extending the rank likelihood for semiparametric estimation. Ann. Appl. Stat. **1**, 265–283 (2007)
8. Grzegorczyk, M.: Being Bayesian about learning Gaussian Bayesian networks from incomplete data. Int. J. Approximate Reasoning **160** (2023). https://doi.org/10.1016/j.ijar.2023.108954
9. Grzegorczyk, M.: Being Bayesian about learning Bayesian networks from ordinal data. Int. J. Approx. Reason. **170** (2024). https://doi.org/10.1016/j.ijar.2024.109205
10. Dobra, A., Lenkoski, A., Rodriguez, A.: Bayesian inference for general Gaussian graphical models with application to multivariate lattice data. J. Am. Stat. Assoc. **106**(496), 1418–1433 (2011)
11. Mohammadi, A., Abegaz, F., Heuvel, E., Wit, E.C.: Bayesian modelling of Dupuytren disease by using Gaussian copula graphical models. J. R. Stat. Soc.: Ser. C: Appl. Stat. **66**(3), 629–645 (2016)

Latent Dirichlet Allocation and Hidden Markov Models to Identify Public Perception of Sustainability in Social Media Data

Luigi Cao Pinna(✉), Claire Miller, and Marian Scott

School of Mathematics and Statistics, University of Glasgow, Glasgow, UK
{luigi.caopinna,Claire.Miller,Marian.Scott}@glasgow.ac.uk
https://www.gla.ac.uk/schools/mathematicsstatistics/staff/luigicaopinna/

Abstract. To help guide a just transition to a sustainable society and onboard the local communities, researchers can identify events of public interest through access to data from community engagement activities and social media content. However, novel analytic methods are required to process and analyse data in unstructured formats (e.g. transcripts, text and images) and to extract useful information for decision-making. This paper proposes an analytics pipeline combining latent Dirichlet allocation and hidden Markov models for automatically detecting multiple latent changepoints in topics over time, without prior knowledge of their occurrence. Analysing social media content (i.e., tweets) related to Glasgow, we identified events that captured social media users' public interest, demonstrating the potential of our method to inform timely and relevant policy making.

Keywords: sustainable society · social media content · latent Dirichlet allocation · multiple latent changepoints

1 Introduction

The transition to a sustainable society is one of the key challenges facing researchers, policymakers and communities today. Key to future sustainable city planning is an understanding of citizens' priorities, and this can be informed by data to aid effective decision-making. The £10.2M NERC-funded GALLANT (Glasgow as a Living Lab Accelerating Novel Transformation) project is acquiring and producing data on Glasgow's environment, ecology, place, people and communities to learn about Glasgow's 'living space', how it is changing, and what effect interventions may have on the future environment, economy, health and wellbeing for the city. Such data are complex and come in quantitative and qualitative forms and as structured and unstructured sources. Examples include deprivation indices, interview transcripts, and photos and text from social media posts. Novel data analytics and data visualisations are essential tools to process and integrate such data to extract useful information to explore sustainable solutions.

J. Einbeck et al. (Eds.): IWSM 2024, CONTRIB.STAT., pp. 14–20, 2024.
https://doi.org/10.1007/978-3-031-65723-8_3

One substantive aspect of GALLANT research is a programme of community engagement. In addition to community consultation within the city, social media data are a potential source of information (carefully considered in the light of clear biases). This paper proposes a novel analytics pipeline to identify events within social media posts and then analyse the corresponding posted text. The main advantages of such a pipeline/framework would be 1) to detect events that capture the public attention and 2) to provide more evidence to aid a deeper understanding of public sentiment. This paper proposes combining a latent Dirichlet allocation (LDA) modelling approach, as a topic modelling framework, with a hidden Markov model [5]. The approach is then used to identify and analyse changepoints in social media data associated with the city of Glasgow. This approach assumes that topic prevalence may change after the estimated changepoint, without requiring additional knowledge regarding the events that caused the topic's shift in position.

2 Methods

LDA allows the extraction of topics from a given text. Specifically, each document d can be described by a mixture of topics z, assuming that each word w could be related to a certain topic. For each document d, LDA assumes the following:

1. Choose $\theta_{(d)} \sim \text{Dirichlet}(\alpha)$, where $\theta_{(d)}$ is the topic distribution for document d, and α indicates the topic's proportion in each document.
2. For each word w_i in document d, $i = 1, \ldots, n$,
   (a) Choose a topic $z_i \sim \text{Multinomial}(\theta_{(d)})$.
   (b) Choose a word $w_i | z_i \sim \text{Multinomial}(\phi_{(z_i)})$, where $\phi_{(z)}$ is the word distribution for topic z.

Rather than directly estimating θ and ϕ, we can use Gibbs sampling for LDA to determine the posterior distribution of the topic's assignment (z) to words (w) as $\phi_{(z)} \sim \text{Dirichlet}(\beta)$ as in [1]. However, we cannot ignore the temporal nature of social media data and assume that the topic proportions of all documents are drawn from a single Dirichlet distribution. We overcome this limitation by assuming that the frequency with which topics are discussed may change over time giving k latent regimes between each latent changepoint. Specifically, we set the concentration parameter α_0 for topic sparsity as predetermined [5] and estimated the vector of probability measure $m(k)$ (i.e., topic prevalence) for each regime k. This has the advantage of detecting changepoints as they emerge while allowing topic identification over the whole time frame, for an easier comparison of topic proportions. The key assumptions of our model are:

1. For each time point t, with $t = 1, 2, \ldots, T$, select a regime $k \sim P(s_t | s_{t-1})$, where s_t is the discrete state at time t. Documents contributing at time t belong to regime k.
2. For each document d in regime k, the collection of which is denoted $\mathcal{D}_k$ with $k \in \mathbb{Z}^+$, $k \leq T$, choose $\theta_{(d)} \sim \text{Dirichlet}(\alpha_0 m(k))$.

This Dirichlet process combined with a hidden Markov model only allows for a one-step forward transition and was used to define any possible number of changepoints from 0 to a maximum of $T-1$. The transition matrix in this model can be represented as:

$$P = \begin{pmatrix} p_{11} & p_{12} & 0 & \cdots \\ 0 & p_{22} & p_{23} & \cdots \\ \vdots & \vdots & \ddots & \vdots \\ \vdots & \vdots & \vdots & \ddots \end{pmatrix} \tag{1}$$

Specifically, from state k, the only possible paths are to remain in the current state k or move to the next one $k+1$ (i.e., $p_{kk} + p_{k,k+1} = 1$). This approach was used, based on the assumption of high topic volatility in social media which rapidly evolves and always tends to progress rather than revert to earlier states. In our model, the transition dynamics between states are governed by the hyperparameters λ and ν. Here, λ controls the tendency to remain in the current state, while ν influences the likelihood of moving to the next state. These hyperparameters are estimated using the Metropolis-Hastings algorithm, with the priors for λ and ν both set using a vague Gamma distribution (1,1), to balance state persistence and transitions in regimes shift dynamics [3].

We then estimate the vector of probability measure $m(k)$, indicating the topic prevalence for each regime k. Thus, the joint distribution of words w and their topic assignments z can be expressed as:

$$P(w, z|\alpha_0 m, \beta, s) = P(w|z, \beta) \prod_{t=1}^{T} \prod_{d \in \mathcal{D}_t} P(z_{(d)}|\alpha_0 m(s_t)), \tag{2}$$

here s defines the sequence of states s_t at each time point t, $z_{(d)}$ defines the topic assignments of words within document d, and $\mathcal{D}_t$ represents the collection of documents at time t. This formulation combines Gibbs sampling for drawing topic assignments z, fixed-point iteration for estimating the probability measure m, and Gibbs sampling to determine the state transitions s, effectively capturing the dynamic changes in topic distributions over time.

3 Data and Analysis Framework

We used the V1.1 free version of the Twitter (X) API, and retrieved 2771 tweets in a 100-mile buffer around the city centre of Glasgow for a sequence of 41 days, from the 1st June till the 11th of July 2023 (Fig. 1), using the query #Glasgow (293 tweets) and Glasgow (2478 tweets) searched directly in the post text.

Punctuation, numbers, stopwords, user's pseudonyms and the search query word 'Glasgow' were removed as not being informative. Additionally, we took the root form of words to minimise their redundancy (e.g., "cities" and "city" were treated as the same entity, and the stemming was performed by using the

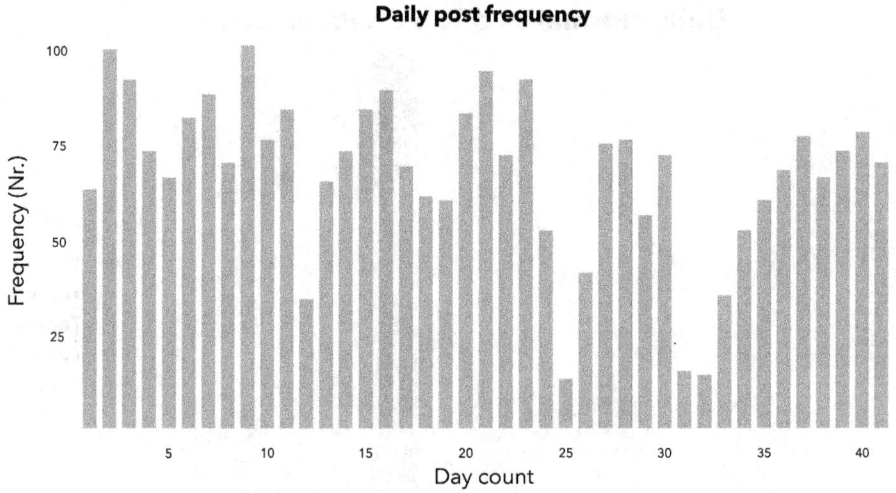

Fig. 1. Daily post frequency (i.e., the daily number of tweets used in our model).

R package *SnowballC* function *wordStem*). Then we removed infrequently used words using sparsity of 0.99, to focus on words that appear in at least 1% of tweets.

The LDA model was applied to detect five main topics, as preliminary analyses showed that identifying more topics led to overlaps among them. Gibbs sampling was used for the LDA model with 1 million burn-in draws. For the hidden Markov model, we split the data into 80/20% for training/testing the model and performed 80000 burn-in draws and 20000 iterations. In this analysis the Dirichlet symmetric hyperprior β for the topic's assignment to word distribution was initialised to 0.5 and optimised with the data; this is done to state whether topics will have a more sparse or uniform distribution over words while being optimised with data to account for highly skewed word frequency distributions of language (i.e., all words are equally likely to be generated from one topic, [4]). The topic sparsity value α_0 was set to 1 (i.e., a low value), suggesting the mild assumption that social media posts having a short amount of text may also contain a low number of topics [4]. Our metrics of likelihood indicated that the model converged.

4 Preliminary Results and Discussions

The model identified three distinct regimes and two changepoints on the 25th and 28th days of the time series (Fig. 2), after which the prevalence of topics changed substantively. As the two changepoints are particularly close, we interpreted them as a transition phase, after which in the third regime, we have a spike in topics 1, 4, 5 and a decrease in topic 2 prevalence (Fig. 2). The proposed model provides clear evidence of the events that capture public opinion (Fig. 3).

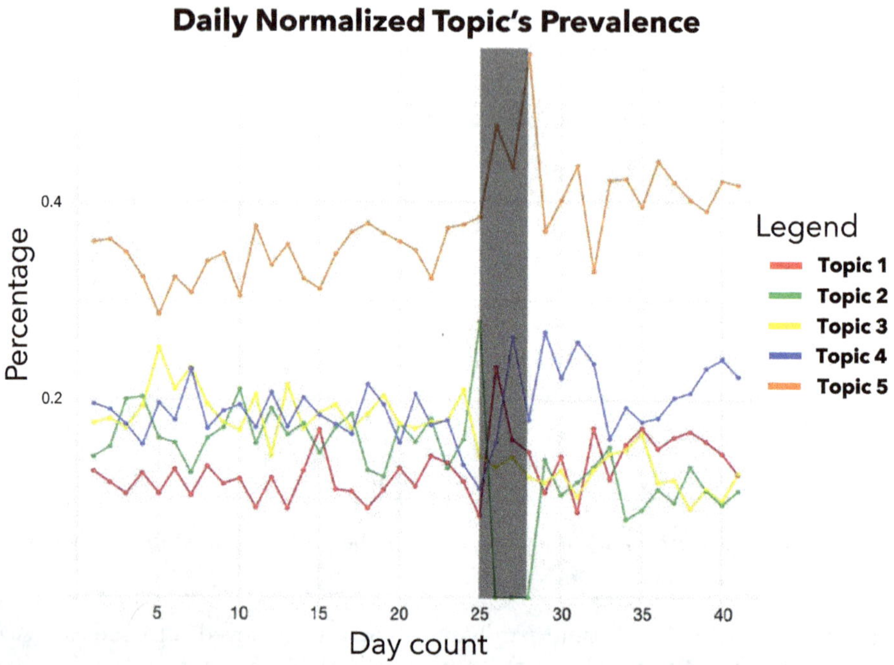

Fig. 2. Topics prevalence normalized by day (i.e., daily topic's prevalence sum to one), showing the two identified changepoints interpreted as a transition phase, and displayed as a grey band in the plot.

By exploring the first five most commonly associated words for each of our five topics we can identify a suggested broad subject: 1 - topic: music events, 2 - topic: sport and games, 3 - topic: support and local community, 4 - topic: travel to work, 5 - topic: evening entertainment. It could be that the third regime and decline in topic 2 may be associated with the school summer holidays and the end of the football season.

Identified changepoints are consistent with those found using alternative methods based on the frequency of the tweets, which suggest a changepoint around the 23th, the 26th and 30th (R package *changepoint* [2]). However, the proposed topic model provides additional information on the topics of interest for the communities and explorations of specific events that improve engagement. Additionally, this method is less sensitive to fluctuations in the number of tweets not accompanied by shifts in topic frequencies, such as on Fridays and weekends.

This approach enables the investigation of human insights from temporal-specific, unstructured data sources, which could be a useful approach as one aspect to inform the development of policies that are both environmentally sustainable and socially beneficial. The main limitations of the proposed methodology are related to the preferential sampling of the V1.1 X API, which only

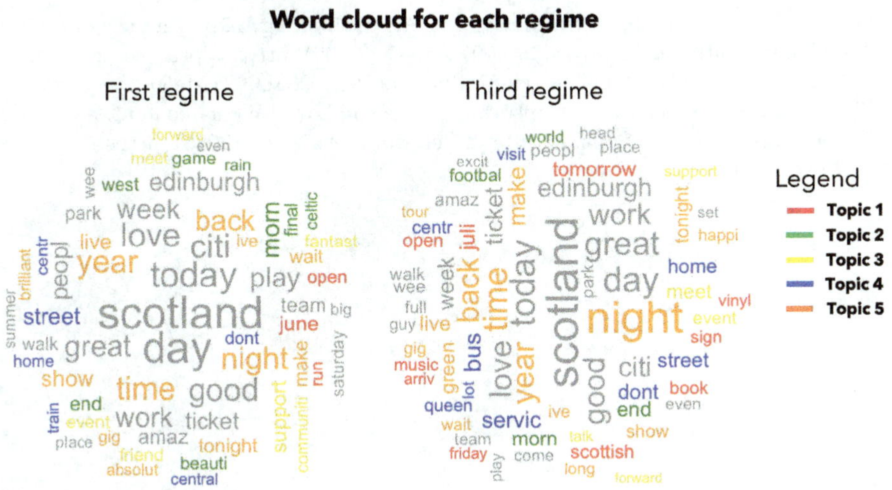

Fig. 3. Word cloud for the first and third regime, presenting words with a higher than 50% frequency, the word's size represents the frequency and the colour refers to the word's topic assignment. Grey words either have multiple topics assigned or lack a clear topic assignment.

retrieved recent or popular posts. Future developments will include complementary analysis on multiple social media platforms and over a longer period. Moreover, we will apply our method in a more controlled scenario, matching the GALLANT community consultation time-frame to explore if engagement activities impacts can be identified on social media platforms.

Acknowledgments. GALLANT is funded by the Natural Environment Research Council as part of the Changing the Environment Programme [grant number NE/W005042/1] (https://www.gla.ac.uk/research/az/sustainablesolutions/ourprojects/gallant/). Special thanks to Cris Hasan, the data analytics and community engagement colleagues for their insights.

References

1. Griffiths, T.L., Steyvers, M.: Finding scientific topics. Proc. Natl. Acad. Sci. **101**(1), 5228–5235 (2004). https://doi.org/10.1073/pnas.0307752101
2. Killick, R., Eckley, I.A.: changepoint: an R package for changepoint analysis. J. Stat. Softw. **58**(3), 1–19 (2014). https://doi.org/10.18637/jss.v058.i03
3. Ko, S.I.M., Chong, T.T.L., Ghosh, P.: Dirichlet process hidden Markov multiple change-point model. Bayesian Anal. **10**(2), 275–296 (2015). https://doi.org/10.1214/14-BA910

4. Wallach, H.M., Mimno, D.M., McCallum, A.: Rethinking LDA: why priors matter. Adv. Neural Inf. Process. Syst. **23**, 1973–1981. (2009). https://proceedings.neurips.cc/paper_files/paper/2009/file/0d0871f0806eae32d30983b62252da50Paper.pdf
5. Zhong, N., Schweidel, D.A.: Capturing changes in social media content: a multiple latent changepoint topic model. Mark. Sci. **39**(4), 827–846 (2020). https://doi.org/10.1287/mksc.2019.1212

Bayesian Approaches to Model Overdispersion in Spatio-Temporal Binomial Data

Mabel Morales-Otero[1] and Vicente Núñez-Antón[2](✉)

[1] Institute of Data Science and Artificial Intelligence (DATAI), University of Navarra, Pamplona, Spain
mmoralesote@unav.es
[2] University of the Basque Country UPV/EHU, Bilbao, Spain
vicente.nunezanton@ehu.eus

Abstract. In this work, we introduce a direct spatio-temporal extension of the spatial conditional overdispersion models for binomially distributed response variables. This proposal incorporates a spatial term similar to the spatial lag of the response variable for each time unit within the linear predictor. These models effectively capture both spatial and temporal correlations inherent in the dataset under study. Furthermore, we introduce temporally varying spatial lag coefficient models, enabling for the possibility of introducing temporal changes in the spatial term. In order to be able to assess the usefulness of our proposals, we apply them to the analysis of low birth weight in Georgia, providing a comparative analysis of the performance of our models to that of the commonly used Knorr-Held's models.

Keywords: Bayesian models · overdispersion · spatio-temporal models

1 Introduction

Spatio-temporal data appear in various fields of study, as researchers often aim to analyse phenomena observed across multiple locations and time periods. Such data commonly exhibit correlations among regions and time units requiring, therefore, a careful consideration when fitting regression models. Spatial conditional overdispersion models, introduced by Cepeda-Cuervo et al. (2018), for spatial count data, offer an innovative modelling approach to be able to address overdispersion and also incorporate spatial dependence by introducing a spatial term into the regression structure for the mean. In this study, we propose alternative extensions for these models to allow for the possibility of fitting spatio-temporal count data when the response variable follows a binomial distribution.

2 Methods

The most commonly applied model to spatio-temporal count data was originally proposed by Knorr-Held (2000). It is commonly used for fitting Poisson

J. Einbeck et al. (Eds.): IWSM 2024, CONTRIB.STAT., pp. 21–27, 2024.
https://doi.org/10.1007/978-3-031-65723-8_4

distributed response variables, but it can also be fitted to binomially distributed responses. In this case, it is assumed that Y_{ij} represents counts for $i = 1, \ldots, n$ regions in $j = 1, \ldots, J$ time periods, and that the number of trials on each region i and time period j, is denoted by n_{ij}. It is also assumed that Y_{ij}, conditioned on the random effects $\nu_i, \eta_i, \delta_j, \phi_j$ and ϵ_{ij}, follows a binomial distribution, with π_{ij} being the probability of success of a trial in region i and time period j. That is, $(Y_{ij}|\nu_i, \eta_i, \delta_j, \phi_j, \epsilon_{ij}) \sim \text{Bin}(n_{ij}, \pi_{ij})$, with regression structure given by:

$$\text{logit}(\pi_{ij}) = \mathbf{x}_{ij}^{\top}\boldsymbol{\beta} + \nu_i + \eta_i + \delta_j + \phi_j + \epsilon_{ij},$$

where $\mathbf{x}_{ij}$ is the $k \times 1$ vector of explanatory variables for the i-th area in the j-th time period, and $\boldsymbol{\beta}$ is the $k \times 1$ vector of unknown regression parameters that needs to be estimated. In addition, ν_i and δ_j are unstructured random effects for space and time (i.e., $\nu_i \sim N(0, \tau_\nu)$, $\tau_\nu > 0$, and $\delta_j \sim N(0, \tau_\delta)$, $\tau_\delta > 0$), respectively, η_i is a spatially structured random effect following an intrinsic conditionally autoregressive (ICAR) distribution and ϕ_j is a temporal effect, following a random walk process of order one (RW1). That is, we assume that the differences $(\phi_j - \phi_{j-1})$ follow a normal distribution, so that $(\phi_j - \phi_{j-1}) \sim N(0, \tau_\phi)$, for $j = 2, \ldots, J$, and $\phi_1 \sim N(0, \tau_\phi)$, with $\tau_\phi > 0$. Finally, ϵ_{ij} is a spatio-temporal interaction term having an unstructured normal prior distribution (i.e. $\epsilon_{ij} \sim N(0, \tau_\epsilon)$, $\tau_\epsilon > 0$). Note that alternative distributions could also be assumed for ϕ_j or ϵ_{ij}, such as a higher order random walk or an autoregressive process. The spatial conditional models have been shown to be quite flexible alternatives for modelling spatial count data (Cepeda-Cuervo et al., 2018; Morales-Otero and Núñez-Antón, 2021). We propose a spatio-temporal extension of these models that includes, for each time period, the spatial term A_{ij} in the regression structure, together with a spatial parameter ρ that will capture the spatial correlation in the data for the whole period under study. This spatial data proposal is similar to the spatial lag of a variable from a logistic link function perspective. Our proposed term is defined so that $A_{ij} = \frac{\hat{\pi}_{\sim ij}}{1-\hat{\pi}_{\sim ij}}$, where $\hat{\pi}_{\sim ij} = \frac{\mathbf{W}_i \mathbf{y}_j}{\mathbf{W}_i \mathbf{n}_j}$, with $\mathbf{W}_i$ being the i-th row of a spatial weights matrix $\mathbf{W}$, corresponding to the i-th region, and $\mathbf{y}_j$ and $\mathbf{n}_j$ being the vector of observations of the response variable and the vector of the number of trials, respectively, for the j-th time period. The term $\hat{\pi}_{\sim ij}$ can be interpreted as the ratio between the weighted average of the number of successes and the number of total cases observed in the neighbours of the i-th region, for each j-th period. Consequently, the term A_{ij} represents this proportion transformed onto the logit scale. Incorporating this term into the regression structure enables us to explore the relationship between the probability of success in a region and time period, π_{ij}, being modelled and this ratio of weighted averages in the neighbouring regions. This allows us to assess the similarity of information between the neighbouring regions and the value of the region itself.

Therefore, we specify a regression structure on the probability of success π_{ij} in the following way:

$$\text{logit}(\pi_{ij}) = \mathbf{x}_{ij}^{\top}\boldsymbol{\beta} + \rho A_{ij} + \nu_i + \delta_j + \phi_j + \epsilon_{ij},$$

where $\mathbf{x}_{ij}$, $\boldsymbol{\beta}$, ρ, A_{ij}, ν_i, δ_j, ϕ_j and ϵ_{ij} are as before. Finally, we also propose the temporally varying spatial lag coefficient model, where we assume that the coefficient for the spatial lag is the sum of a fixed coefficient, ρ_0, and a random coefficient, ρ_j, which varies according to the time units $j = 1, \ldots, J$. More specifically, we propose different specifications for the temporal varying coefficient, such as an unstructured normal distribution, a random walk process or an autoregressive process. The estimated value obtained for ρ_0 would represent the strength of the spatial dependence among the regions for the whole time period under study, whereas the estimated values obtained for ρ_j would indicate whether the spatial association increases or decreases with time. This would allow us to examine the variability of the coefficient of the spatial lag from one time unit with regard to the others.

In models incorporating random effects as discussed, non-identifiability issues are a known concern. In order to avoid these problems, we can impose a sum to zero constraint on the spatially structured random effect following the ICAR model as well as on the temporally structured random effect following a RW1 process. Note that, if we assume an unstructured normal prior distribution for the interaction term, no constraint is necessary for this component (Schrödle, B. and Held, L., 2011). Additionally, in the case of the proposed spatio-temporal conditional model, the spatially structured random effect is being replaced by a fixed effect given by the spatial term, eliminating the need for imposing the constraint for this particular case.

3 Application

We have studied a dataset containing the number of live births on each of the $n = 159$ counties in the state of Georgia, USA, for $J = 10$ years, from 2010 up to 2019 (i.e., variable NB) and on the counts of infants with low birth weight (i.e., variable LBW) in these counties, for the same time period. These data have been obtained from the Online Analytical Statistical Information System (OASIS) database of the Georgia Department of Public Health (DPH). Low birth weight, defined as less than 2500 g, is linked to higher neonatal mortality rates and a heightened risk of various health issues and chronic diseases. Our analysis examines a recent dataset, in contrast to previous studies by Lawson (2008) and Blangiardo et al. (2013), which focused on similar datasets from earlier years identifying spatio-temporal correlation in their studies. With this information, we can compute the proportion of low weight births over the total number of births in each county and year, generating the spatial distribution that can be observed in the maps shown in Fig. 1. Here, we can see that there is a certain concentration of high values in the southwestern regions of the state, which becomes more pronounced from the year 2016 onwards.

We have fitted the spatio-temporal model proposed by Knorr-Held (2000), where we assume that the variables LBW_{ij}, conditioned on the random effects $\nu_i, \eta_i, \delta_j, \phi_j$ and ϵ_{ij}, follows a binomial distribution, where NB_{ij} is the number of trials on each region and time period. That is, $(\text{LBW}_{ij} | \nu_i, \eta_i, \delta_j, \phi_j, \epsilon_{ij}) \sim$

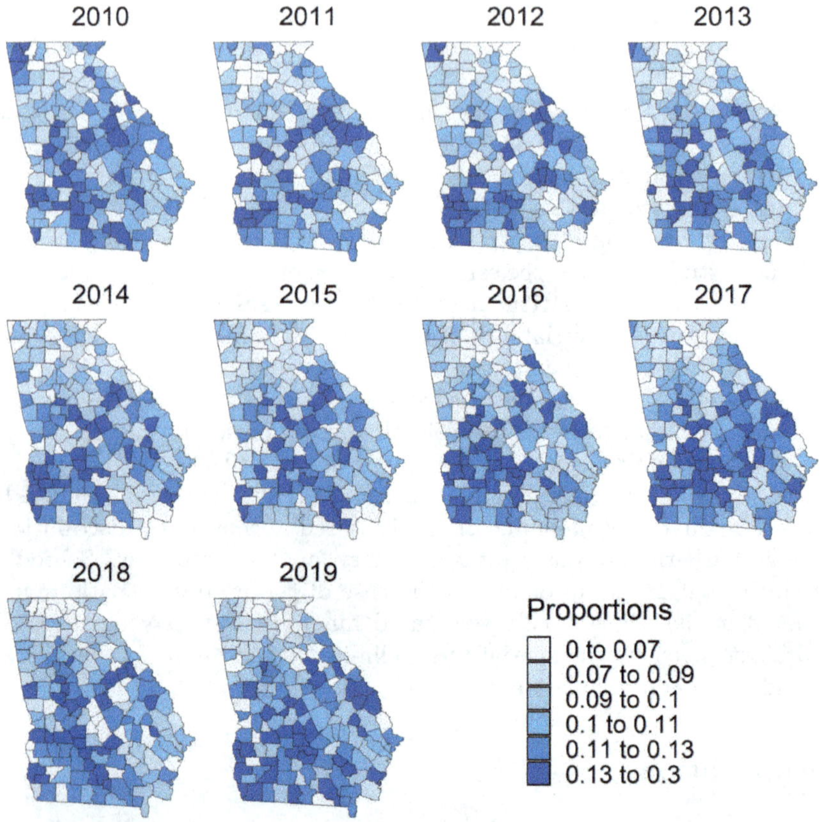

Fig. 1. Spatial distribution of the proportion of low birth weight (LBW) in Georgia by counties and year.

$\text{Bin}(\text{NB}_{ij}, \pi_{ij})$, for $i = 1, \ldots, n$ and $j = 1, \ldots, J$, with π_{ij} modelled so that:

$$\text{logit}(\pi_{\text{ij}}) = \beta_0 + \nu_{\text{i}} + \eta_{\text{i}} + \delta_{\text{j}} + \phi_{\text{j}} + \epsilon_{\text{ij}}, \tag{1}$$

where β_0 is a standard global intercept and the remaining terms are as before. In addition, we have also fitted our proposed spatio-temporal conditional model, where we assume that $(\text{LBW}_{ij}|\text{LBW}_{\sim ij}, \nu_i, \delta_j, \phi_j, \epsilon_{ij}) \sim \text{Bin}(\text{NB}_{ij}, \pi_{ij})$, for $i = 1, \ldots, n$ and $j = 1, \ldots, J$, with π_{ij} modelled in the following way:

$$\text{logit}(\pi_{\text{ij}}) = \beta_0 + \rho \text{A}_{\text{ij}} + \nu_{\text{i}} + \delta_{\text{j}} + \phi_{\text{j}} + \epsilon_{\text{ij}}, \tag{2}$$

where all the terms are as before. Finally, we have also fitted the proposed temporally varying spatial lag coefficient model, where we assume that $(\text{LBW}_{ij}|\text{LBW}_{\sim ij}, \nu_i, \delta_j, \phi_j, \epsilon_{ij}) \sim \text{Bin}(\text{NB}_{ij}, \pi_{ij})$, for $i = 1, \ldots, n$ and $j = 1, \ldots, J$, with π_{ij} modelled in the following way:

$$\text{logit}(\pi_{\text{ij}}) = \beta_0 + (\rho_0 + \rho_{\text{j}}) \text{A}_{\text{ij}} + \nu_{\text{i}} + \delta_{\text{j}} + \phi_{\text{j}} + \epsilon_{\text{ij}}, \tag{3}$$

where $\rho_j \sim N(0, \tau_\rho)$, with $\tau_\rho > 0$, and all the remaining terms are as before.

All the models have been fitted in R-INLA and we have assumed that the spatial structure of the data under study is represented by a spatial weights matrix $\mathbf{W}$, following the order one contiguity criterion. Additionally, in our assumed Bayesian framework, we have specified noninformative prior distributions. In particular, normal priors with large variances for the intercept (i.e., $\beta_0 \sim N(0, 1 \times 10^{-5})$) and also, for the spatial parameters ρ and ρ_0 (i.e., $\rho \sim N(0, 1 \times 10^{-5})$ and $\rho_0 \sim N(0, 1 \times 10^{-5})$). For the precision parameters of the random effects (i.e., for $\psi_\nu = 1/\tau_\nu$, $\psi_\eta = 1/\tau_\eta$, $\psi_\delta = 1/\tau_\delta$, $\psi_\phi = 1/\tau_\phi$, $\psi_\epsilon = 1/\tau_\epsilon$ and $\psi_\rho = 1/\tau_\rho$), we have assumed vague gamma priors, so that $\psi_{(\cdot)} \sim G(1 \times 10^{-4}, 1 \times 10^{-4})$. Furthermore, we have performed a sensitivity analysis in order to properly assess the values specified for the prior distributions of the precision parameters estimated in the models fitted in this study. Model comparison has been carried out by computing the Deviance Information Criterion (DIC) (Spiegelhalter et al., 2002) and Widely Applicable Information Criterion (WAIC) (Watanabe, 2010). The model with the lowest DIC or WAIC values is typically considered the best fitting one. DIC is based on the posterior mean of the deviance statistic, while WAIC is calculated from the expected log pointwise predictive density. These are both penalized by measures of model complexity.

Results obtained after fitting the models in Eqs. (1) and (2) to the low birth weight in Georgia data are reported in Table 1.

After fitting the model in Eq. (3), we obtained a value for the global spatial parameter of $\hat{\rho}_0 = 2.1318$ (SD $= 0.4519$), with a credible interval of $(1.2442, 3.0178)$ and information criteria values of DIC $= 10295$ and WAIC $= 10324$. The estimates obtained for ρ_j, which represent the temporal variation of the spatial correlation with respect to the one given by ρ_0, can be better assessed by examining Fig. 2. In this plot, the red curve represents the estimated mean value of ρ_j and the green bands, its 95% credible intervals, for the years under study. The remaining estimates are very similar to those obtained from the spatio-temporal conditional model included in Table 1.

Table 1. Results obtained after fitting the Knorr-Held and the spatio-temporal conditional models to the low birth weight in Georgia data.

	Knorr-Held			Spatio-temporal conditional		
	Mean	SD	CI	Mean	SD	CI
β_0	−2.205	(0.012)	(−2.228, −2.182)	−2.451	(0.053)	(−2.554, −2.348)
ρ	–	–	–	2.124	(0.443)	(1.254, 2.993)
τ_ν	0.012	(0.004)	(0.005, 0.021)	0.035	(0.005)	(0.027, 0.045)
τ_η	0.060	(0.021)	(0.030, 0.113)	–	–	–
τ_δ	2.66e−04	(3.00e−04)	(3.17e−05, 0.001)	2.17e−04	(2.43e−04)	(3.13e−05, 8.46e−04)
τ_ϕ	5.85e−04	(5.11e−04)	(9.47e−05, 0.002)	3.35e−04	(3.59e−04)	(2.80e−05, 0.001)
τ_ϵ	0.003	(7.54e−04)	(0.002,0.005)	0.004	(7.84e−04)	(0.002, 0.005)
	DIC = 10294, WAIC = 10325			DIC = 10296, WAIC = 10325		

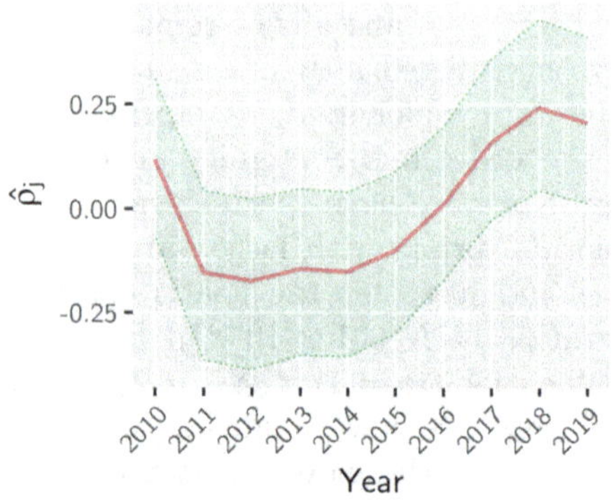

Fig. 2. Estimated mean and its credible interval, obtained for ρ_j after fitting the considered temporally varying spatial lag coefficient model.

4 Conclusions

We have proposed spatial conditional overdispersion models extensions for fitting spatio-temporal binomial count data and applied them to the study of low birth weight in Georgia. Our proposed models yielded similar goodness-of-fit when compared to the Knorr-Held model. However, they provided valuable additional insights about the type and strength of the spatial autocorrelation present in the data, with the positive spatial autocorrelation present in the data being appropriately captured. Furthermore, we applied the temporally varying spatial lag coefficient model to the same dataset, which additionally allowed us to investigate the temporal variation of the spatial autocorrelation coefficient. The analysis illustrated in Fig. 2, revealed a decreasing trend from 2011, followed by an increase from 2014, which slightly declined again from 2018. These findings suggest that the strongest spatial dependence occurred in 2018, while the weakest was observed approximately between 2011 and 2014, which is consistent with the pattern that was observed in the maps shown in Fig. 1. This comprehensive understanding of spatial dynamics enhances the interpretability and utility of our proposed models, distinguishing them as valuable tools for analysing spatio-temporal binomial count data.

Acknowledgements. This research has been partially funded by Ministerio de Ciencia e Innovación (MCIN, Spain), Agencia Estatal de Investigación (AEI/10.13039/501100011033/) and Fondo Europeo de Desarrollo Regional (FEDER) "Una manera de hacer Europa" under the I+D+i research grant PID2020-112951GB-I00 and by the Department of Education of the Basque Government (UPV/EHU Econometrics Research Group) under research grant IT-1508-22.

References

Blangiardo, M., Cameletti, M., Baio, G., Rue, H.: Spatial and spatio-temporal models with R-INLA. Spat. Spat.-Temp. Epidemiol. **4**, 33–49 (2013)

Cepeda-Cuervo, E., Córdoba, M., Núñez-Antón, V.: Conditional overdispersed models: application to count area data. Stat. Methods Med. Res. **27**, 2964–2988 (2018)

Knorr-Held, L.: Bayesian modelling of inseparable space-time variation in disease risk. Stat. Med. **19**, 2555–2567 (2000)

Lawson, A.: Bayesian Disease Mapping: Hierarchical Modeling in Spatial Epidemiology, 3rd edn. Chapman & Hall/CRC Press, Boca Raton (2008)

Morales-Otero, M., Núñez-Antón, V.: Comparing Bayesian spatial conditional overdispersion and the Besag-York-Mollié models: Application to infant mortality rates. Math. (Spec. Issue Spat. Stat. Appl.) **9**, 282 (2021)

Schrödle, B., Held, L.: Spatio-temporal disease mapping using INLA. Environmetrics **22**, 725–734 (2011)

Spiegelhalter, D.J., Best, N.G., Carlin, B.P., Van Der Linde, A.: Bayesian measures of model complexity and fit. J. Roy. Stat. Soc. - Ser. B **64**, 583–639 (2002)

Watanabe, S.: Asymptotic equivalence of Bayes cross validation and widely applicable information criterion in singular learning theory. J. Mach. Learn. Res. **11**, 3571–3594 (2010)

Elicitation of Priors for Intervention Effects in Educational Trial Data

Qing Zhang[1](✉), Germaine Uwimpuhwe[1], Dimitris Vallis[1,2], Akansha Singh[1], Tahani Coolen-Maturi[1], and Jochen Einbeck[1]

[1] Durham University, Durham, UK
{qing.zhang,germaine.uwimpuhwe,akansha.singh,tahani.maturi, jochen.einbeck}@durham.ac.uk, dimitris.vallis@kcl.ac.uk
[2] The Policy Institute, King's College London, London, UK

Abstract. Effect sizes for educational interventions are commonly small, and hence decisions to re-grant efficacy trials (small trials with homogeneous populations under idealized conditions) as effectiveness trials (larger trials with heterogeneous populations) are often based on limited evidence from the efficacy trial itself. However, supplementary evidence may be available on how (past) effectiveness trials with similar outcomes tend to perform. This work proposes a Bayesian approach of making use of such evidence for re-granting decisions.

Keywords: Randomized controlled trial · Multilevel model · Meta-analysis

1 Introduction

We introduce a Bayesian approach to support re-granting decisions for efficacy trials. By harvesting prior information from past effectiveness trials, and feeding this information in form of a prior distribution on the intervention parameter into a multilevel model, we aim to gain principled evidence on the effect size which would likely have been observed if the efficacy trial had been be run under the less idealized conditions of an effectiveness trial. The Education Endowment Foundation (EEF) established in 2011 have commissioned more than 200 educational efficacy and effectiveness trials in England. Two case studies funded by the EEF have been considered, involving re-granting decisions for the 'Lexia® Core5® Reading' and 'Maths Count' efficacy trials, to which we refer in brief as "Lexia trial" and "Maths trial" henceforth. For each case study, a series of 'similar' EEF effectiveness trials has been identified, their effect sizes obtained, and combined through a fixed-effect meta-analysis. The combined effect size was then used to inform the prior distribution in a Bayesian multilevel model for the estimation of the posterior. These analyses demonstrate how incorporating prior information can lead to more precise estimates of intervention effects, which, despite often resulting in smaller posterior effect sizes, lead to narrower

J. Einbeck et al. (Eds.): IWSM 2024, CONTRIB.STAT., pp. 28–33, 2024.
https://doi.org/10.1007/978-3-031-65723-8_5

confidence intervals[1] and a greater likelihood of identifying significant intervention effects.

2 Methodology

In accordance with the multi-site design of the efficacy trial to be re-granted (here, Lexia or Maths), a multilevel model can be defined following Singh et al. [2] as

$$Y_{ij} = \beta_0 + \beta_1 P_{ij} + \beta_2 T_{ij} + b_{0j} + b_{2j} T_{ij} + \epsilon_{ij}. \tag{1}$$

Here, Y_{ij} and P_{ij} represent the post-test and pre-test score for pupil i in school j, respectively, b_{0j}, b_{2j} school-specific (random) intercept and slope terms, and β_2 the intervention effect with prior distribution

$$\pi(\beta_2) = N(\mu, \sigma^2), \tag{2}$$

where typically μ and σ^2 need to be informed by a collection of K past effectiveness trials. A complication is that the outcome measures of the past effectiveness trials, and the efficacy trial at hand, may be different, so that the absolute scale of β_2 would be meaningless. This requires the outcome measure of the efficacy trial to be standardized (mean zero, unit variance). We consider two approaches to adjust the results from the K trials to this standardized scale. In the first approach, we re-fit a Bayesian multilevel model of type (1) with standardized outcomes to each trial $k = 1, \ldots, K$, yielding full posterior treatment distributions with mean μ_k and variance σ_k^2, which are then meta-analyzed to obtain $\mu = \frac{\sum_k w_k \mu_k}{\sum_k w_k}$, where $w_k = 1/\sigma_k^2$. In the second approach, we manually extract the intervention effects, in form of effect sizes, from the evaluation reports of the effectiveness trials, and then meta-analyze these effect sizes. The rationale for this approach is provided in Sect. 3.

3 Manual Elicitation of Priors from Evaluation Reports

For simplicity of presentation, we consider only a single past effectiveness trial, with estimated intervention effect $\hat{\beta}$ (obtained from a non-standardised analysis of the data) and standard error $\text{se}(\hat{\beta})$. Denote by $\hat{\sigma}_T^2$ the estimated total variance (usually, unconditional) from that trial. This defines the effect size $ES = \hat{\beta}/\hat{\sigma}_T$, with standard error $\text{se}(ES)$ (Hedges [1]). Effect size is a common measure used to estimate intervention effects in educational trials. These values will usually be provided in trial evaluation reports. Recall that the objective is to find a prior for the intervention parameter of the efficacy trial to be re-granted, denoted β_2 in (1). We denote this parameter now by β^* and assume that the analysis of

[1] This is technically a 'credible interval' but for ease of presentation we will use the term 'confidence interval' irrespective of whether it has been obtained in a Bayesian or frequentist way.

this efficacy trial will be carried out using standardised data. Accordingly, we denote by $\hat{\beta}^*$, $\hat{\sigma}_T^{*2}$ and ES^* an estimate of the intervention effect, the total unconditional variance, and the effect size, for the efficacy trial. The task is to elicit suitable values of μ^* and σ^* which can be used to specify a prior distribution $\pi(\beta^*) = N(\mu^*, \sigma^{*2})$. The key insights are as follows: If the outcome variable is standardised, then the true total variance exactly equals 1 so that one will have $\hat{\sigma}_T^{*2} \approx 1$. Since effect size is a dimensionless concept it is reasonable to assert that $ES = ES^*$. Combining these, one has $\hat{\beta}^* \approx ES^* = ES$. Hence, the effect size estimate from the evaluation report can be used as the prior mean for the standardised Bayesian analysis of the efficacy trial. In order to specify the prior variance, we note that

$$\text{se}(ES^*) = \text{se}(\hat{\beta}^*/\widehat{\sigma}_T^*) = \sqrt{\text{var}(\hat{\beta}^*/\widehat{\sigma}_T^*)} \gtrsim \sqrt{\text{var}(\hat{\beta}^*)} = \text{se}(\hat{\beta}^*), \tag{3}$$

where the property at $\gtrsim$ follows from results in Goodman [3]. That is, the variance of $\hat{\beta}^*/\widehat{\sigma}_T^*$ will tend to be a bit larger than that of $\hat{\beta}^*$ (since the denominator, while approximately equal to 1, will still induce additional variation). Derivation (3) implies that $\text{se}(\hat{\beta}^*) \lesssim \text{se}(ES^*)$ and hence it is reasonable to use $\text{se}(ES^*)$ as an upper bound for $\text{se}(\hat{\beta}^*)$, to represent our prior uncertainty about $\hat{\beta}^*$. Finally, we follow analogous reasoning as above to assert that $\text{se}(ES) = \text{se}(ES^*)$. In summary, following the extraction of an effect size ES and its standard error, $\text{se}(ES)$, from an evaluation report, one has the remarkably simple result

$$\pi(\beta^*) = N(ES, \text{se}(ES)^2) \tag{4}$$

as the prior for our efficacy trial. While this will remain valid irrespectively of whether the past effectiveness trial has been using standardised or non-standardised data, it is important to recall that the analysis of the efficacy trial always needs to use standardised data. It also needs noting that $\text{se}(ES)$ will often not be given in the evaluator's report, but will instead need to be inferred from a reported 95% confidence interval for the effect size, $CI_{ES} = (\underline{ES}, \overline{ES})$, via $\text{se}(ES) = (\overline{ES} - \underline{ES})/(1.96 \times 2)$.

In some special situations one may not be able to use (4), e.g. because the evaluation reports do not provide effect sizes and standard errors. Apart from such rare cases, Eq. (4) will generally be usable, and can equally be used for a meta-analyzed effect size arising from a collection of trials.

4 Results

Figure 1 displays the fixed-effect meta-analyses that were performed on all collected priors using inverse-variance weighting to generate the combined prior for both the manual and Bayesian methodologies within the Lexia and Maths efficacy trials. The priors are represented by squares, and the horizontal lines correspond to the 95% confidence intervals (CI). Larger squares indicate a greater weight in the meta-analysis. For the Lexia trial, the manual priors ranged from

-0.06 to 0.13 with a combined prior of 0.061. The heterogeneity among the studies was low ($I^2 = 2\%$), indicating a high level of consistency across studies. The Bayesian priors showed a slightly reduced combined prior of 0.031, with no observed heterogeneity ($I^2 = 0\%$). For the Maths trial, the manual priors varied more significantly, ranging from −0.01 to 0.27 with a combined prior of −0.000. Heterogeneity was substantial ($I^2 = 64\%$), reflecting variability in the study outcomes. Bayesian priors showed a combined prior of 0.036 with moderate heterogeneity ($I^2 = 56\%$).

Application of the methodologies to the two efficacy trials is provided in Tables 1 and 2. We see that the priors based on the two elicitation approaches are similar. Employing the priors obtained from re-fitted Bayesian model, one finds that despite reducing posterior means, the posterior precision has increased, indicating, in the case of Lexia, increased support towards a positive re-granting decision.

The application of meta-analyzed priors resulted in considerably shifted posterior estimates compared to those obtained using non-informative priors. This discrepancy elucidates the substantial influence that the choice of prior can exert on the posterior treatment effect within a Bayesian analytical framework. The employment of a non-informative prior, often representing a state of relative agnosticism regarding prior knowledge, yields a posterior distribution that is more influenced by the data from the current analysis. Conversely, informative priors, particularly those derived from meta-analytical methods, can markedly temper the posterior estimates, thus manifesting a more moderated effect size that is informed by a broader base of pre-existing evidence. Such moderation is observable in the decreased mean and standard deviation of the posterior estimates, suggesting that the informative priors contribute to a more nuanced and potentially more reliable estimation of treatment effects.

Table 1. Meta-analyzed priors from manual computation and resulting from refitted Bayesian models.

Trial	Priors	Meta-analysed ES CI_{ES}	Prior	
			Mean	S. Dev.
Lexia	Manual	0.061 $(-0.001, 0.124)$	0.061	0.032
	Bayesian	0.031 $(-0.028, 0.089)$	0.031	0.030
Maths	Manual	−0.000 $(-0.019, 0.019)$	−0.000	0.010
	Bayesian	0.036 $(-0.025, 0.097)$	0.036	0.031

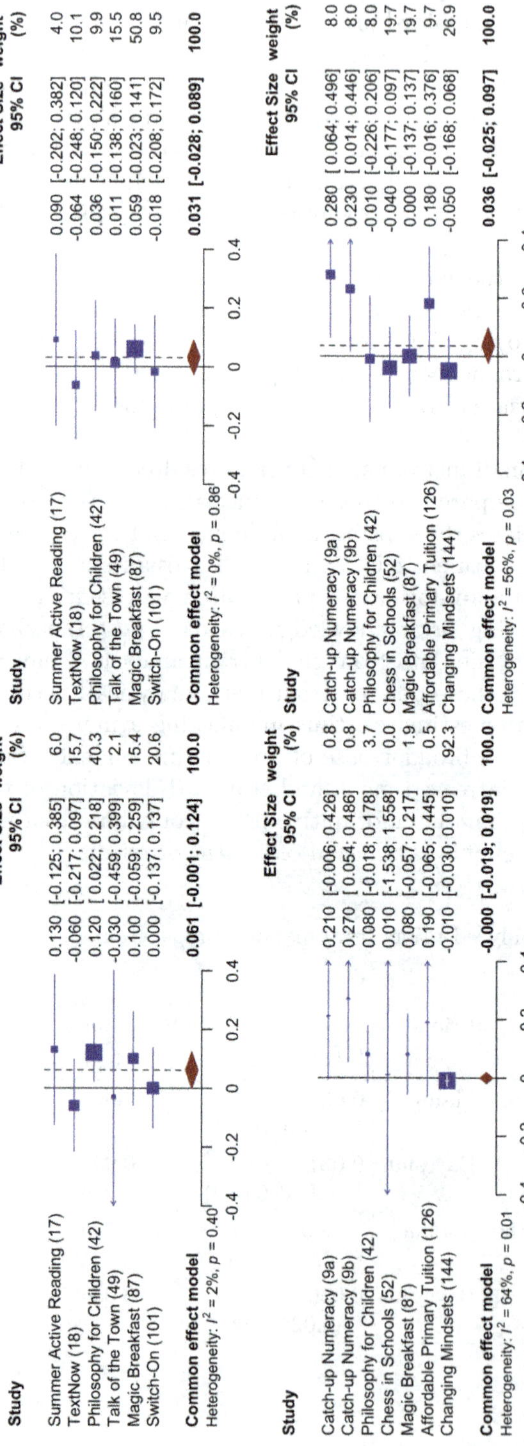

Fig. 1. Meta-analyses of manual versus Bayesian priors across two trials (Upper panel: Lexia trial; lower panel: Maths trial; left column: manual priors; right column: Bayesian priors)

Table 2. Prior and posterior intervention means and standard deviations for the intervention parameter β_2, using non-informative priors, and priors resulting from re-fitted and meta-analyzed Bayesian model estimates.

Trial	Priors source	Prior		Posterior	
		Mean	S. Dev.	Mean	S. Dev.
Lexia	Non-Informative	0.000	100.000	0.078	0.066
	Meta-analysis	0.031	0.030	0.038	0.027
Maths	Non-Informative	0.000	100.000	0.203	0.130
	Meta-analysis	0.036	0.031	0.046	0.030

Acknowledgments. Special thanks to the EEF for funding this research. We would like to thank FFT for enabling access to EEF's data archive. This work was produced using statistical data from ONS. The use of the ONS statistical data in this work does not imply the endorsement of the ONS in relation to the interpretation or analysis of the statistical data. This work uses research datasets which may not exactly reproduce National Statistics aggregates.

References

1. Hedges, L.V.: Effect sizes in cluster-randomized designs. J. Educ. Behav. Stat. **32**, 341–370 (2007)
2. Singh, A., Uwimpuhwe, G., Li, M., Einbeck, J., Higgins, S., Kasim, A.: Multi-site educational trials: estimating the effect size and its confidence intervals. Int. J. Res. Method Educ. **45**, 18–38 (2021)
3. Goodman, L.A.: The variance of the product of K random variables. J. Am. Stat. Assoc. **57**, 55–60 (1962)

Addressing Covariate Lack in Unit-Level Small Area Models Using GAMLSS

Lorenzo Mori(✉) and Maria Rosaria Ferrante

Department of Statistical Sciences "Paolo Fortunati", University of Bologna, Bologna, Italy
{lorenzo.mori7,maria.ferrante}@unibo.it

Abstract. The primary goal of this study is to estimate the Theil index using a unit-level Small Area Estimation (SAE) model. This has lead two primary challenges in the unit-level SAE field: the identification of individual covariates and the reduction of computational burden. We propose a unit-level Simplified SAE model based on Generalized Additive Models for Location, Scale and Shape (GAMLSS), which is specified without covariates and is able to reduce variability in comparison with the direct estimator. The performance of the proposed model used to estimate the Theil index is evaluated based on design-based simulations. An application to the Italian Regions, distinguish between Urban, Peri-Urban and Rural areas, conclude the paper.

Keywords: GAMLSS · Atkinson index · Computational burden

1 The Core of the Problem

Small Area Estimation (SAE) techniques are tools for generating reliable estimates in scenarios where sample sizes within specific domains or areas are insufficient. These methods aim to reduce estimate variability by incorporating information from neighboring areas and auxiliary data sources that are typically free from sampling error.

Unit-level models present two main challenges: the availability of individual-level auxiliary information without sampling errors and the increased computational effort, which becomes more pronounced for non-Normal and/or non-linear estimates. Securing individual-level auxiliary information, even from national statistical institutes, is often hindered by confidentiality restrictions. The relationship between covariate inclusion and computational burden is noteworthy. Monte Carlo (MC) approximation and parametric bootstrap techniques, essential for estimating outcome parameters and variability measures, respectively, are computationally intensive, particularly in unit-level models. Each iteration of MC estimation and parametric bootstrap necessitates the prediction of outcome variable values for non-sampled units based on estimated regression parameters and auxiliary information. This process significantly escalates computational time, particularly in unit-level models with large populations.

J. Einbeck et al. (Eds.): IWSM 2024, CONTRIB.STAT., pp. 34–40, 2024.
https://doi.org/10.1007/978-3-031-65723-8_6

In the following, we propose to use a Simplified SAE method defined using Generalized Additive Models for Location, Scale and Shape (referred to as Simplified SAE-GAMLSS), feasible without covariates and able to reduce the computational times when compared with SAE-GAMLSS. For an introduction to GAMLSS and the specifics of SAE-GAMLSS, which employs the MC to obtain estimates and a parametric bootstrap for the Mean Square Error (MSE) estimation, we mainly refer to [6,8].

2 The Proposal

Suppose we have a finite population Ω of N units divided into J sub-populations $\Omega_1, \ldots, \Omega_J$, called areas of size $N_1, \ldots, N_J$, where $N = \sum_{j=1}^{J} N_j$. Identifying with Y_{ij} the target variable and with y_{ij} the observation for unit $i = 1, \ldots, n$ and area $j = 1, \ldots, J$. In the SAE context, the aim is to estimate area parameters in the form of $H_j = \zeta(Y_{ij})$ where $\zeta(\cdot)$ is a real measurable function. Design-based estimates of these area parameters are obtained using data from the sample s of size n drawn from the population Ω with sub-sample $s_j = s \cap \Omega_j$ from area j of size n_j, where $n = \sum_{j=1}^{J} n_j$. Assume a generic PDF $f(Y_{ij})$ with at most four different parameters μ, σ, ν and τ each of which is defined in terms of an intercept and a random effect, i,e. covariates are not available. In this case a GAMLSS is:

$$
\begin{cases}
g_{\mu}(\mu_j) = \beta^{\mu} + \gamma_j^{\mu} \\
g_{\sigma}(\sigma_j) = \beta^{\sigma} + \gamma_j^{\sigma} \\
g_{\nu}(\nu_j) = \beta^{\nu} + \gamma_j^{\nu} \\
g_{\tau}(\tau_j) = \beta^{\tau} + \gamma_j^{\tau}
\end{cases}
\tag{1}
$$

where g_k's are link-functions and γ_j^k random effects for $k = (\mu, \sigma, \nu, \tau)$. This formulation indicates that each parameter is only influenced by the random effects of the area. Unlike the SAE-GAMLSS approach, we use a penalized weighted likelihood function to estimate (1), incorporating sample weights w_i. By using sample weights, we effectively include information from informative sampling designs without exacerbating issues for non-informative ones. Two key observations are noteworthy: (i) most indicators can be expressed as integrals of a transformation of a PDF, and (ii) when the PDF's parameters are determined solely by an intercept and a random effect, all units within a given area share the same predicted value. This implies that $\widehat{H}_j$ of $H_j = \zeta(Y_{ij})$ can be obtained by solving an integral:

$$
\widehat{H}_j = E[\zeta(Y_{ij})] = \int_a^b \zeta(Y_{ij}) f(Y_{ij}) dY_i, \quad j = 1, \ldots, J \tag{2}
$$

Here, a and b denote the limits of the integral, chosen depending on the index. Notably, the Theil index (T_j) has a closed-form expressions derived from (2) for various probabilistic distributions suitable for household income/consumption.

These closed-form expressions play a central role in the Simplified SAE-GAMLSS. Instead of using MC approximation, we leverage the closed form of the index leading to a more rapid estimation process.

In Table 1, we present closed-form expressions of T_j for various distributions.

Let us consider, for example, the Log-Normal distribution. In this specific case, T_j is a function of the scale parameter only. By estimating Eq. 1, we are able, thanks to the random effects, to estimate the Theil index for all areas without using covariates and without burdening the model by incorporating random effects in the μ parameter as well.

Table 1. Theil index for classical income/consumption distribution ($\Gamma(\cdot)$ is the Gamma function and $\Psi(\cdot)$ is the Digamma function)

Distribution	Theil index
Exponential	$1-\mu_j^{-1}$
GB2	$\frac{\Psi(\nu_j+1/\sigma_j)-\Psi(\tau_j-1/\sigma_j)}{\sigma_j} - \frac{\log(\Gamma(\nu_j+1/\sigma_j)\Gamma(\tau_j-1/\sigma_j))}{\Gamma(\nu_j)\Gamma(\tau_j)}$
Log-Normal	$\sigma_j^2/2$
Pareto	$\log(1-1/\sigma_j)+(\sigma_j-1)^{-1}$
Weibull	$\sigma_j^{-1}\Psi(1+1/\sigma_j)-\log(\Gamma(1+1/\sigma_j))$

To estimate the MSE of the Theil index, we propose to use a non-parametric bootstrap based on the methodology outlined by [9].

2.1 Non-parametric Bootstrap

Keeping in mind the results obtained by [4] and by [7] for the non-parametric bootstrap with clustered data and following the idea of [9], we propose a non-parametric bootstrap to estimate the MSE that uses specific bootstrap sample weights. The use of specific sample weights is required by the weighted penalized likelihood function used to estimate GAMLSS. In the following we distinguish sampled units i, $i=1,\ldots,n_j$, in area j of size n_j and sample weights w_i for the sampled households. Using the superscript h for all the "elements" linked to households we have: n_j^h units, $i^h=1,\ldots,n_j^h$, in area j of size $n_j^h : n_j^h \leq n_j$ and sample weights w_{i^h}. For simplicity, we denote $H_j(Y_{ij})$ as H_j and $\widehat{H}_j(Y_{ij})$ as $\widehat{H}_j$. The MSE of $\widehat{H}_j$ is defined as:

$$MSE_j = E[(\widehat{H}_j - H_j)^2] \quad \text{for} \quad j=1,\ldots,J \tag{3}$$

and can be estimated based on the following steps:

1. Split the data-set into j sub data-sets one for each area.
2. For each sub data-set re-sample n_j^h-1 households with replacement.

3. Create a bootstrap sample data binding the sub data-sets together, call S^*, and assign each unit a re-weighting adjustment factor equal to:

$$G_{i^h} = \frac{n_j^h}{n_j^h - 1} \times Hs_{i^h} \tag{4}$$

where Hs_{i^h} is the number of times the household i^h is selected in the resample.
4. Compute the bootstrap sampling weight as:

$$w^*_{i^h} = G_{i^h} w_{i^h}$$

5. Account for the calibration by calibrating the weights $w^*_{i^h}$ on the totals X_{tot}. This leads to the bootstrap calibrated weights:

$$w^c_{i^h} = w^*_{i^h}(1 + x^T_{i^h}\lambda^*_t)$$

with

$$\lambda^*_t = \left(\sum_{i^h in S^*} w^*_{i^h} x_{i^h} x^T_{i^h}\right)^{-1} \left(X_{tot} - \sum_{i^h \in S^*} w^*_{i^h} x_{i^h}\right)$$

6. Expand the sample S^* from households to units and fit the model.
7. Obtain the bootstrap estimator of H_j through the proposed method and denote it as $\hat{H}^*_j$.
8. Repeat steps [2–7] a large number of times, say B times.

Let $\hat{H}^*_j(b)$ the estimator obtained in b-th replicate of the bootstrap procedure, $b = 1, \ldots, B$, the bootstrap mean square-error estimator of $\hat{H}_j$ is given by:

$$\widehat{MSE}_B(\hat{H}_j) = \frac{1}{B-1} \sum_{b=1}^{B} \left[\hat{H}^*_j(b) - \frac{1}{B} \sum_{b=1}^{B} \hat{H}^*_j(b)\right]^2 \tag{5}$$

The bootstrapping procedure deserves some explanation. First, we use households rather than individuals as resampling units ([1,5]) because classical consumption and income surveys usually use households as sample units. The definition of a specific individual weight is not necessary because the most common surveys report data for all household units, i.e., within the same household, the individual weights for each unit are (often) equal to the household weight. Second, between steps 4 and 5, a correction for non-response can be applied to the weights. Thirdly, but even more important than the previous points, the calibration of the weights requires the knowledge of some totals. We use as a known total only the total number of households in the population, i.e., N^h. This methodology is notably faster than the usual parametric bootstrap.

3 Simulation Results

In this simulation the Household Budget Survey (HBS) plays the role of a pseudo-population which is kept fixed. This survey, conducted by the Italian Statistical Institute, is based on a sample of approximately 18000 households, representative of all Italian households. We set up a simulation based on 49 small areas (NUTS 2) subdivided into urban, peri-urban and rural areas. The target index is the Theil index computed using the equivalized consumption expenditure. The sample size ranges from a minimum of 2 to a maximum of 68 and the sample design mimic the original one. We include in the simulation, in addition to the Direct estimator, a SAE-GAMLSS (with as covariates: sex, age, education level and primary source of income) and a Simplified SAE-GAMLSS assuming for both a Log-Normal distribution.

The main aims of this simulation are to evaluate if Simplified SAE-GAMLSS performs better than Direct estimator and what is the gap, paid in terms of reliability, between SAE-GAMLSS and Simplified SAE-GAMLSS.

In order to compare results, we consider indicators that evaluate both accuracy in terms of variability and bias. The following measures of performance averaged over areas are used: average absolute relative bias (AARB), average coefficient of variation (ACV) and average relative root mean square error (ARRMSE). Table 2 summarises all previously reported measures of performance. Examining the AARB, it becomes clear that SAE-GAMLSS consistently has the lowest AARB, followed by Simplified SAE-GAMLSS and finally by the Direct estimator that as known can be heavily biased for such low sample size ([3]). Regarding the reliability measures (ACV, ARRMSE), Table 2 shows that, as expected, the ACV of direct estimates is the highest. SAE-GAMLSS significantly reduces the variability of the estimates. Again as expected, Simplified SAE-GAMLSS performs worse than SAE-GAMLSS but better than Direct.

From these initial results, it is evident that Simplified SAE-GAMLSS performs worse than SAE-GAMLSS but consistently produces better results compared to the Direct estimator, establishing itself as a valid alternative in case of inaccessible covariates. Furthermore, is able to reduce the computational times of SAE-GAMLSS by more than 80%.

Table 2. Measures of Performance (results in %)

	Direct	SAE-GAMLSS	Simplified SAE-GAMLSS
Theil index			
AARB	3.00	1.30	2.57
ACV	40.66	10.16	20.09
ARRMSE	4.48	1.32	3.07

4 Application and Concluding Remarks

In this section we use the Simplified SAE-GAMLSS to estimate the Theil index for foreigners and Italian citizens in 49 different areas. The areas are defined as the Italian NUTS 2 (20 administrative Regions), each of which is further subdivided into three subgroups: urban, peri-urban and rural (not all areas have all three groupings). This definition is in line with the HBS variables. Urban areas are metropolitan centers, peri-urban areas are cities with more than 50000 inhabitants and those included in the metropolitan areas but outside the center. All other areas are rural. The migrants in question are regular migrants who already have a residence permit. Those in an irregular status, those waiting for a permit or those who own property in Italy without having a residence are not included in the sample and are therefore not considered in this discussion. The dependent variable is the equivalised expenditure recorded in the HBS.

The HBS sample size allows reliable estimates of the Theil index only for Italian citizens. Due to the small sample sizes, the estimates for foreigners are unreliable. For those reasons we use the direct estimator for Italians and the Simplified SAE-GAMLSS for Foreigners. The mean CV, using those two estimators, is 7.307% and 18.751% respectively. Note as using the direct estimator also for Foreigners the mean CV is around 30%.

Figure 1 shows the estimated values for Italians and for foreigners in Italy. At a first glance, one immediately notices significant disparities in inequalities between foreigners and Italians. Let us begin with the urban areas. The Theil index for migrants is more than 3% points higher than that of native-born individuals in this area. Moving to peri-urban areas, estimates indicate that differences between the two groups are less pronounced. Among foreigners, the indicators follow a similar trajectory from North to South as in urban areas, but, on average, indicators are around 2.5% points lower. For Italians, differences are less conspicuous, with indicators only 2% lower. Additionally, the gap between the two groups is narrower. the Theil index is, on average, 2.8% points higher for foreigners. In rural areas, indicators are nearly equal to those in peri-urban areas for Italians. However, for foreigners the inequality increase by approximately 1% point.

In our opinion, these findings mark a preliminary stride towards crafting location-specific policies aimed at fostering equity. The resultant maps unveil significant disparities across the designated areas. Undoubtedly, the Southern regions of Italy, particularly the rural areas of Calabria and Apulia, demand heightened attention. These regions have gained notoriety for migrant exploitation within the agricultural sector. Furthermore, as highlighted by [2], approximately 20 settlements in Apulia lack basic utilities and services, existing as makeshift outdoor dwellings. Our findings echo the conclusions drawn by other scholars, underscoring the imperative need for decisive policies to address this plight. Calabria, alongside Apulia, likely confront similar challenges albeit, warranting equivalent attention.

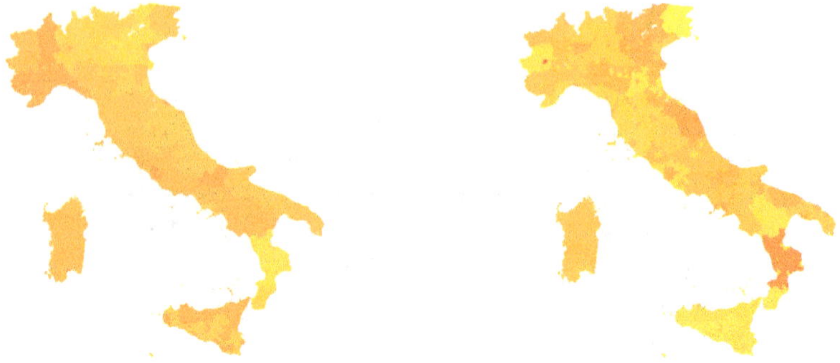

(a) Theil index, Italian (b) Theil index, foreigners

Fig. 1. Estimates of the Theil index for Foreigners and Italians

References

1. Bessonneau, P., Brilhaut, G., Chauvet, G., Garcia, C.: With replacement bootstrap variance estimation for household surveys: Principles, examples and implementation. Working paper, Statistic Canada hal-02514797f (2020)
2. Busetta, A., Mendola, D., Wilson, B., Cetorelli, V.: Measuring vulnerability of asylum seekers and refugees in Italy. J. Ethn. Migr. Stud. **47**(3), 596–615 (2021)
3. De Nicoló, S., Ferrante, M.R., Pacei, S.: Small-sample bias correction of inequality estimators in complex surveys. J. Official Stat., 1–24 (2024). (In Press)
4. Field, C.A., Welsh, H.A.: Bootstrapping clustered data. J. R. Stat. Soc. Ser. B Stat Methodol. **69**(3), 369–390 (2007)
5. Luus, R., Neethling, A., De Wet, T.: Effectiveness of weighting and bootstrap in the estimation of welfare indices under complex sampling: theory and methods. S. Afr. Stat. J. **46**(1), 85–114 (2012)
6. Mori, L., Ferrante, M.R.: Small area estimation under unit-level generalized additive models for location, scale and shape. ArXiv preprint (2023)
7. Ng, E.S.-W., Grieve, R., Carpenter, J.R.: Two-stage nonparametric bootstrap sampling with shrinkage correction for clustered data. Stand Genomic Sci. **13**(1), 141–164 (2013)
8. Rigby, R.A., Stasinopoulos, D.M.: Generalized additive models for location, scale and shape. J. R. Stat. Soc.: Ser. C: Appl. Stat. **54**(3), 507–554 (2005)
9. Rust, K., Rao, J.N.K.: Variance estimation for complex surveys using replication techniques. Stat. Methods Med. Res. **5**(3), 283–310 (1996)

Optimism Correction of the AUC with Complex Survey Data

Amaia Iparragirre[1(✉)] and Irantzu Barrio[1,2(✉)]

[1] Univesity of the Basque Country UPV/EHU, Leioa, Spain
{amaia.iparragirre,irantzu.barrio}@ehu.eus
[2] BCAM - Basque Center for Applied Mathematics, Leioa, Spain

Abstract. Special statistical techniques are required to develop valid prediction models for complex survey data. Recently, a weighted estimator has been proposed to estimate the area under the receiver operating characteristic curve in this context. However, the proposed estimator has shown an optimistic behaviour. Thus, the goal of this work is to analyze the performance of replicate weights methods to correct for the optimism of the AUC in the context of complex survey data.

Keywords: area under the receiver operating characteristic curve (AUC) · complex survey data · optimism correction · Replicate weights

1 Introduction

Complex survey data (CSD) is usually obtained by sampling a population of interest for the survey following complex sampling design techniques such as stratification or clustering. The units that finally end up in the sample are assigned a sampling weight, which indicates the number of units that the sampled unit represents in the finite population. Given the special characteristics of CSD, statistical techniques accounting for the sampling design should be considered to develop good prediction models.

This work focuses on logistic regression models and the discrimination ability of these. In particular, Iparragirre et al. (2023b) proposed a weighted estimator to estimate the area under the receiver operating characteristic curve (AUC) of logistic regression models in the context of CSD [1]. Even though this estimator corrects for the bias produced by ignoring the sampling design, the authors regarded that the weighted estimator of the AUC offered slightly greater estimates than the true AUC, in the same line as has been observed for simple random samples [2]. Hence, the goal of this work is to analyze the validity of "replicate weights" techniques such as Rescaling Bootstrap [3] and design-based cross-validation [4] to correct for this optimism. For this purpose, a simulation study has been conducted considering different complex sampling designs, and the AUCs corrected by means of replicate weights methods have been compared to the true population AUCs.

J. Einbeck et al. (Eds.): IWSM 2024, CONTRIB.STAT., pp. 41–47, 2024.
https://doi.org/10.1007/978-3-031-65723-8_7

2 Methods

Given a finite population, U, and a sample $S \subset U$ obtained based on a complex design sampling scheme, the vector of regression coefficients $\boldsymbol{\beta}$ for the logistic regression model is estimated ($\hat{\boldsymbol{\beta}}$) based on the pseudo-likelihood function in Eq. (1):

$$PL(\boldsymbol{\beta}) = \prod_{i \in S} p_i^{y_i w_i} (1 - p_i)^{(1-y_i)w_i}, \tag{1}$$

and the probability of event estimated for each unit in S can be computed following Eq. (2):

$$\hat{p}_i = e^{\hat{\boldsymbol{\beta}}^t \boldsymbol{x}_i} / (1 + e^{\hat{\boldsymbol{\beta}}^t \boldsymbol{x}_i}), \tag{2}$$

where $\forall i \in S$ y_i indicates the value of the dichotomous response variable, $\boldsymbol{x}_i$ its vector of covariates and w_i the corresponding sampling weight. Iparragirre et al. (2023b) [1] proposed estimating the AUC (apparent AUC, hereinafter) of the fitted model following Eq. (3):

$$\widehat{AUC}_w^{\text{app}} = \frac{\sum_{i_0 \in S_0} \sum_{i_1 \in S_1} w_{i_0} w_{i_1} \psi(\hat{p}_{i_0}, \hat{p}_{i_1})}{\sum_{i_0 \in S_0} \sum_{i_1 \in S_1} w_{i_0} w_{i_1}}, \tag{3}$$

where,

$$\psi(\hat{p}_{i_0}, \hat{p}_{i_1}) = I(\hat{p}_{i_0} < \hat{p}_{i_1}) + 0.5 I(\hat{p}_{i_0} = \hat{p}_{i_1}), \tag{4}$$

and S_0 and S_1 indicate the subsets of the units without and with the event of interest, respectively (i.e., $\forall i_0 \in S_0$ $y_{i_0} = 0$ and $\forall i_1 \in S_1$ $y_{i_1} = 1$, note that $S = S_0 \cup S_1$). However, this estimator may be optimistic when the same data is used to fit the model and estimate its discrimination ability. Therefore, in this work, we propose using the Rescaling Bootstrap (RB) or the design-based cross-validation (dCV) replicate weights methods for the optimism correction of $\widehat{AUC}_w^{\text{app}}$. The validity of those methods for this purpose has been analyzed by means of a simulation study.

3 Simulation Study

Population Generation: A finite population U of $N = 10\,000$ units is generated with information on $p = 5$ covariates and 2 design variables following a Gaussian distribution. The response variable for the population units is randomly generated by following Bernoulli's distribution based on their probability of event, for which the vector of regression coefficients has been pre-defined. Several strata and clusters within strata have been defined in the finite population, considering the information on the design variables. A more detailed explanation regarding the population generation can be seen elsewhere [1].

Sampling Process: Three different scenarios have been considered for different sampling designs: one-stage stratified sampling (SH), two-stage stratified cluster sampling without any cluster-level covariates (SC.0), and two-stage stratified cluster sampling with a cluster-level covariate (SC.1). In SC.0 and SC.1,

$a_h = 2$ clusters per stratum are randomly selected in the first stage. A predefined number of units are sampled from each stratum (SH) or cluster (SC.0 and SC.1).
Set-Up: For $r = 1, \ldots, 500$, obtain the sample S^r and the sampling weights w_i^r, $\forall i \in S^r$ following the corresponding sampling design and sampling scheme each time. Fit the model to S^r ($\hat{\boldsymbol{\beta}}^r$), obtain $\hat{p}_i^r, \forall i \in S^r$ and estimate the apparent AUC following Eq. (3): $\widehat{AUC}_w^{r,\text{app}}$. Estimate the corrected AUCs using one of the following methods, $\forall r = 1, \ldots, 500$:

Rescaling Bootstrap (RB)

1. Based on S^r, obtain bootstrap resamples $S^{r(b)}$, $\forall b = 1, \ldots, B$ and the corresponding replicate weights $w_i^{*,r(b)}$ [4]. Then, $\forall b = 1, \ldots, B$:
   (a) Fit the model to $S^{r(b)}$ by Eq. (1) and obtain $\hat{\boldsymbol{\beta}}^{r(b)}$ and $\hat{p}_i^{r(b)}, \forall i \in S^{r(b)}$. Estimate the AUC ($\widehat{AUC}_w^{r(b)}$) in $S^{r(b)}$ following eqs. (3) and (4), considering $\hat{p}_i^{r(b)}, \forall i \in S^{r(b)}$:

$$\widehat{AUC}_w^{r(b)} = \frac{\sum_{i_0 \in S_0^{r(b)}} \sum_{i_1 \in S_1^{r(b)}} w_{i_0}^{*,r(b)} w_{i_1}^{*,r(b)} \psi(\hat{p}_{i_0}^{r(b)}, \hat{p}_{i_1}^{r(b)})}{\sum_{i_0 \in S_0^{r(b)}} \sum_{i_1 \in S_1^{r(b)}} w_{i_0}^{*,r(b)} w_{i_1}^{*,r(b)}}, \quad (5)$$

   where $S^{r(b)} = S_0^{r(b)} \cup S_1^{r(b)}$.
   (b) Apply the coefficients $\hat{\boldsymbol{\beta}}^{r(b)}$ estimated in (a) to S^r and obtain $\hat{p}_{i,S^r}^{r(b)}, \forall i \in S^r$ following Eq. (2). Estimate the AUC ($\widehat{AUC}_{w,S^r}^{r(b)}$) in S^r following eqs. (3) and (4), considering $\hat{p}_{i,S^r}^{r(b)}, \forall i \in S^r$:

$$\widehat{AUC}_{w,S^r}^{r(b)} = \frac{\sum_{i_0 \in S_0^r} \sum_{i_1 \in S_1^r} w_{i_0}^r w_{i_1}^r \psi(\hat{p}_{i_0,S_0^r}^{r(b)}, \hat{p}_{i_1,S_1^r}^{r(b)})}{\sum_{i_0 \in S_0^r} \sum_{i_1 \in S_1^r} w_{i_0}^r w_{i_1}^r}, \quad (6)$$

   where $S^r = S_0^r \cup S_1^r$.
2. Estimate the optimism of the resamples and correct the AUC:

$$O^r = \frac{1}{B} \sum_{b=1}^{B} (\widehat{AUC}_w^{r(b)} - \widehat{AUC}_{w,S^r}^{r(b)}),$$

$$\widehat{AUC}_w^{r,\text{RB}} = \widehat{AUC}_w^{r,\text{app}} - O^r. \quad (7)$$

Two different techniques to define bootstrap resamples have been considered: the one proposed by Rao and Wu (1988) [3] (RB, hereinafter) and the one proposed by Canty and Davison (1999) [5] (RBn).

Design-Based Cross-Validation (dCV)

Define K subsets randomly splitting the sample S^r into K disjoint groups as proposed in [4]. The whole process is repeated L times with a different sample split each time. For $k = 1, \ldots, K$ and $l = 1, \ldots, L$, form the training set excluding the kth subset ($S_{\text{train}}^{r(l,k)}$, with the corresponding replicate weights $w_{\text{train}}^{*,r(l,k)}$) and fit the model with Eq. (1) ($\hat{\boldsymbol{\beta}}^{r(l,k)}$). Apply $\hat{\boldsymbol{\beta}}^{r(l,k)}$ to the corresponding test set $S_{\text{test}}^{r(l,k)}$ formed by the kth subset (with replicate weights $w_{\text{test}}^{*,r(l,k)}$) and estimate the probabilities for those units following Eq. (2): $\hat{p}_i^{r(l,k)}$, $\forall i \in S_{\text{test}}^{r(l,k)}$. Note that each unit is set to the test set only once. Thus, for each unit, only one probability is estimated based on the corresponding training model (in each split l). Two different ways of estimating the AUC have been considered. On the one hand, by means of the so-called average strategy, the AUC of each test set $S_{\text{test}}^{r(l,k)}$ is estimated first following eqs. (3) and (4) (let us denote as $\widehat{AUC}_w^{r(l,k)}$ this AUC):

$$\widehat{AUC}_w^{r(l,k)} = \frac{\sum_{i_0 \in S_{\text{test},0}^{r(l,k)}} \sum_{i_1 \in S_{\text{test},1}^{r(l,k)}} w_{\text{test},i_0}^{*,r(l,k)} w_{\text{test},i_1}^{*,r(l,k)} \psi(\hat{p}_{i_0}^{r(l,k)}, \hat{p}_{i_1}^{r(l,k)})}{\sum_{i_0 \in S_{\text{test},0}^{r(l,k)}} \sum_{i_1 \in S_{\text{test},1}^{r(l,k)}} w_{\text{test},i_0}^{*,r(l,k)} w_{\text{test},i_1}^{*,r(l,k)}}, \tag{8}$$

where $S_{\text{test}}^{r(l,k)} = S_{\text{test},0}^{r(l,k)} \cup S_{\text{test},1}^{r(l,k)}$. The AUC based on the split l is the average of K estimated AUCs, and the final AUC ($\widehat{AUC}_w^{r,\text{dCV.av}}$) is the average of L estimated AUCs based on each of the splits, i.e.,

$$\widehat{AUC}_w^{r,\text{dCV.av}} = \frac{1}{L}\sum_{l=1}^{L}\left[\frac{1}{K}\sum_{k=1}^{K}\widehat{AUC}_w^{r(l,k)}\right]. \tag{9}$$

On the other hand, the pooling strategy estimates a unique AUC considering all the estimated probabilities in each test set $S_{\text{test}}^{r(l,k)}$, that is, the AUC is estimated for the whole S^r following eqs. (3) and (4), and considering the estimated probabilities based on the corresponding training model $\hat{p}_i^{r(l,k)}, \forall i \in S^r$. Let us denote this AUC as $\widehat{AUC}_w^{r,\text{dCV.pool}(l)}$:

$$\widehat{AUC}_w^{r,\text{dCV.pool}(l)} = \frac{\sum_{i_0 \in S_0^r} \sum_{i_1 \in S_1^r} w_{i_0}^r w_{i_1}^r \psi(\hat{p}_{i_0}^{r(l,k)}, \hat{p}_{i_1}^{r(l,k)})}{\sum_{i_0 \in S_0^r} \sum_{i_1 \in S_1^r} w_{i_0}^r w_{i_1}^r}. \tag{10}$$

Finally, the cross-validated AUC based on the pooling strategy ($\widehat{AUC}_w^{r,\text{dCV.pool}}$) is defined as follows:

$$\widehat{AUC}_w^{r,\text{dCV.pool}} = \frac{1}{L}\sum_{l=1}^{L}\widehat{AUC}_w^{r,\text{dCV.pool}(l)}. \tag{11}$$

The extreme case of the pooling cross-validation method would be equivalent to defining $K = a$ subsets, being $a = \sum_{h=1}^{H} a_h$, the total number of sample clusters. This method is usually denoted as leave-one-cluster-out cross-validation or Jackknife Repeated Replication (JKn, hereinafter).

True AUC: Extend $\hat{\boldsymbol{\beta}}^r$ to U, obtain $\hat{p}_i$, $\forall i \in U$ following Eq. (2) and estimate the true population AUC ($\widehat{AUC}_{\text{pop}}^r$) as in Eq. (12),

$$\widehat{AUC}_{\text{pop}}^r = \frac{1}{N_0 N_1}\sum_{i_0 \in U_0}\sum_{i_1 \in U_1}\left[I(\hat{p}_{i_0} < \hat{p}_{i_1}) + 0.5 I(\hat{p}_{i_0} = \hat{p}_{i_1})\right], \tag{12}$$

where N_0 and N_1 are the sizes of the population subsets U_0 (formed with the units without the event of interest, i.e., $\forall i_0 \in U_0,\ y_{i_0} = 0$) and U_1 (formed with the units with the event of interest, i.e., $\forall i_1 \in U_1,\ y_{i_1} = 1$), being $U = U_0 \cup U_1$. $\forall m \in \{\text{app}, \text{RB}, \text{RBn}, \text{dCV.av}, \text{dCV.pool}, \text{JKn}\}$, define the difference between the AUC estimates and the true population AUC as in Eq. (13),

$$\text{diff}^{r,m} = \widehat{AUC}_w^{r,m} - \widehat{AUC}_{\text{pop}}^{r}. \tag{13}$$

dCV methods have been carried out with $K = 10$ subsets and $L = 20$ replicates, while in RB and RBn $B = 200$ bootstrap resamples have been considered.

3.1 Results

Results of the simulation study are shown in Fig. 1, in which the differences between the different AUC estimates and the true population AUC are calculated as in Eq. (13) for the three scenarios considered.

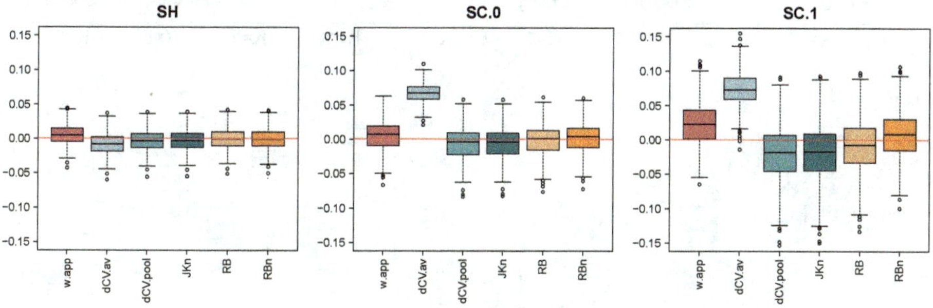

Fig. 1. Differences between the apparent and corrected AUCs, and the true population AUCs across $r = 1, \ldots, 500$ samples, for the three scenarios considered.

In addition, in order to analyze the performance of the differences between averaging and pooling strategies of dCV under two-stage sampling designs (SC.0 and SC.1), we analyzed the methods' performances for a different number of clusters sampled from each stratum (a_h) for $K = 10$ subsets, and a different number of subsets (K) for $a_h = 2$ clusters sampled from each stratum. The results are shown in Figs. 2 and 3, respectively.

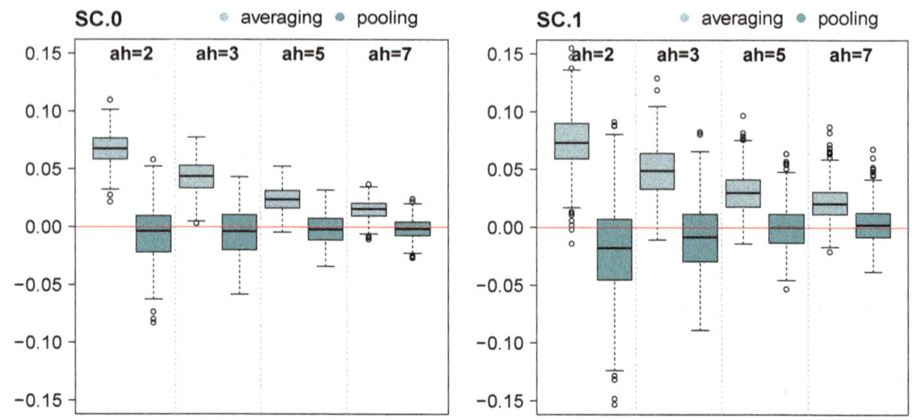

Fig. 2. Comparison between the differences of the averaging and pooling dCV ($K = 10$) estimates to the true population AUC across $r = 1, \ldots, 500$ samples, when $a_h \in \{2, 3, 5, 7\}$ clusters have been sampled from each stratum.

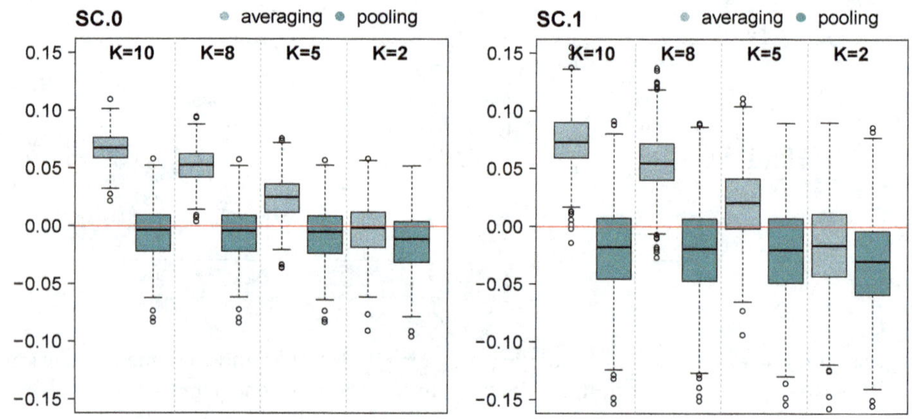

Fig. 3. Comparison between the differences of the averaging and pooling dCV estimates for $K \in \{10, 8, 5, 2\}$ subsets to the true population AUC across $r = 1, \ldots, 500$ samples, when $a_h = 2$ clusters have been sampled from each stratum.

4 Conclusions

The performance of the apparent estimate of the AUC, as well as the AUC correction methods (replicate weights methods), depends on the scenario. In the scenario based on the one-stage stratified sampling design (SH), all the methods perform quite properly, and no bias is observed. In contrast, both variability and optimism of the apparent AUC are greater in scenarios based on two-stage sampling designs (SC.0 and SC.1), and some differences can also be observed between analyzed correction methods. In particular, the performance of the averaging and pooling dCV methods differ considerably in those scenarios, being the pooling technique the one that best corrects for the optimism of the AUC under the analyzed scenarios. The performance of the averaging strategy completely depends on the number of clusters sampled from each stratum and/or the number of subsets K defined. In general, as either the selected number of clusters per stratum increases or the number of subsets K decreases, the difference between averaging and pooling strategies decreases. As an example, for the same number of subsets $K = 5$, the difference between the averaging and pooling strategies is, on average, 0.031 for $a_h = 2$, while when $a_h = 5$ are selected, this difference decreases to 0.010 in the scenario SC.0; in scenario SC.1, those differences decrease from 0.042 to 0.012 (numerical results not shown). However, in practice, the number of sampled clusters is previously specified and cannot be selected; thus, selecting a proper number of subsets K is crucial for the proper performance of the averaging dCV method. Regarding bias, the pooling strategy offers more constant results, but in contrast, it has greater variability than the averaging strategy. The performance of the RB and RBn methods has been good in all the scenarios that have been analyzed, and no major differences have been observed.

Therefore, we recommend using RB, RBn, or pooling dCV methods to prevent the possible optimism of the apparent estimates of the AUC when developing logistic regression models for real survey data derived from complex sampling designs. However, more analysis is required in order to better study the performance of different methods under other scenarios, specifically when greater optimism of the apparent AUC appears.

The replicate methods used in this work are implemented in the R package wROC, available at https://github.com/aiparragirre/wROC/.

References

1. Iparragirre, A., Barrio, I., Arostegui, I.: Estimation of the ROC curve and the area under it with complex survey data. Stat **12**(1), e635 (2023)
2. Iparragirre, A., Barrio, I., Rodríguez-Álvarez, M.X.: On the optimism correction of the area under the receiver operating characteristic curve in logistic prediction models. SORT - Stat. Oper. Res. Trans. **43**(1), 145–162 (2019)
3. Rao, J., Wu, C.: Resampling inference with complex survey data. J. Am. Stat. Assoc. **83**(401), 231–241 (1988)
4. Iparragirre, A., Lumley, T., Barrio, I., Arostegui, I.: Variable selection with LASSO regression for complex survey data. Stat **12**(1), e578 (2023)
5. Canty, A.J., Davison, A.C.: Resampling-based variance estimation for labour force surveys. Statistician **48**, 379–391 (1999)

Statistical Models for Patient-Centered Outcomes in Clinical Studies

Gillian Heller[1(✉)], Andrew Forbes[2], and Stephane Heritier[2]

[1] NHMRC Clinical Trials Centre, University of Sydney, Sydney, Australia
gillian.heller@sydney.edu.au

[2] School of Public Health and Preventive Medicine, Monash University, Melbourne, Australia

Abstract. Days alive and out of hospital is recommended as a patient-centered outcome in perioperative clinical studies. It is defined as the number of days, out of the first M postoperative days, that the patient has been discharged from hospital, or zero if the patient dies within M days of surgery. This composite measure presents statistical challenges in its unusual distributional shape, and its inability to distinguish between the qualitatively different outcomes of death, and a hospital stay longer than M days. We propose a mixed binary-continuous model that overcomes these difficulties, and illustrate its use on a clinical trial of a drug administered in cardiac surgery.

Keywords: distributional regression · censoring · hospital length of stay · GAMLSS · patient-centered outcomes

1 Introduction

Traditionally, outcomes of clinical studies have typically been defined as: time to event: death/cardiac event/cancer recurrence; or numeric measures: blood pressure/tumour size/number of falls; or categorical measures: death/disease recurrence (yes/no). More recently, there have been moves to define outcomes which are *patient-centered.* A consultative process to investigate patient-centered outcomes for studies involving surgery (perioperative trials) resulted in the recommendation for the use of three measures: a health-related quality of life measure (EuroQol 5 Dimension); a functional-status measure (WHO Disability Assessment Schedule); and a life-impact measure, days alive and out of hospital (DAOH) at 30 days after surgery [4]. This latter measure is predicated on the belief that, following surgery, patients want to: (1) survive; and (2) go home as soon as possible. We focus on the modelling of this measure. This is a composite outcome which captures both death and surgery-related morbidity and, because of its general nature, enables comparison between studies. The nature of the DAOH outcome presents some statistical modelling challenges, which we investigate.

J. Einbeck et al. (Eds.): IWSM 2024, CONTRIB.STAT., pp. 48–54, 2024.
https://doi.org/10.1007/978-3-031-65723-8_8

2 A Statistical Model for DAOH

The DAOH outcome is defined as

1. Discharge to home within M days: DAOH = M - LOS
2. Discharge to home after M days: DAOH = 0
3. Death at any time within M days: DAOH = 0

where LOS = hospital length of stay and M is a given cutoff e.g. M = 30. An example of DAOH is given in Fig. 1, which shows the histogram of DAOH30 for the ATACAS study [6]. This outcome is: continuous; left-skewed; and bounded above at M=30 and below at zero. It is characterised by a spike at zero, for which there are two sources: those originating from patients with LOS>M; and those from patients who died within M days of surgery.

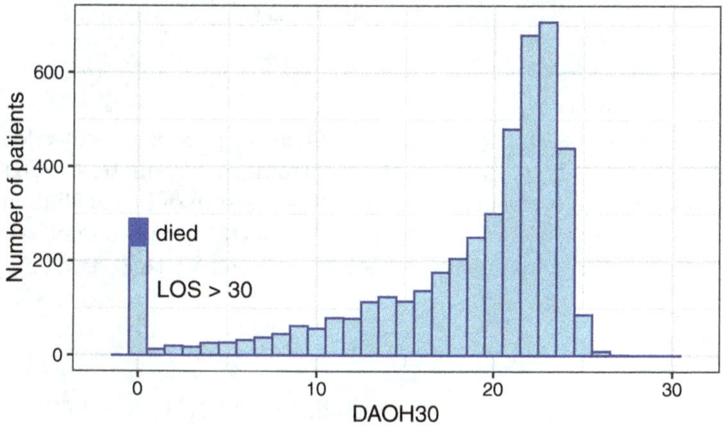

Fig. 1. Histogram of DAOH30 for the ATACAS study.

This results in the composite outcome

$$\text{DAOH} = \begin{cases} 0 & \text{if patient died within M days of surgery} \\ \max(\text{M} - \text{LOS}, 0) & \text{otherwise.} \end{cases}$$

This outcome presents modelling complexities. The continuous component of DAOH is left-censored at zero, bounded above at M, and generally left-skewed. For modeling, choices of left-skewed, bounded continuous distributions are very limited. We have a far greater choice of response distribution if we consider, equivalently, the distribution of the original variable LOS, right-skewed and right-censored at M. The **gamlss** package [9], which was used for estimation, has numerous such response distributions available.

Not distinguishing between the two sources of zero, which are qualitatively different, is questionable so we prefer to separate them in the modelling. An alternative definition of the composite outcome which distinguishes the two sources, and reverses the continuous component, is

$$y = \begin{cases} -1 & \text{if patient died within M days of surgery} \\ \min(\text{LOS, M}) & \text{otherwise.} \end{cases}$$

(The choice of $y = -1$ is arbitrary; any value outside [0, M] could be chosen.) The response distribution is written as the mixed probability function

$$f(y|\pi, \boldsymbol{\theta}) = \begin{cases} \pi & \text{for } y = -1 \\ (1-\pi) \cdot f_1(y|\boldsymbol{\theta}) & \text{for } 0 \leq y \leq M \\ 0 & \text{otherwise} \end{cases} \tag{1}$$

where π is the probability of death within M days, and $f_1(y|\boldsymbol{\theta})$ is the censored pdf of the LOS component. For the "mortality sub-model", we define the indicator variable

$$y_0 = \begin{cases} 1 & \text{if } y = -1 \\ 0 & \text{otherwise} \end{cases}$$

having $y_0 \sim \text{Bernoulli}(\pi)$.

We now develop a statistical model in which we propose a suitable distribution $f_1(\cdot|\boldsymbol{\theta})$, and specify models for the distribution parameters $(\pi, \boldsymbol{\theta})$. As the log-likelihood function for (1) can be written as the sum of log-likelihoods for the continuous "LOS sub-model" and the binary "mortality sub-model", MLEs are obtained by separately maximising the log-likelihoods for these two components.

3 Analysis

The ATACAS study is a randomized controlled trial (RCT, $n = 4{,}631$) of tranexamic acid administered to patients undergoing cardiac surgery. "Tranexamic acid reduces the risk of bleeding among patients undergoing cardiac surgery, but it is unclear whether this leads to improved outcomes. Furthermore, there are concerns that tranexamic acid may have prothrombotic and proconvulsant effects" [6]. Besides treatment group and basic demographics (age, sex, BMI), a number of baseline covariates are available for analysis as predictors, shown in Table 1.

3.1 Results

Model selection involves the choice of (1) the distribution of LOS; and (2) the covariates in the equations for the parameters of the chosen distribution for the LOS sub-model; and the covariates in the mortality sub-model.

Distribution choice for LOS: After initial data exploration, the distribution choice was conditioned on the covariates age and heart failure, for the first two distribution parameters. Candidate distributions considered were right-censored versions of all distributions with support on $\mathbb{R}_+$, in the **gamlss** package, as well as the log-transformed sinh-arcsinh (SHASH) distribution [7]. The BIC was used for selection, which resulted in the choice of the logSHASH distribution. This

Table 1. Baseline covariates in ATACAS study.

Variable	Description
country	Australia, Canada, Hong Kong, Europe, NZ, UK
asa	ASA Physical status (1=healthy, ..., 6=brain-dead)
heart failure	prior history of heart failure (yes/no)
prior MI	prior history of myocardial infarction (yes/no)
diabetes status	yes/no
respiratory disease	yes/no
smoking history	current or previous history (yes/no)
surgery type	coronary artery bypass/OPCAB

is defined as the distribution of y, where $w = \log y \sim \text{SHASH}(\theta_1, \theta_2, \theta_3, \theta_4)$. The SHASH is a four-parameter continuous distribution with support on $\mathbb{R}$, location parameter median$(w) = \theta_1$ and shape/scale parameters θ_2, θ_3 and θ_4. Hence the logSHASH$(\theta_1, \theta_2, \theta_3, \theta_4)$ distribution has support on $\mathbb{R}_+$, with location parameter median$(y) = \exp(\theta_1)$ and shape/scale parameters θ_2, θ_3 and θ_4.
Covariate selection: Regression equations for the distribution parameters of (1) are specified as

$$\begin{aligned} \log\left[\pi_i/(1-\pi_i)\right] &= \boldsymbol{x}_{i\pi}^\top \boldsymbol{\beta}_\pi \\ g_k(\theta_k) &= \boldsymbol{x}_{ik}^\top \boldsymbol{\beta}_k \qquad \text{for } k = 1, \ldots, 4 \end{aligned}$$

where the $g_k(\cdot)$ are appropriate link functions; and the covariate vectors $\boldsymbol{x}_\pi$, $\boldsymbol{x}_1, \ldots, \boldsymbol{x}_4$ may be overlapping or distinct.

Covariate selection was performed using best subset regression [3], implemented using weights in the penalty matrix of ridge regression, in the `ri()` function in **gamlss**. This resulted in the covariates shown in Table 2. Note that no covariates were selected for either θ_2 or θ_4; and treatment was not significant in either the binary or continuous component of the model. For assessment of model fit, worm plots [10] are shown in Fig. 2; these indicate good fits of the two sub-models.

Our decision to separate the deaths from the LOS≥M zeroes is vindicated by the fact that only age, heart failure, country and respiratory disease are predictive for death (π), whereas a range of other covariates are predictive for LOS ($\boldsymbol{\theta}$).

3.2 Model Interpretation

We would usually be interested in quantifying the effect of treatment on the DAOH30 outcome; however, treatment is not significant in either sub-model. As an illustration of the interpretability of the model, we examine instead the effect of age, which is significant in both sub-models. Separating the interpretation of each sub-model's age coefficients is problematic, because of (1) the simultaneous

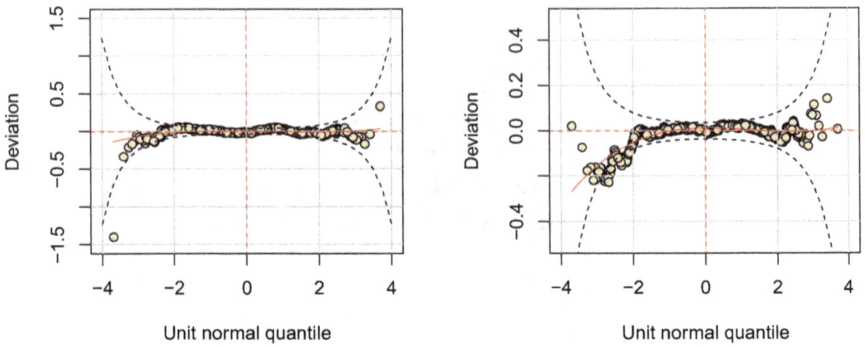

Fig. 2. Worm plots for the LOS sub-model (left) and mortality sub-model (right).

Table 2. Selection of covariates in ATACAS study.

Covariate	Distribution parameter				
	π	θ_1	θ_2	θ_3	θ_4
age	✓	✓		✓	
sex		✓			
BMI		✓			
country	✓	✓		✓	
ASA		✓			
heart failure	✓	✓			
prior MI		✓			
diabetes status		✓			
respiratory disease	✓	✓			
smoking history		✓			
surgery type		✓			

effect of age on the two sub-models; and (2) within the LOS sub-model, the simultaneous effect of age on two distribution parameters (θ_1 and θ_3). We adopt the approach of [8], which is appropriate in the case where a covariate appears in the model equations of more than one distribution parameter. The effect of the covariate is visualised by comparing the probability density functions of the outcome, at selected covariate values. As an illustration we show the fitted pdf of DAOH30, for age at (approximately) its lower and upper quartiles: 60 and 75 years (Fig. 3). This enables the assessment of the effect of age on both the distribution of hospital stay (or days at home), and mortality. Clearly older age (75 years) is associated with the negative outcomes of higher mortality, and fewer days at home, compared with younger age (60 years).

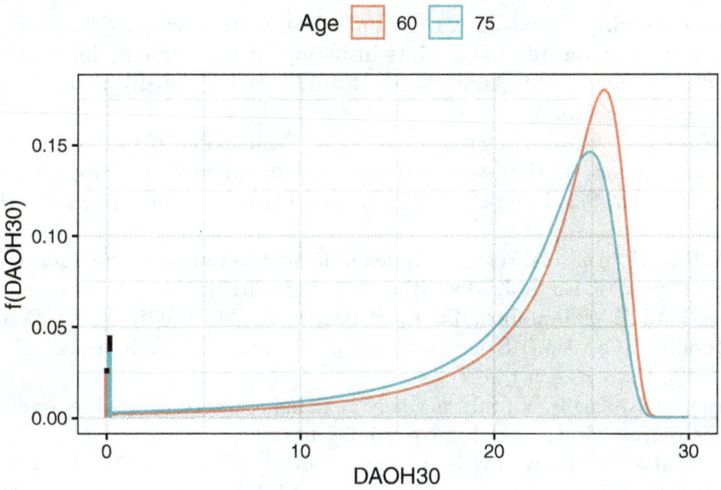

Fig. 3. Fitted pdfs of DAOH30, for age at 60 and 75 years. The probability of death is shown as zeroes (in black).

4 Discussion

As the DAOH outcome is used in the context of RCTs, we need to be aware of the problem of the non-causal interpretation of treatment in a RCT with such an outcome. The issue is that in the LOS sub-model, only subjects having DAOH>0 are included, with the consequence that randomisation is compromised and it is no longer valid to give a causal interpretation of the effect of treatment in the LOS part. However a fitted density for treatment, as given for age in Fig. 3, would have a valid graphical interpretation of its overall effect.

The separation of the two sources of zeroes is an important feature of this modelling approach. Mortality is modelled separately by [1], although their overall modelling approach is quite different to ours; it is not treated separately in the quantile regression approach, which is a popular method for the analysis of DAOH (e.g., [2,5]).

References

1. Boyle, L., Lumley, T., Cumin, D., et al.: Using days alive and out of hospital to measure surgical outcomes in New Zealand: a cross-sectional study. BMJ Open **13**(7), e063787 (2023). https://doi.org/10.1136/bmjopen-2022-063787
2. Delaney, A., Tian, D.H., Higgins, A., et al.: The association between days alive and out of hospital and health-related quality of life in patients with sepsis. CHEST Critical Care **1**(3) (2023). https://doi.org/10.1016/j.chstcc.2023.100024
3. Hastie, T., Tibshirani, R., Friedman, J.H.: The Elements of Statistical Learning: Data Mining, Inference, and Prediction, 2nd edn. Springer, New York (2009)

4. Moonesinghe, S.R., Jackson, A.I.R. et al.: Systematic review and consensus definitions for the Standardised endpoints in perioperative medicine initiative: patient-centred outcomes. Br. J. Anaesthesia **123**(5), 664–670 (2019). https://doi.org/10.1016/j.bja.2019.07.020
5. M'Pembele, R., Roth, S., Stroda, A. et al.: Validation of days alive and out of hospital as a new patient-centered outcome to quantify life impact after heart transplantation. Sci. Rep. **12**, 18352 (2022). https://doi.org/10.1038/s41598-022-21936-4
6. Myles, P.S., Smith, J.A., et al.: Tranexamic acid in patients undergoing coronary-artery surgery. N. Engl. J. Med. **376**, 136–148 (2017)
7. Rigby, R.A., Stasinopoulos, D.M., Heller, G.Z., De Bastiani, F.: Distributions for Modeling Location, Scale, and Shape: Using GAMLSS in R. Chapman & Hall/CRC, Boca Raton (2019)
8. Stadlmann, S., Kneib, T.: Interactively visualizing distributional regression models with distreg.vis. Stat. Model. **22**(6), 527–545 (2022)
9. Stasinopoulos, D.M., Rigby, R.A., Heller, G.Z., Voudouris, V., De Bastiani, F.: Flexible Regression and Smoothing: Using GAMLSS in R. Chapman & Hall/CRC, Boca Raton (2017)
10. van Buuren, S.V., Fredriks, M.: Worm plot: a simple diagnostic device for modelling growth reference curves. Stat. Med. **20**(8), 1259–1277 (2001)

Bayesian Hidden Markov Models for Early Warning

Daniele Tancini(✉), Francesco Bartolucci, and Silvia Pandolfi

Department of Economics, University of Perugia, IT, Perugia, Italy
daniele.tancini@dottorandi.unipg.it,
{francesco.bartolucci,silvia.pandolfi}@unipg.it

Abstract. We show how Bayesian hidden Markov models may be employed to build early warning systems of particular risky events. The adopted model formulation assumes that every binary response variable depends only on the latent state further to the lagged covariates and response. A Markov chain Monte Carlo algorithm is proposed for estimation and forecasting, where the latter is based on the optimisation of the F-score. An application referred to banking crisis of countries based on an unbalanced panel dataset is used as an illustration.

Keywords: Discrete latent variable models · F-score · forecasting · Markov chain Monte Carlo

1 Introduction

Early Warning Systems (EWSs) are general and flexible tools largely employed to promptly generate meaningful warning signals of certain risky events in several fields, such as financial crises; for recent references see [1]. They are useful in predicting extreme events with a certain level of reliability, so as to enable policy makers to prepare appropriate responses aimed at limiting potential damages. The typical context of application is with longitudinal data, where repeated observations of the same units, which may be individuals, countries or firms, are collected at different time occasions. A widely used approach to build an EWS relying on data about previous events is based on classification tools, such as logistic regression [2] and k-nearest neighbors, which are very popular in the machine learning literature [3].

In order to improve the performance of standard EWSs based on the logistic model, we propose to use a Bayesian hidden Markov model (HMM) with covariates [4]. HMMs rely on a sequence of discrete latent variables for each unit that follows a Markov chain of first order, so that each unit- and time-specific binary response variable for the crisis is assumed to depend on the underlying latent variable and the lagged covariates and response. These models extend logistic models as they allow accounting for unobserved heterogeneity in a dynamic fashion. Moreover, certain problems of logistic models with individual fixed effects [1] are avoided.

J. Einbeck et al. (Eds.): IWSM 2024, CONTRIB.STAT., pp. 55–61, 2024.
https://doi.org/10.1007/978-3-031-65723-8_9

In order to estimate the adopted model and at the same time make forecasting, we propose a Markov chain Monte Carlo (MCMC) algorithm that relies on a data augmented scheme [5]. This algorithm is based on performing, at each iteration, different steps consisting in drawing new values of latent variables, parameters, and also choosing an optimal value of the cut-off on the basis of the F-score, which is suitable for the forecasting of rare events [6].

We evaluate the performance of the proposed approach by means of a real data application based on an unbalanced longitudinal dataset of 129 countries followed for the period from 1983 to 2017. The binary response variable corresponds to systemic banking crisis events defined as in [7]. As covariates, we consider certain macroeconomic indicators, such as real GDP growth rate, the logarithm of per capita GDP, inflation, and the real interest rate, which are publicly available as International Financial Statistics, issued by the International Monetary Fund, or as World Development Indicators, from the World Bank.

In the following, we first illustrate the adopted model and then, in Sect. 3, we outline the MCMC algorithm for estimation and forecast. Finally, in Sect. 4 we outline the real data application.

2 Model

With reference to n units observed at T time occasions, let Y_{it} denote the binary response variable for the crisis event, with $i = 1, \dots, n$ and $t = 1, \dots, T$. Also let $\boldsymbol{x}_{it}$ denote a corresponding vector of covariates that are supposed to be observed also for the time preceding the first observation.

The proposed modelling approach assumes that, for every unit i, the response variables Y_{it} are conditionally independent given the lagged covariates and responses, in addition to a sequence of latent variables $U_{i1}, \dots, U_{iT}$ that follows a Markov chain with state space $\{1, \dots, k\}$, initial probabilities $\pi_u = p(U_{i1} = u)$, $u = 1, \dots, k$, and transition probabilities $\pi_{uv} = p(U_{it} = v | U_{i,t-1} = u)$, $t = 2, \dots, T$, $u, v = 1, \dots, k$. In a Bayesian framework, we assume that

$$\log \frac{p(Y_{it} = 1 | U_{it} = u, \boldsymbol{x}_{i,t-1}, y_{i,t-1}, \alpha_u, \boldsymbol{\beta}, \gamma)}{p(Y_{it} = 0 | U_{it} = u, \boldsymbol{x}_{i,t-1}, y_{i,t-1}, \alpha_u, \boldsymbol{\beta}, \gamma)} = \alpha_u + \boldsymbol{x}'_{i,t-1}\boldsymbol{\beta} + y_{i,t-1}\gamma, \quad (1)$$

where α_u is an intercept depending on the underlying latent state, while $\boldsymbol{\beta}$ and γ are regression coefficients.

The adopted Bayesian framework has the advantage of providing regularised parameter estimates that are particularly useful in terms of forecasting. Then, we assume that *a priori* the vector of initial probabilities $\boldsymbol{\pi}$ with elements π_u, $u = 1, \dots, k$, has a Dirichlet distribution with parameters $\boldsymbol{d}$; similarly, each row $\boldsymbol{\pi}_u$ of the transition matrix $\boldsymbol{\Pi}$ with elements π_{uv}, $v = 1, \dots, k$, follows a Dirichlet distribution with parameters $\boldsymbol{d}_u$.

We configure the hyper-parameters for $\boldsymbol{\Pi}$ according to a prior assumption favouring a higher persistence in the same state. This implies an expectation that the probabilities along the diagonal of the transition probability matrix are higher compared to the off-diagonal ones. For the vector of regression parameters

α_u, $u = 1, \ldots, k$, we consider a multivariate normal distribution with parameters $\boldsymbol{\mu}$ and $\boldsymbol{\Sigma}$, where $\boldsymbol{\Sigma} = \sigma_u \boldsymbol{I}$.

Finally, for the vector $\boldsymbol{\beta}$ and the parameter γ, we use the spike and slab lasso formulation proposed in [8]. In particular, we consider the marginalised formulation

$$\beta_p|\phi_p \sim \phi_p \psi_1(\beta_p) + (1 - \phi_p)\psi_0(\beta_p), \tag{2}$$

with $p = 1, \ldots, P$, where P is number of predictors. In this case $\psi_0(\cdot)$ and $\psi_1(\cdot)$ are two Laplace (double exponential) densities defined as $\psi_1(\beta_p) = \frac{\lambda_1}{2} e^{-\lambda_1|\beta_p|}$, with λ_1 small, and $\psi_0(\beta_p) = \frac{\lambda_0}{2} e^{-\lambda_0|\beta_p|}$, with λ_0 large. Clearly, when $\lambda_0 \to \infty$ we have a point mass in 0, while $\psi_1(\beta_p) \propto c > 0$ as $\lambda_1 \to 0$. We also assume that $\phi_p \sim \mathcal{B}eta(a, b)$, where we fix $a = b = 1$.

In the proposed formulation we choose $\lambda_1 = 1$, while we consider a sequence of L increasing values of λ_0, denoted by $\lambda_0^1, \ldots, \lambda_0^L$, with $\lambda_0^1 = 1$, for an MCMC warm-in period, starting each β_p at 0. Notice that Eq. (2) defines a mixture of double-exponential distributions, which performs simultaneous variable selection and parameter estimation. Different hyper-parameters for a and b can also be considered, such as $a = b = \frac{1}{2}$, in order to induce *a priori* a more concentration of ϕ_p on 0 or 1.

We denote by $p(\boldsymbol{\beta}|\boldsymbol{\phi})$ the prior $\prod_{p=1}^{P} p(\beta_p|\phi_p)$, where $p(\beta_p|\phi_p)$ is the mixture defined in Eq. (2), and by $p(\boldsymbol{\phi})$ the prior $\prod_{p=1}^{P} p(\phi_p)$, corresponding to a product of independent Beta distributions. We include the same spike and slab prior also on γ, denoting by ϕ_γ the probability of the mixture and assuming that $\phi_\gamma \sim \mathcal{B}eta(a, b)$, with $a = b = 1$.

We assume *a priori* independence between parameters, so that

$$\begin{aligned} p(\boldsymbol{\beta}, \boldsymbol{\phi}, \boldsymbol{\alpha}, \boldsymbol{\pi}, \boldsymbol{\Pi}, \boldsymbol{U}, \gamma, \phi_\gamma|\boldsymbol{X}, \boldsymbol{Y}) \propto\ & p(\boldsymbol{Y}|\boldsymbol{U}, \boldsymbol{\beta}, \boldsymbol{\alpha}, \gamma, \boldsymbol{X}) p(\boldsymbol{U}|\boldsymbol{\pi}, \boldsymbol{\Pi}) p(\boldsymbol{\beta}|\boldsymbol{\phi}) \times \\ & \times p(\boldsymbol{\phi}) p(\boldsymbol{\alpha}) p(\gamma|\phi_\gamma) p(\phi_\gamma) p(\boldsymbol{\pi}) p(\boldsymbol{\Pi}), \end{aligned} \tag{3}$$

where $\boldsymbol{U}$ denotes the vector of all latent variables, $\boldsymbol{X}$ the matrix of all covariates and lagged responses, and $\boldsymbol{Y}$ that of all responses.

3 Markov Chain Monte Carlo Algorithm

The proposed MCMC algorithm is a Gibbs-within-Metropolis. Based on the assumptions defined in model (3), it is possible to obtain closed forms for the full conditionals involved. In particular, we have

$$\boldsymbol{\pi}|\cdots \sim \mathcal{D}(d_1 + \sum_{i=1}^{n} \mathbb{I}(U_{i1} = 1), \ldots, d_k + \sum_{i=1}^{n} \mathbb{I}(U_{i1} = k))$$

and

$$\boldsymbol{\pi}_{u,\cdot}|\cdots \sim \mathcal{D}(d_{u,1} + \sum_{i,t} \mathbb{I}(U_{i,t-1} = u, U_{it} = 1), \ldots, d_{u,k} + \sum_{i,t} \mathbb{I}(U_{i,t-1} = u, U_{it} = k)),$$

for $t = 2, \ldots, T$ and $u = 1, \ldots, k$, where $\mathcal{D}$ denotes a Dirichlet distribution and $\mathbb{I}(\cdot)$ an indicator function. Furthermore, we have

$$p(U_{it} = u|\cdots) \propto \pi_{u_{i,t-1},u} p(y_{it}|U_{it} = u, \boldsymbol{x}_{i,t-1}, y_{i,t-1}, \alpha_u, \boldsymbol{\beta}, \gamma)\pi_{u,u_{i,t+1}},$$

for $t = 2, \ldots, T-1$, while different forms are provided for $t = 1$ and $t = T$. Regarding the other parameters, we consider random walk Metropolis-Hastings (RWMH) steps. In particular, for each α_u, we generate a new value as $\alpha_u^* = \alpha_u + \epsilon$, where $\epsilon \sim \mathcal{N}(0, \sigma_{\alpha_u})$, and we accept it with probability

$$1 \wedge \frac{p(\boldsymbol{Y}|\boldsymbol{U}, \boldsymbol{\beta}, \alpha_u^*, \boldsymbol{\alpha}_{-u}, \gamma, \boldsymbol{X})p(\alpha_u^*)}{p(\boldsymbol{Y}|\boldsymbol{U}, \boldsymbol{\beta}, \alpha_u, \boldsymbol{\alpha}_{-u}, \gamma, \boldsymbol{X})p(\alpha_u)},$$

where $\boldsymbol{\alpha}_{-u}$ denotes the vector $\boldsymbol{\alpha}$ once removed α_u. We propose RWMH steps also for any β_p, ϕ_p, γ and ϕ_γ, taking into account the transformation $f(\phi) = \log \frac{\phi}{1-\phi}$, because we need to map ϕ from $[0, 1]$ to $\mathbb{R}$. Notice that for each ϕ also the ratio of the Jacobians is involved.

Regarding the optimisation of the cut-off value, we recall that this is used for prediction according to the following rule:

$$\hat{y}_{it} = \mathbb{I}(p_{it} > c), \quad i = 1, \ldots, n, \ t = 1, \ldots, T, \tag{4}$$

where c is the cut-off and $p_{it} = p(Y_{it} = 1|U_{it} = u_{it}, \boldsymbol{x}_{i,t-1}, y_{i,t-1}, \alpha_u, \boldsymbol{\beta}, \gamma)$ is the probability of the risky event computed on the basis of Eq. (1). At each iteration (after warm-in) we evaluate the cut-off based on the F-score [6], obtaining a collection of $c^{(r)}$ values, where $r = l, \ldots, R$ is the iteration starting after a warm-in of $l-1$ iterations.

Using the sampling obtained from the MCMC algorithm, we consider to optimise the cut-off on the basis of the parameters sampled from the posterior distribution, taking into account the variability of the distribution itself. This interpretation of c is more in line with the Bayesian framework where the parameters are random variables. Relying on the set of the cut-off obtained, we can also provide a collection of predictions based on the proposed HMM.

Regarding the last step, that is, the prediction of the new value of the response variable, for given values of the parameters and supposing to know the value of the last latent variable, namely $u_{iT}^{(r)}$, the forecasting probability $p_{i,T+1}^{(r)}$ is obtained as

$$p_{i,T+1}^{(r)} = \sum_{v=1}^{k} \pi_{u_{iT}^{(r)} v}\, p(Y_{i,T+1} = 1|U_{i,T+1} = v, \boldsymbol{x}_{iT}, y_{iT}, \alpha_u^{(r)}, \boldsymbol{\beta}^{(r)}, \gamma^{(r)}). \tag{5}$$

Then, to perform a prediction for the next crisis event, we have to use the cut-off value selected as in the previous step. Finally, based on Eq. (4) we obtain a collection of prediction $\hat{y}_{i,T+1}^{(r)}$ for $i = 1, \ldots, n$.

4 Real Data Application

We assess the effectiveness of our proposed method through a practical application using real-world data from a longitudinal dataset spanning 129 countries over the period from 1983 to 2017 [1]. Our analysis focuses on identifying systemic banking crisis events, as defined in [7], using a binary response variable. Additionally, we incorporate $P = 7$ macroeconomic indicators as covariates; see [1] for detail. To ensure data quality, we preprocess the dataset to address potential measurement errors and missing values. Subsequently, we refine our analysis by selecting a subset of the dataset comprising consecutive years from 1984 to 2016 and including only countries experiencing at least one default event.

The preprocessing leads to a total of 76 defaults out of 660 observations, indicating an unbalanced dataset. We partition the dataset into training and testing sets; in particular, the training set encompasses all countries from 1984 to 2004, while the testing set spans from 2005 to 2016. For model selection, we examine a series of models starting with $k = 2$, incrementally introducing additional latent components. To compare these models, we employ the leave-one-out cross-validation (LOO) proposed in [9] and implemented in the R package **loo**. We provide point estimates and standard errors of the expected log pointwise predictive density (elpd_loo), the effective number of parameters (p_loo) and the LOO information criterion (looic), where looic $= -2 \times$ elpd_loo. As starting model we consider $k = 2$ and we compare the looic estimates, introducing additional latent components. We select the final model on the basis of the lowest looic value. Table 1 summarises the results obtained.

Table 1. Model selection based on LOO. In evidence the final model selected.

k	Estimate$_{(\text{SE})}$		
	elpd_loo	p_loo	looic
2	$\mathbf{-144.8}_{(15.9)}$	$\mathbf{37.8}_{(6.8)}$	$\mathbf{289.5}_{(31.9)}$
3	$-150.0_{(16.1)}$	$53.0_{(7.2)}$	$300.0_{(32.1)}$
4	$-348.3_{(35.8)}$	$262.3_{(28.5)}$	$696.5_{(71.6)}$

The final model selected is with $k = 2$, identifying two latent components, which can be interpreted in terms of a risky level, in particular a lower and higher level of risk.

We provide the estimation (conditional expectation) of the parameters in Table 2, including also diagnostics on the samples obtained from the MCMC based on the Monte Carlo standard errors (MCSE) calculated by using the batch means estimator [10] and the $\hat{R}$ proposed in [11] and implemented in the **rstan** package.

From Table 2 we observe that $U_{it} = 1$ denotes the higher level and $U_{it} = 2$ denotes the lower level of risk. Furthermore, we observe a higher prevalence to

Table 2. Parameters estimated for the period 1984–2004.

Parameter	Estimate$_{(\text{MCSE})}$	$\hat{R}$
α_1	$0.403_{(0.091)}$	1.011
α_2	$-1.014_{(0.054)}$	1.000
γ	$3.416_{(0.027)}$	1.002
β_1	$-0.130_{(0.013)}$	1.009
β_2	$-0.285_{(0.018)}$	1.017
β_3	$0.012_{(0.001)}$	1.010
β_4	$-0.014_{(0.004)}$	1.025
β_5	$0.000_{(0.001)}$	1.006
β_6	$0.006_{(0.007)}$	1.023
β_7	$-0.012_{(0.007)}$	1.025
π_1	$0.375_{(0.010)}$	1.002
$\pi_{1,1}$	$0.757_{(0.008)}$	1.005
$\pi_{2,2}$	$0.810_{(0.006)}$	1.001

remain in the same state and an initial risky probability associated to $\pi_1 = p(U_{i1} = 1)$ lower than $\pi_2 = p(U_{i1} = 2)$.

Using the sampling obtained from the MCMC, we optimise the cut-off on the basis of F-score and the parameters sampled from the posterior distribution, taking into account the variability of the distribution itself. In Fig. 1 we represent the collection of cut-off values obtained using the MCMC for the model with $k = 2$, considering the period 1984–2004.

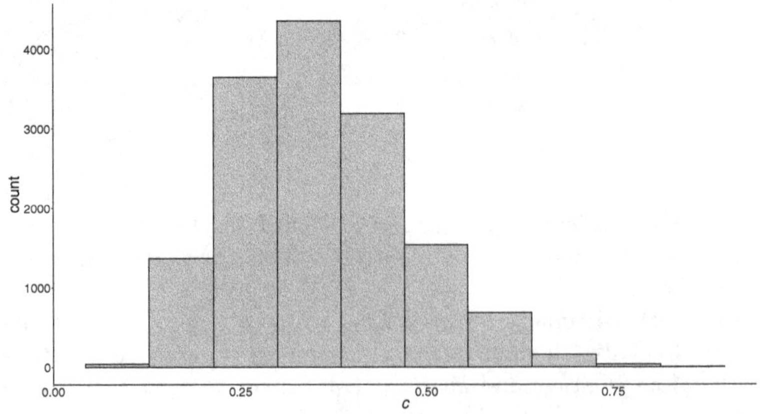

Fig. 1. Histogram representing the collection of $c^{(r)}$ obtained for the period 1984–2004.

Based on Eq. (5) it is possible to obtain the forecasting probability, which is then used in Eq. (4) with the optimal cut-off $c^{(r)}$ in order to obtain the collection of prediction $\hat{y}_{i,T+1}^{(r)}$, from which we can get the final prediction $\hat{y}_{i,T+1}$ as the maximum a posteriori.

Acknowledgments. F. Bartolucci and S. Pandolfi acknowledge the financial support from the grant "Hidden Markov Models for Early Warning Systems" of Ministero dell'Università e della Ricerca (PRIN 2022TZEXKF) funded by European Union - Next Generation EU.

References

1. Pigini, C.: Penalized maximum likelihood estimation of logit-based early warning systems. Int. J. Forecast. **37**, 1156–1172 (2021)
2. Filippopoulou, C., Galariotis, E., Spyrou, S.: An early warning system for predicting systemic banking crises in the eurozone: a logit regression approach. J. Econ. Behav. Organ. **172**, 344–63 (2020)
3. Murphy, K.P.: Probabilistic Machine Learning: An Introduction. MIT press, Cambridge (2022)
4. Bartolucci, F., Farcomeni, A., Pennoni, F.: Latent Markov Models for Longitudinal Data. CRC Press, Boca Raton (2013)
5. Tanner, M.A., Wong, W.H.: The calculation of posterior distributions by data augmentation. J. Am. Stat. Assoc. **82**, 528–540 (1987)
6. Davis, J., Goadrich, M.: The relationship between precision- recall and ROC curves. In: Proceedings of the 23rd International Conference on Machine Learning, pp. 233–240. ACM (2006)
7. Laeven, L., Valencia, F.: Systemic banking crises revisited. IMF working paper 18/206, International Monetary Fund (2018)
8. Ročková, V., George, E.I.: The spike-and-slab lasso. J. Am. Stat. Assoc. **113**, 431–444 (2018)
9. Vehtari, A., Gelman, A., Gabry, J.: Practical Bayesian model evaluation using leave-one-out cross-validation and WAIC. Stat. Comput. **27**, 1413–1432 (2017)
10. Flegal, J.M., Jones, G.L.: Batch means and spectral variance estimators in Markov chain Monte Carlo. Ann. Stat. **38**, 1034–1070 (2010)
11. Vehtari, A., Gelman, A., Simpson, D., Carpenter, B., Bürkner, P.C.: Rank-normalization, folding, and localization: an improved $\hat{R}$ for assessing convergence of MCMC (with discussion). Bayesian Anal. **16**, 667–718 (2021)

A Bayesian Markov-Switching for Smooth Modelling of Extreme Value Distributions

Vincenzo Gioia(✉), Gioia Di Credico, and Francesco Pauli

Department of Economic, Business, Mathematical and Statistical Sciences "Bruno de Finetti", University of Trieste, Trieste 34127, Italy
https://www.units.it/persone/index.php/from/abook/persona/35148

Abstract. Markov-switching models are attractive for analysing time series that exhibit different stochastic processes along different periods, and where the regime-switching is controlled by an unobservable Markovian process. Model flexibility can be enhanced considering regime-specific distributions, whose distributional parameters may be modelled using smooth functions of covariates. Here, we propose a two-state Markov-switching model using full Bayesian inference and accounting for extreme value modelling. The proposal is illustrated by analysing energy prices.

Keywords: distributional regression · energy price modelling · regime-switching

1 Introduction

Markov-switching models combine different parametric specifications by introducing a latent variable that determines which regime applies to each observation. This has proven useful in applications to model phenomena showing different behaviours in different time periods. We focus on the tail behaviour and propose a model with two regimes in which one is Gaussian and the second may be an extreme value distribution. In both regimes flexible smooth regression models are considered [1,5]. We exploit a full Bayesian approach to inference including smooth modelling of the distributional parameters of the generalized extreme value distributions and we illustrate the proposal through an application to energy price modelling.

2 Markov-Switching Model Settings

Let y_t, $t = 1, \dots, T$, be the realisations of an observable stochastic process, Y_t, and consider a two-state unobservable stochastic process S_t, such that $S_t \in \{1, 2\}$. We assume that the Y_t's are conditionally independent given S_t, and $Y_t | S_t = s_t \sim \mathcal{D}_{s_t}\left(\boldsymbol{\theta}^t_{s_t}\right)$, where $\mathcal{D}_{s_t}(\cdot)$ represents a parametric distribution

J. Einbeck et al. (Eds.): IWSM 2024, CONTRIB.STAT., pp. 62–67, 2024.
https://doi.org/10.1007/978-3-031-65723-8_10

family, with density $f_{Y_t|S_t}(\cdot)$, and $\boldsymbol{\theta}^t_{s_t}$ is the related q_{s_t}-dimensional distributional parameter. The components of the distributional parameter vectors are related to the linear predictors through a suitable link function

$$g_{s_t r}\left(\theta^t_{s_t r}\right) = \eta^t_{s_t r} = \sum_k h_{k s_t r}\left(x^t_k\right), \quad r = 1, \ldots, q_{s_t}, \tag{1}$$

where $h_{k s_t r}(\cdot)$ can be a linear or smooth function of the covariate x^t_k. By considering a reduced rank linear-basis expansion for the smooth effects in (1), the linear predictors turn out to be expressed as $\eta^t_{s_t r} = \boldsymbol{x}^t_{\eta_{s_t r}} \boldsymbol{\beta}_{\eta_{s_t r}}$, where $\boldsymbol{x}^t_{\eta_{s_t r}}$ and $\boldsymbol{\beta}_{\eta_{s_t r}} = \left(\beta_{\eta_{s_t r,1}}, \beta_{\eta_{s_t r,2}}, \ldots\right)^\top$ are, respectively, a row vector of covariate information and the corresponding regression parameter.

The latent process, which determines the membership of each observation to the two regimes, is ruled by a first-order Markov chain. Then, given an initial vector of probabilities $\boldsymbol{\pi}^0$, where $\pi^0_{s_j} = \Pr(S_0 = s_j)$, the evolution over time of the unobservable stochastic process is properly described by the 2×2 transition probability matrix $\boldsymbol{\delta}^t$, whose elements are $\delta^t_{jk} = \Pr(S_t = k|S_{t-1} = j)$, for $j, k = 1, 2$. Here, we model the probability of switching regimes using the logit link function, thus facilitating their modelling as a function of covariates; see [2] for an example of semi-parametric modelling. Then, we assume that the linear predictors involved in modelling $\text{logit}(\delta^t_{jk})$, with $j \neq k$, are parametrised by the vectors $\boldsymbol{\beta}_{\delta_{12}}$ and $\boldsymbol{\beta}_{\delta_{21}}$.

Let $\boldsymbol{\beta} = (\boldsymbol{\beta}^\top_{\eta_{11}}, \boldsymbol{\beta}^\top_{\eta_{21}}, \boldsymbol{\beta}^\top_{\eta_{12}}, \boldsymbol{\beta}^\top_{\eta_{22}}, \ldots, \boldsymbol{\beta}^\top_{\delta_{12}}, \boldsymbol{\beta}^\top_{\delta_{21}})^\top$ the p-dimensional parameter vector. Leveraging the Hamilton's filter [3], the log-likelihood is

$$\ell(\boldsymbol{\beta}) = \sum_{t=1}^T \log f_{Y_t}(y_t|\tilde{\mathcal{I}}_t; \boldsymbol{\beta}) = \sum_{t=1}^T \log \left\{ \sum_{j,k=1}^2 \delta^t_{jk} \pi^{t-1}_j f_{Y_t|S_t}\left(y_t|s_t = k; \boldsymbol{x}^t_{s_t}, \boldsymbol{\beta}_{s_t}\right) \right\},$$

where $\pi^t_j = \sum_{k=1}^2 \delta^t_{kj} \pi^{t-1}_k f_{Y_t|S_t}(y_t|s_t = j; \boldsymbol{x}^t_{s_t}, \boldsymbol{\beta}_{s_t}) / f_{Y_t}(y_t|\tilde{\mathcal{I}}_t; \boldsymbol{\beta})$ is the filtered state probability, that is $\pi^t_{s_t} = \Pr(S_t = s_t|\mathcal{I}_t; \boldsymbol{\beta})$, for $t \geq 1$. Above, we denoted with $\mathcal{I}_t$ the set of all information available up to time t, with $\tilde{\mathcal{I}}_t = \mathcal{I}_t \setminus \{y_t\}$, and with $\boldsymbol{x}^t_{s_t}$ and $\boldsymbol{\beta}_{s_t}$ the vectors of covariate information and regression parameters involved in modelling the regime-specific distributional parameters. We carry out full Bayesian inference considering, where possible, data-scaled weakly informative priors for the intercepts, while we adopt normal priors for the regression coefficients associated with linear and smooth effects of the covariates. The amount of regularisation on the smooth terms is controlled by half student-t priors on the inverse of the smoothing parameter [8]. The model simulations are performed using the No-U-Turn Sampler extension to the Hamiltonian Monte Carlo, as implemented in the probabilistic programming language `Stan`.

3 Application to Energy Prices in Spain

We consider data on energy prices in Spain, analysed by [1] and available in the `R` package `MSwM` [6]. The data span the period from January 2002 to October 2008, only covering working days. We consider as response variable the daily average energy prices (Cent/kwh) and, as in [1], we only focus on the oil price information (`Oil`, Euro/barrel) as a predictor. We assume the Gaussian distribution for modelling the energy prices under the regime labelled as 1, while we vary the distribution of regime 2 involving Gaussian (thereafter `Gaussian - Gaussian`), Gumbel (`Gaussian - Gumbel`), and Fréchet (`Gaussian - Fréchet`). Here, we denote with μ and σ, respectively, the location and scale parameter of these distributions, while ξ is the shape parameter of the Fréchet distribution. For all the regime-specific distributions we model the location parameters as

$$\mu_{s_t}^t = \eta_{s_t 1}^t = h_{s_t 1}(\texttt{Oil}_t), \quad t = 1, \ldots, 1784, \; s_t = 1, 2, \tag{2}$$

where $h(\cdot)$ is a P-spline-based function of the covariate `Oil`, built using ten basis functions. Then, for $s_t = 1, 2$, we consider increasingly complex specifications for $\eta_{s_t 2}^t$, that is the linear predictors involved in modelling the (log-) scale parameters

$$\begin{aligned}
\texttt{Setting 1}: \quad & \log \sigma_{s_t}^t = \beta_{\eta_{s_t 2,1}}, \\
\texttt{Setting 2}: \quad & \log \sigma_{s_t}^t = \beta_{\eta_{s_t 2,1}} + \beta_{\eta_{s_t 2,2}} \texttt{Oil}_t, \\
\texttt{Setting 3}: \quad & \log \sigma_{s_t}^t = h_{s_t 2}(\texttt{Oil}_t),
\end{aligned}$$

where $h(\cdot)$ is specified as in (2), while we model via intercepts both $\eta_{s_t 3}^t = \log \xi_{s_t}^t = \beta_{\eta_{s_t 3,1}}$ under Fréchet regime ($s_t = 2$) and the logit transition probabilities, that is $\text{logit}(\delta_{jk}^t) = \beta_{\delta_{jk,1}}$, for $j, k = 1, 2$, with $j \neq k$.

Table 1 reports the leave-one-out information criterion (LOOIC) for all the combinations of regimes distributional assumptions and scale parameter modelling settings. We chose LOOIC as per [9], noticing that the Watanabe-Akaike information criterion was almost equal. The results highlight the gain achieved by modelling the scale parameters using a smooth function of `Oil` and, under this setting, there is marginal evidence of adopting the Gumbel distribution for regime 2.

Table 1. LOOIC. Underline indicates the best model.

MODEL	`Setting 1`	`Setting 2`	`Setting 3`
`Gaussian - Gaussian`	4068	4017	3705
`Gaussian - Gumbel`	3921	3901	<u>3686</u>
`Gaussian - Fréchet`	3931	3912	3704

Figure 1 reports for the `Gaussian - Gumbel` case under `Setting 3` the posterior conditional mean and standard deviation estimates with 95% credible intervals, by considering 0.5 as a cut-off probability for determining the membership to the two regimes. Under both regimes, the estimated posterior conditional means capture the upward trending patterns between `Oil` and energy prices.

However, the data points belonging to regime 2 exhibit a pronounced non-linear relationship, which is well-encompassed by modelling both the location and the (log-) scale parameter through a smooth effect of `Oil`. Further, the shape of the estimated posterior standard deviations provides information on the volatility of energy prices as a function of `Oil`. Overall, the volatility under regime 1 is less affected by `Oil` values and it is estimated to be lower than regime 2. In contrast, regime 2 is characterised by higher volatility for low and intermediate values of `Oil`. However, the high volatility for low levels of `Oil` is attributable to an exceptional event that occurred at the beginning of 2002.

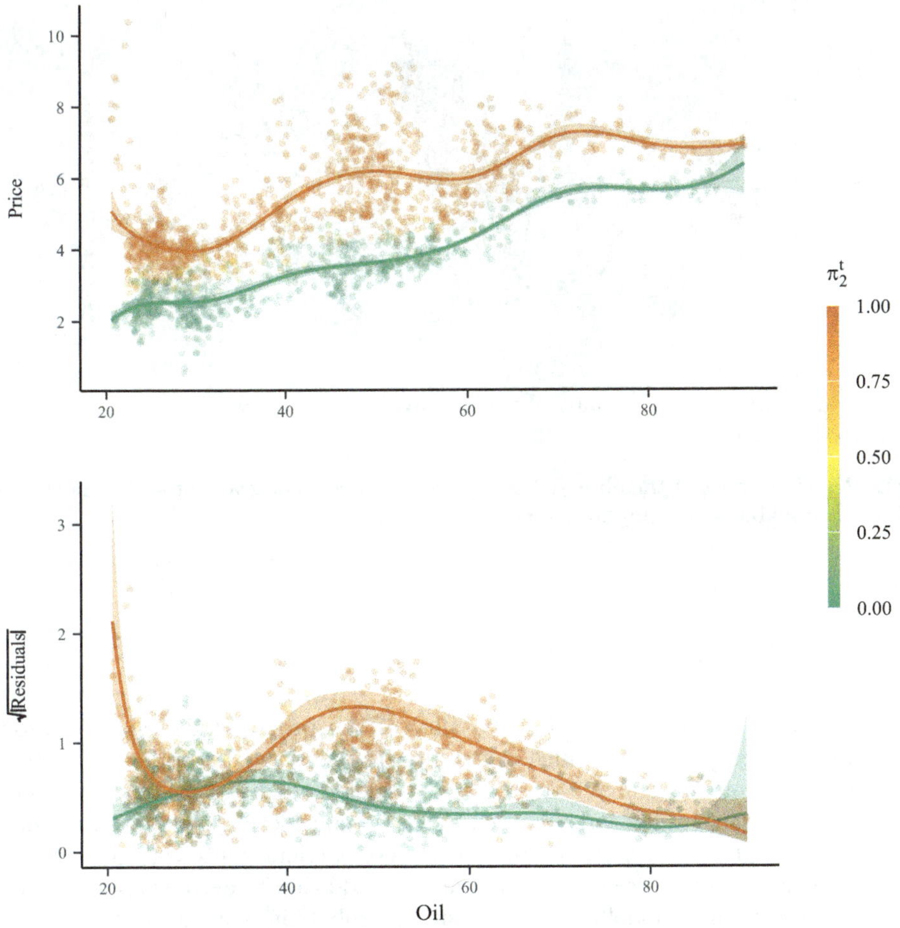

Fig. 1. Posterior conditional mean (top) and standard deviation (bottom) estimates with 95% credible intervals for the two regimes, using 0.5 as a cut-off probability for determining the regime-membership. The color gradient scale reports the filtered probability of being in regime 2 (Gumbel).

Figure 2 reports the evolution of the energy prices over the observed period, along with the probability of being in regime 2. Except for a short period in 2004, the filtered state probabilities allow discerning the membership to the two regimes, which correspond to a more stable and an unstable energy price market, respectively. By jointly interpreting the information from Fig. 1 and Fig. 2, the periods associated with regime 2 are mainly characterised by higher prices and volatility, compared to those well-depicted by regime 1.

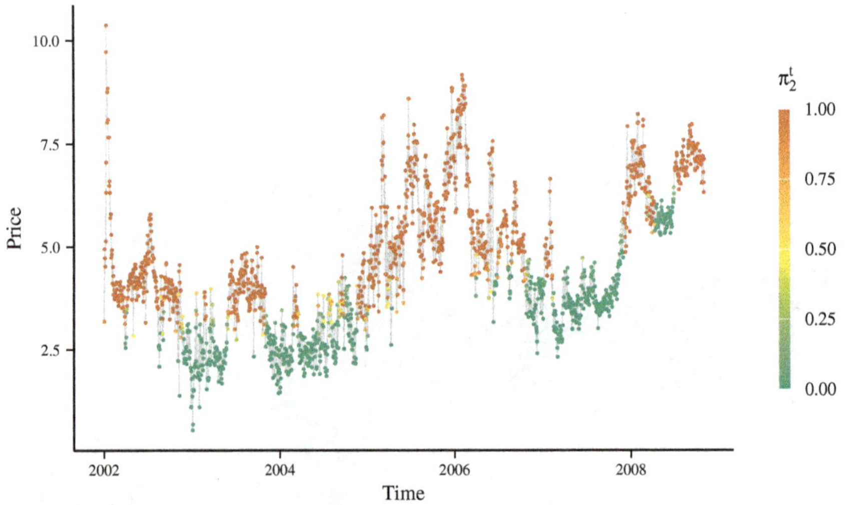

Fig. 2. Time series of the observed energy prices. The color gradient scale reports the filtered probability of being in regime 2 (Gumbel).

4 Conclusions

The results so far illustrate the capability of the proposed Bayesian Markov-switching regression model, which contributes to the recent developments by [1,4] in the framework of generalized additive models and distributional regression models, respectively. We enhance flexibility by considering a regime that may follow an extreme value distribution, which is of particular interest, for instance, in analysing economic or climate outcomes. In addition to accounting for multi-state processes and modelling the transition probabilities using covariates, the following research streams can be outlined: (i) Extend previous findings by [7] in the context of heat waves dynamics; (ii) Nest the Markov-switching model into multivariate modelling; (iii) Enhance interpretability of the covariates effect on a output of interest; see, e.g., [10]. Finally, an R package implementing the Markov-switching for extreme value modelling is currently under development.

References

1. Adam, T., Mayr, A., Kneib, T.: Gradient boosting in Markov-switching generalized additive models for location, scale, and shape. Econom. Stat. **22**, 3–16 (2022). https://doi.org/10.1016/j.ecosta.2021.04.002
2. Feldmann, C.C., Mews, S., Langrock, R.: Modelling time-of-day variation in hidden Markov models using cyclyc P-splines. In Bergherr, E., Groll, A., and Mayr, A. (eds.): Proceedings of the 37th International Workshop of Statistical Modelling, pp. 131–134. TU Dortmund University, Dortmund, Germany (2023). https://iwsm2023.statistik.tu-dortmund.de/storages/iwsm2023-statistik/r/dokumente/IWSM_2023_Conference_Proceedings.pdf
3. Hamilton, J.D.: Regime switching models. In: Durlauf, S.N., and Blume, L.E. (eds.) Macroeconometrics and Time Series Analysis. The New Palgrave Economics Collection, pp. 202–209. Palgrave Macmillan, London, UK (2010). https://doi.org/10.1057/9780230280830_23
4. Langrock, R., Kneib, T., Glennie, R., Michelot, T.: Markov-switching generalized additive models. Stat. Comput. **27**(1), 259–270 (2017). https://doi.org/10.1007/s11222-015-9620-3
5. Laurini, F., Pauli, F.: Smoothing sample extremes: the mixed model approach. Comput. Stat. Data Anal. **53**(11), 3842–3854 (2009). https://doi.org/10.1016/j.csda.2009.04.005
6. Sanchez-Espigares, J.A., Lopez-Moreno A.: MSwM: fitting Markov switching models. R package version 1.5 (2021). https://CRAN.R-project.org/package=MSwM
7. Shaby, B.A., Reich, B.J., Cooley, D., Kaufman, C.G.: A Markov-switching model for heat waves. Ann. Appl. Stat. **10**(1), 74–93 (2016). https://doi.org/10.1214/15-AOAS873
8. Umlauf, N., Klein, N., Zeileis, A.: BAMLSS: Bayesian additive models for location, scale, and shape (and beyond). J. Comput. Graph. Stat. **27**(3), 612–627 (2018). https://doi.org/10.1080/10618600.2017.1407325
9. Vehtari, A., Gelman, A., Gabry, J.: Practical Bayesian model evaluation using leave-one-out cross-validation and WAIC. Stat. Comput. **27**(5), 1413–1432 (2017). https://doi.org/10.1007/s11222-016-9696-4
10. Xu, S.G., Reich, B.J.: Bayesian nonparametric quantile process regression and estimation of marginal quantile effects. Biom. **79**(1), 151–164 (2023). https://doi.org/10.1111/biom.13576

Derivatives of the Log of a Determinant

Paul H. C. Eilers[1(✉)] and Martin P. Boer[2]

[1] Erasmus MC, Rotterdam, The Netherlands
p.eilers@erasmusmc.nl
[2] Wageningen University and Research, Wageningen, The Netherlands

Abstract. We present an efficient way to calculate effective model dimensions, using automated differentiation of the Cholesky algorithm. The method is illustrated with two examples using P-splines: adaptive smoothing and smoothing of over-dispersed counts.

Keywords: Choleksy Decomposition · Sparse Linear Algebra · Automated Differentiation · Effective Model Dimension

1 Introduction

The title says it all: we discuss derivatives of the logarithm of a determinant. They occur naturally when estimating mixed models or using penalized regression. They can be computed in an elegant, explicit way, which is very efficient when working with sparse matrices. It has been implemented in the R package `LMMsolver` [1]. We explain the theory and apply it to a adaptive smoothing and to smoothing of over-dispersed counts.

2 Theory

The partial derivative of the logarithm of the determinant of a positive definite matrix A is given by Harville [6]:

$$\frac{\partial \log |A|}{\partial \lambda} = \mathrm{tr}(A^{-1}\frac{\partial A}{\partial \lambda}). \tag{1}$$

If the matrix A is sparse, there is an efficient way to calculate the partial derivative. First, it uses the Cholesky decomposition $A = LL'$, where L is a sparse lower triangular matrix. The next step is automated differentiation of the Cholesky algorithm, as described by Smith [11], and will be explained in more detail below.

First we introduce some notation. Let m be the number of observations and n the length of a, the vector of B-spline coefficients. Let B be a $m \times n$ B-splines basis, with $\mu = Ba$, and $P = D'D$ be a d-th order difference penalty matrix; ϕ and ψ are precision parameters, with variances $\sigma^2 = 1/\phi$ and $\tau^2 = 1/\psi$. The effective model dimension is defined as [4]

$$ED = \mathrm{tr}[B(\phi B'B + \psi P)^{-1}\phi B'] = \mathrm{tr}[(\phi B'B + \psi P)^{-1}\phi B'B]. \tag{2}$$

J. Einbeck et al. (Eds.): IWSM 2024, CONTRIB.STAT., pp. 68–74, 2024.
https://doi.org/10.1007/978-3-031-65723-8_11

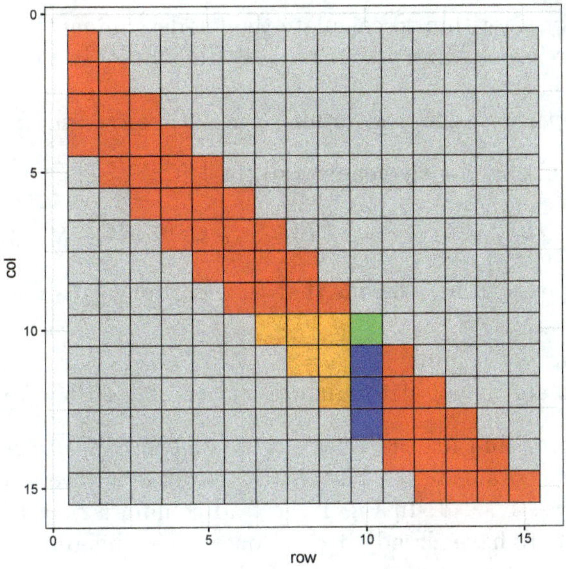

Fig. 1. Example of Cholesky Decomposition of the matrix $\phi B'B+\psi P = LL'$, where L is a lower triangular matrix. The grey entries are zero's. In the figure it is assumed that the current column to be updated is $j = 10$. The left-looking Cholesky decomposition first updates the lead-column $j = 10$ with the elements in orange, next calculates the pivot in green, and finally updates the elements in blue. Reverse differentiation of the Cholesky decomposition first updates the elements in blue, next the pivot in green, and finally adjusts the orange elements for column $j = 10$.

Using Eq. (1) the effective dimension can be written as the derivative of a log of a determinant, multiplied with the precision parameter ϕ

$$ED = \text{tr}[(\phi B'B + \psi P)^{-1}\phi B'B] = \phi \frac{\partial \log |\phi B'B + \psi P|}{\partial \phi}. \tag{3}$$

Since $\phi B'B + \psi P$ is sparse, the effective dimension ED can be calculated efficiently using automated differentiation of the Cholesky algorithm [11], without calculating the inverse of $\phi B'B + \psi P$.

The Cholesky decomposition of a positive definite matrix is well known, and efficient functions are available in most programming languages. However, using the differentiation of the Cholesky algorithm is less known. We will start with an algorithm for the Cholesky decomposition, and then show that differentiation is relatively easy.

Figure 1 shows an example of the Cholesky decomposition L for the matrix $\phi B'B + \psi P$ with $n = 15$ cubic P-splines and 2-nd order penalties. The matrix L is a banded lower-triangle. We use a left-looking Cholesky algorithm, where columns are updated with elements to the left. In Fig. 1 this is illustrated for lead column $j = 10$, and the orange non-zero elements on the left.

The Cholesky algorithm to calculate the log-determinant consists of the following steps, for lead column $j = 1, 2, \ldots, n$, and shown in Fig. 1 for $j = 10$.

Cholesky decomposition and calculation of the log-determinant:

1 Update lead column j with elements to the left

$$L_{i,j} = L_{i,j} - L_{i,k} \cdot L_{j,k}, \quad j < i \leq n, 1 \leq k < j,$$

where the equal sign here means that the value of $L_{i,j}$ is updated.
2 Define pivot $L_{j,j} = L_{j,j}^{1/2}$.
3 Update the current column j: $L_{i,j} = L_{i,j}/L_{j,j}$, $j < i \leq n$.
4 If $j = n$, calculate the log-determinant: $\log |\phi B'B + \psi P| = 2 \sum_{i=1}^{n} \log L_{i,i}$.

Given the algorithm for the Cholesky decomposition, backward differentiation can be easily obtained [11]. The algorithm works in reverse order, with lead column $j = n, n-1, \ldots, 1$. In Fig. 1 the lead column is $j = 10$, which implies that columns $j > 10$ have already been updated. The differentiation is in reverse order, therefore starting at step 4.

Backwards Differentiation of the Cholesky decomposition:

4 For $j = n$, initialize the $n \times n$ matrix F, by differentiating the expression for the log-determinant:

$$F_{i,i} = 2/L_{i,i}, \ 1 \leq i \leq n, \quad F_{i,k} = 0, i \neq k.$$

3 Update the current column j:

$$F_{i,j} = F_{i,j}/L_{j,j}, \quad F_{j,j} = F_{j,j} - L_{i,j} \cdot F_{i,j}, \quad j < i \leq n$$

2 Differentiation for the pivot: $F_{j,j} = \frac{1}{2} F_{j,j}/L_{j,j}$.
1 Update elements to the left of lead column j:

$$F_{i,k} = F_{i,k} - F_{i,j} \cdot L_{j,k}, \ F_{j,k} = F_{j,k} - F_{i,j} \cdot L_{i,k}, \ j < i \leq n, 1 \leq k < j.$$

Finally, with $K = B'B$, the effective dimension can be calculated as

$$ED = \phi \sum_{i,j} F_{i,j} K_{i,j}. \tag{4}$$

All calculations are sparse, and therefore computation time is linear in n, the number of B-splines. An alternative algorithm by Hutchinson and de Hoog [7] and used in by Frasso and Eilers [5] to calculate the effective dimension could also be used, but it is only available for one-dimensional P-splines. The method based on Automated Differentiation of the Cholesky algorithm can be extended to more general cases and has been implemented in `LMMsolver` [1].

So far we have shown the advantages of using sparse matrix algebra to calculate the effective dimension. We will extend this idea a bit further, to algorithms to estimate the P-splines parameters and the penalties. From [1] and [2] it follows that minus two times the restricted log-likelihood is defined by (ignoring some constants)

$$Q = -m \log \phi + \phi ||y - Ba||^2 - (n - d) \log \psi + \psi a'Pa + \log |\phi B'B + \psi P|, \quad (5)$$

where a is given by

$$(\phi B'B + \psi P)a = \phi B'y. \quad (6)$$

Using the sparse Cholesky Decomposition $LL' = \phi B'B + \psi P$ Eqs. (5) and (6) can be solved in an efficient way.

Using (1) we obtain

$$\frac{\partial Q}{\partial \phi} = -m/\phi + ||y - Ba||^2 + \text{tr}[(\phi B'B + \psi P)^{-1}B'B], \quad (7)$$

and

$$\frac{\partial Q}{\partial \psi} = -(n - d)/\psi + a'Pa + \text{tr}[(\phi B'B + \psi P)^{-1}P]. \quad (8)$$

In (7) we recognize the effective dimension ED, defined in (2).

Setting the partial derivative wrt ϕ to zero we get

$$\phi = (m - ED)/||y - Ba||^2 \quad \text{or} \quad \sigma^2 = ||y - Ba||^2/(m - ED), \quad (9)$$

a familiar result. In (8) we have

$$\text{tr}[(\phi B'B + \psi P)^{-1}P] = \text{tr}[(\phi B'B + \psi P)^{-1}\psi P]/\psi \quad (10)$$

But, with $G = \phi B'B + \psi P$,

$$\text{tr}[G^{-1}\psi P] = \text{tr}[G^{-1}(G - \phi B'B)] = \text{tr}[I - G^{-1}\phi B'B] = n - ED. \quad (11)$$

After simplification we arrive at

$$\psi = (ED - d)/(a'Pa) \quad \text{or} \quad \tau^2 = a'Pa/(ED - d), \quad (12)$$

also a familiar result. By repeatedly solving Eqs. (6), (9) and (12) we find the proper estimates of coefficients and precision parameters.

Assume that we have multiple penalties which overlap, meaning that every penalty can involve all parameters. We write $\mathcal{P}_\psi = \sum_k \psi_k P_k$, with $P_k = D'H_kD$, where H_k are semi-positive matrices, assumed to be sparse.

Using the P-splines sparse mixed model formulation introduced by Boer [1] [2], it can be shown that the deviance Q is defined by:

$$Q = -m \log \phi + \phi ||y - Ba||^2 - \log |\mathcal{H}_\psi| + a'P_\psi a + \log |\phi B'B + \mathcal{P}_\psi|, \quad (13)$$

where a is given by

$$(\phi B'B + \mathcal{P}_\psi)a = \phi B'y, \quad \text{and} \quad \mathcal{H}_\psi = \sum_k \psi_k H_k. \quad (14)$$

The partial derivatives of (13) wrt ψ_k are

$$\frac{\partial Q}{\partial \psi_k} = -\text{tr}[\mathcal{H}_\psi^{-1} H_k] + a' P_k a + \text{tr}[G^{-1} P_k], \tag{15}$$

where $G = \phi B'B + \mathcal{P}_\psi$. The last term in (15) can be interpreted as the effective dimension again and we find for ϕ the same result as in (9). We arrive at the following result:

$$\psi_k = \frac{f_k - g_k}{a' P_k a}, \quad f_k = \text{tr}[\mathcal{H}_\psi^{-1} \psi_k H_k] \quad \text{and} \quad g_k = \text{tr}[G^{-1} \psi_k P_k]. \tag{16}$$

We can interpret $f_k - g_k$ as the effective dimension connected to penalty matrix P_k. Both f_k and g_k can be calculated efficiently using automated differentiation of the Cholesky algorithm for $\mathcal{H}_\psi$ and $\mathcal{P}_\psi$, respectively.

With B a B-spline basis matrix and one penalty, $P = D'D$, we have the standard case of P-splines smoothing. We are not limited to that. With B a tensor product of two B-splines bases and P_1 and P_2 difference penalties on the coefficients, the theory holds for two-dimensional smoothing too.

The pattern is that the derivative of the log of a determinant leads directly to a matrix equation and the trace of its solution. That trace can be interpreted as a partial effective dimension. The package `LMMsolver` reverses the pattern: it computes the derivative and so finds the effective dimension. Even for large problems this can be done very efficiently, in time and memory use, with automatic differentiation. The package uses `C++` and `Rcpp` to make computations fast. It combines the automatic differentiation of the Cholesky algorithm [11] with a sparse implementation using supernodal left-looking Cholesky factorization [8]. Boer [1] presents further details. The `LMMsolver` package can handle quite general mixed models, but it also offers smoothing in one, two or three dimensions right out of the box.

3 Applications

Rodriguez-Alvarez et al. [10] present SOP, an algorithm and R package for fitting mixed models with overlapping penalties. One of the examples is adaptive one-dimensional smoothing of a signal with a strongly varying frequency. The penalty is $P = \sum_{k=1}^{q} \lambda_k D' \text{diag}(v_k) D$, with v_k column k of a relatively small B-spline basis matrix, as shown in the middle panel of Fig. 1. There we simulated $y_i = \sin(4/(x + 0.1)) + 1.5$ plus normal noise and computed the smooth fit with $n = 1000$ and $q = 10$. Using the `SOP` R-package we get essentially the same fit, the new sparse algorithm being at least ten times faster.

Our second example concerns smoothing of over-dispersed counts. Perperoglou and Eilers [9] proposed penalized individual random effects (PRIDE) for this purpose. The data, shown as vertical bars in Fig. 2, are the reported number of male deaths in Greece in 1960. All ages above 84 are excluded because the form one group in the data. Strong digit preference (for multiples of 5) is apparent. The thin blue line shows they result of applying `LMMsolver` to the raw data,

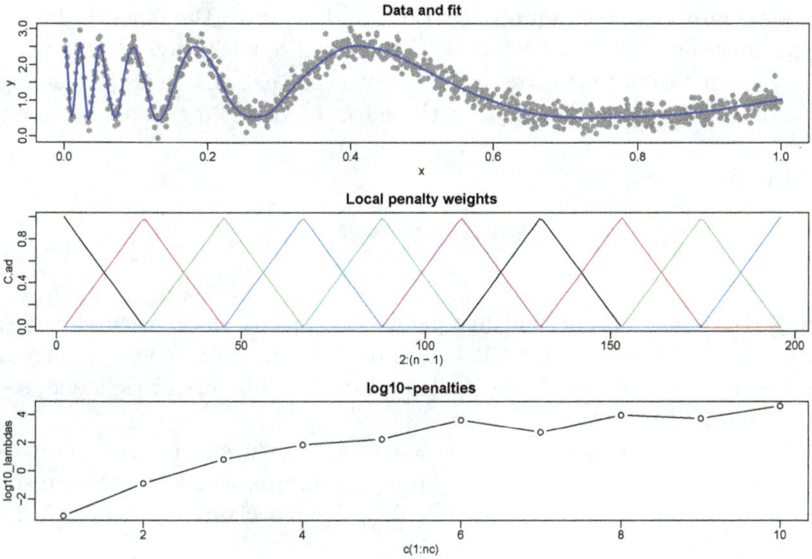

Fig. 2. Upper panel: simulated data and fit, adaptive smoothing using 200 cubic B-splines. Middle panel: The linear B-splines basis for the penalties. Lower panel: The log10-penalties for the linear B-splines basis.

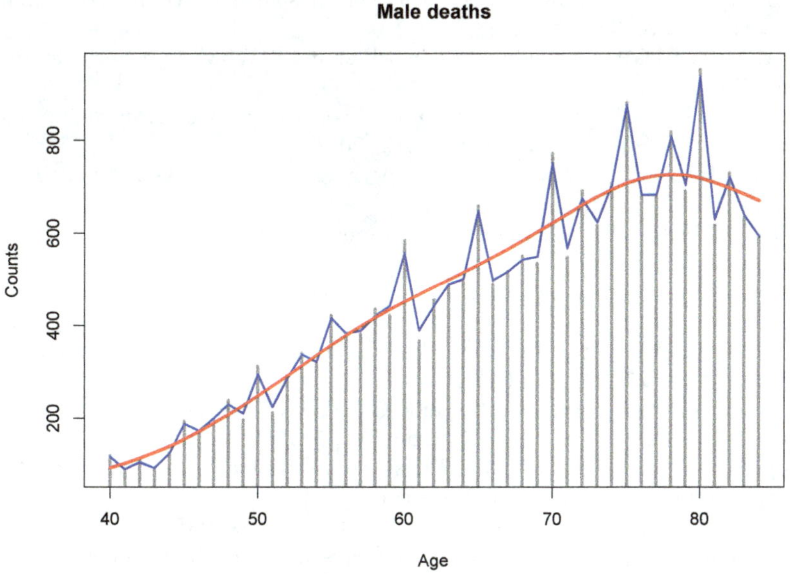

Fig. 3. Smoothing of (a part of) the age distribution of male deaths in Greece in 1960. The vertical bars show the counts and the thin blue line the result standard generalized linear P-splines smoothing. The red thick line is based on the PRIDE model, with a random effect for each year of age.

assuming conditional Poisson distributions and using 45 B-splines and a second order penalty. The fitted curve follows the data quite faithfully. That is not what we want when estimating a trend. The reason is that the Poisson distribution implies that the variance is equal to the mean, which is far from true for these data.

The PRIDE model is

$$\eta_i = \log(\mu_i) = \sum_j \alpha_j B_j(x_i) + u_i.$$

To the extra parameters in u a ridge penalty is applied. In [9] a search algorithm based on AIC was used to tune it to the data. Using `LMMsolver`, with u as an extra random effect, we easily get the solution, showing a realistic trend, see the thick red line in Fig. 3.

PRIDE approximates digit preference, a systematic effects, as random effect. This appears to work well. A more principled approach is to introduce specific fixed effects for numbers ending with 0 or 5. See Camarda et al. [3] for an extensive analysis.

References

1. Boer, M.P.: Tensor product P-splines using a sparse mixed model formulation. Stat. Model. **23**, 465–479 (2023)
2. Boer, M.P.: REML for two-dimensional P-splines. IWSM 2024 Springer Proceedings (2024)
3. Camarda, C.G., Eilers, P.H.C., Gampe, J.: Modelling trends in digit preference patterns. J. R. Stat. Soc. C **66**, 893–918 (2017)
4. Eilers, P.H.C., Marx, B.D.: Flexible smoothing with B-splines and penalties. Stat. Sci. **11**, 89–121 (1996)
5. Frasso, G., Eilers, P.H.C.: L-and V-curves for optimal smoothing. Stat. Model. **15**, 91–111 (2015)
6. Harville, D.A.: Matrix Algebra from a Statistician's Perspective. Taylor & Francis (1998)
7. Hutchinson, M.F., de Hoog, F.R.: Smoothing noisy data with spline functions. Numer. Math. **47**, 99–106 (1985)
8. Ng, E.G., Peyton, B.W.: Block sparse Cholesky algorithms on advanced uniprocessor computers. SIAM J. Sci. Comput. **14**, 1034–1056 (1993)
9. Perperoglou, A., Eilers, P.H.C.: Penalized regression with individual deviance effects. Comput. Stat. **25**, 341–361 (2010)
10. Rodríguez-Alvarez, M.X., Durban, M., Lee, D.J., Eilers, P.H.: On the estimation of variance parameters in non-standard generalised linear mixed models: Application to penalised smoothing. Stat. Comput. **29**, 483–500 (2019)
11. Smith, S.P.: Differentiation of the Cholesky algorithm. J. Comput. Graph. Stat. **4**, 134 (1995)

Monitoring Viral Infections in Severe Acute Respiratory Syndrome Patients in Brazil

João Flávio Andrade Silva[1(✉)], Rafael Izbicki[2], Leonardo S. Bastos[3], and Guilherme P. Soares[4]

[1] Interinstitutional Graduate Program in Statistics UFSCar-USP (PIPGEs), Federal University of São Carlos and University of São Paulo, São Carlos, Brazil
joaoflavio@usp.br

[2] Department of Statistics, Federal University of São Carlos, São Carlos, Brazil

[3] Scientific Computing Program, Fundação Oswaldo Cruz, Rio de Janeiro, Brazil

[4] Institute of Mathematical and Computer Sciences, University of São Paulo, São Carlos, Brazil

Abstract. We introduce a novel methodology for estimating the distribution of viruses in Severe Acute Respiratory Syndrome (SARS) patients in Brazil, addressing significant challenges for data in that country, such as data delays and the absence of negative test results. By employing a probabilistic classifier, our approach offers precise, adaptable estimates across various demographic characteristics and regions of the country without the need for predefined groups. Comparative analyses demonstrate the effectiveness of the model. This methodology significantly contributes to public health by enhancing disease monitoring and supporting targeted prevention strategies.

Keywords: Severe Acute Respiratory Syndrome · Epidemiological Modeling · Machine Learning · Virus Distribution · Public Health Surveillance

1 Introduction

Severe Acute Respiratory Syndrome (SARS) is a serious condition caused by various infectious agents, notably highlighted by the COVID-19 pandemic. Beyond coronavirus, common causes also include influenza and respiratory syncytial viruses. Epidemiological data is crucial for public health analyses to understand viral distribution and infectious disease spread. Since its implementation in Brazil in 2009, SARS surveillance mandates the collection and reporting of all hospitalized cases and/or deaths due to respiratory viruses [1].

The Brazilian Ministry of Health provides records of Severe Acute Respiratory Syndrome, which contain epidemiological information about the incidence of this syndrome in the country. These records include dates, locations, demographic characteristics, and identification of the causative viruses. Typically, this information is shared weekly through an open data portal [2].

J. Einbeck et al. (Eds.): IWSM 2024, CONTRIB.STAT., pp. 75–80, 2024.
https://doi.org/10.1007/978-3-031-65723-8_12

Our goal is to monitor efficiently the predominant viruses causing SARS across all Brazilian municipalities for patients of any age. Figure 1 illustrates the results of our approach by showing the estimated distribution of viruses during the first 43 weeks of 2022 for the municipality of São José dos Campos in patients aged 1 year. This tool enables continuous monitoring, assisting healthcare professionals in identifying patterns of viral spread to support prevention and control strategies.

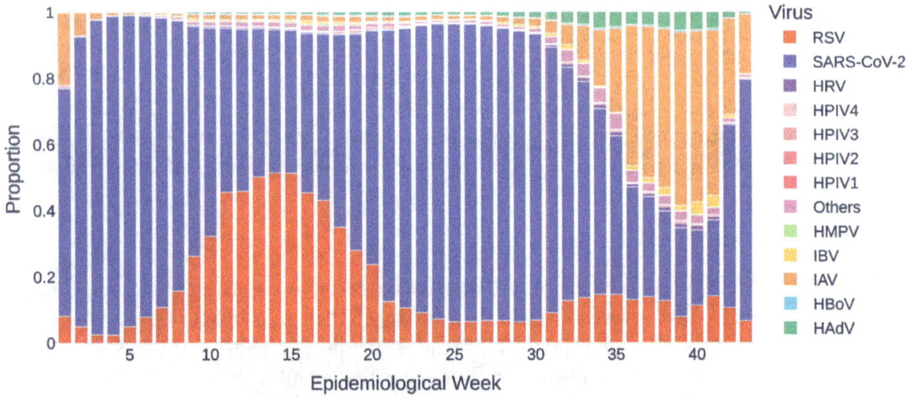

Fig. 1. Estimated distribution of viruses in patients aged 1 year in São José dos Campos during the first 43 weeks of 2022.

To achieve these goals, we need to address many challenges:

1. Information Delays: Delays in data availability arise from the time required for it to pass through several stages, from an individual's first symptom perception to system reporting with virus identification. This includes seeking medical care, undergoing testing, obtaining results, and entering the results into the system [3].
2. Incomplete Data on Negative Tests: The database records a virus only if the test result is positive, except for influenza. This leads to a lack of data on negative test results: the data does not distinguish individuals with negative results from those not tested for a given virus.
3. Data Sparsity in Some Regions: Information collection and availability vary significantly across different areas. For example, in São José dos Campos, as shown in Fig. 1, gathering enough data on 1-year-old patients is highly unlikely. This data sparsity can result from factors such as lower population density, limited healthcare resources, or infrequent reporting in these specific demographics.

To circumvent issues 1 and 2, we estimate the proportion of new infections for each virus among individuals with SARS who have tested positive for at least one virus. This approach helps bypass the limitations of missing negative data and reduces the impact of delays in data availability.

Estimating these proportions is complicated further by data sparsity in certain regions, issue 3. This is typically addressed by aggregating data across various regions and age groups, which unfortunately leads to a loss of information. To overcome this, our methodology models the proportion through the probability of observing a specific virus, conditioned on specific covariates.

2 Methodology

Our dataset is denoted by $\mathbb{D} = \{(X_i, Y_i)\}_{i=1}^n$, where X_i consists of input variable vectors containing information about the i-th individual. This information includes the epidemiological week of the first symptoms, the patient's age, geographical coordinates (latitude and longitude of the city, state, and region), and the population size of the notifying municipality. The target variable, Y_i, indicates which virus the patient's test result was positive for: Severe Acute Respiratory Syndrome Coronavirus 2, Influenza A/B Virus, Respiratory Syncytial Virus, Human Parainfluenza Virus 1/2/3/4, Human Adenovirus, Human Metapneumovirus, Human Bocavirus, Human Rhinovirus, and/or Others (other viruses or unspecified). The dataset only contains patients who tested positive for at least one virus. Refer to Table 1 for a sample representation of the dataset $\mathbb{D}$.

Table 1. Example illustrating the structure of dataset $\mathbb{D}$.

Virus	Epid. Week 1st Sympt.	Patient's Age	City		State		Region		Population Size
			Lat.	Long.	Lat.	Long.	Lat.	Long.	
IAV	1	68	−23.87	−47.99	−23.54	−46.63	−21.64	−43.53	32,062
SARS-CoV-2	3	56	−23.54	−46.63	−23.54	−46.63	−21.64	−43.53	12,200,180
SARS-CoV-2	4	72	−10.91	−37.07	−10.91	−37.07	−7.31	−37.99	605,309
RSV	5	0.17	−16.82	−49.24	−16.67	−49.25	−17.12	−51.98	500,760
HMPV	12	2	−23.54	−46.63	−23.54	−46.63	−21.64	−43.53	12,200,180
SARS-CoV-2	26	46	−23.59	−48.05	−23.54	−46.63	−21.64	−43.53	166,959
IAV	42	8	−25.42	−49.27	−25.42	−49.27	−27.68	−49.68	1,871,789
Others	46	68	−14.67	−40.47	−12.97	−38.51	−7.31	−37.99	23,290
SARS-CoV-2	47	43	−30.03	−51.22	−30.03	−51.22	−27.68	−49.68	1,404,269
RSV	48	0.83	−23.54	−46.63	−23.54	−46.63	−21.64	−43.53	12,200,180

Our goal is to estimate the proportion of patients who test positive for a specific virus among positive patients, conditioned on x. We approach this task as a multiclass classification problem, where the variable y represents the different viruses being considered. The proportion is modeled by the conditional probability, denoted as $\mathbb{P}_Y(y \mid X)$, which indicates the likelihood of a patient testing positive for a specific virus given the value of x. To estimate this probability, we employ a probabilistic classifier, denoted as $\hat{g}(\cdot)$, obtained based on the data in

$\mathbb{D}$. For the function $\hat{g}(\cdot)$, we chose the Gradient Boosting Machine (GBM) model based on decision trees, mathematically expressed as

$$\hat{g}(x) = \sum_{k=1}^{K} \alpha_k h_k(x),$$

where K is the total number of trees, $h_k(x)$ is the prediction of the k-th decision tree, and α_k is the learning rate, adjusting each tree's contribution [4].

The choice of a tree-based estimator is due to its effective partitioning of the covariate space. It allows detailed analysis across geographical and temporal dimensions and interaction with other relevant variables, eliminating the need for predefined groups and offering a more flexible and precise data analysis approach.

We highlight the creation of the Python package PySRAG, developed by our team [5]. This package provides a comprehensive set of tools essential for analyzing and processing data related to SARS in Brazil. This package includes functionalities for data preprocessing, feature engineering, and training classification models, thus facilitating the application of the proposed method.

3 Results

We conducted a comparative analysis of the proportion of SARS-CoV-2 among individuals with SARS who have tested positive for at least one virus in São Paulo during the first 26 weeks of 2022, utilizing the proposed methodology, baseline (observed proportion, in the data immediately after its first release, and thus subject to updates, in the state for each epidemiological week), and ground truth (observed proportion, in the latest data set available for 2022, in the municipality for each epidemiological week and specific age group). We found that the estimates generated by our methodology better approximated the ground truth curve (Fig. 2).

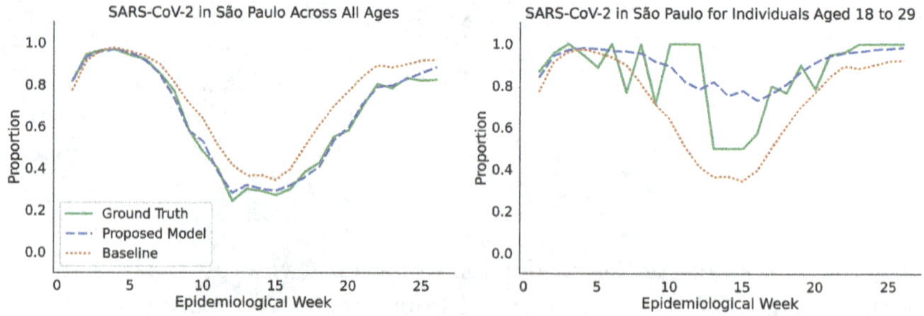

Fig. 2. Comparison of SARS-CoV-2 proportion curves among individuals with SARS who have tested positive for at least one virus in São Paulo using ground truth, the proposed model, and baseline. The curve of the proposed model most accurately reflects the ground truth.

In another analysis, we used 60 datasets from 2022 released weekly, focusing on each dataset's most recent 14 epidemiological weeks. We compared the estimates from our proposed methodology to those from the baseline method, obtained with subsamples of 10% of the data and evaluated on the remaining 90% of the database. Our methodology proved to be more effective, particularly for the SARS-CoV-2 and RSV viruses, as indicated by lower Brier scores [6]. The Brier score evaluates the accuracy of probabilistic predictions by quantifying the squared differences between predicted probabilities and actual outcomes, where a lower score signifies more accurate probability estimates. For viruses with low proportions, such as HPIV 1/2/3/4, the superiority of our methodology was less pronounced, suggesting that in cases with few occurrences, simpler methods may be equally effective (Fig. 3).

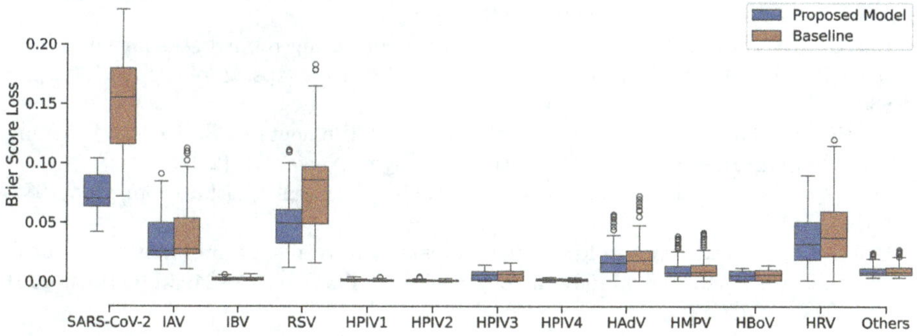

Fig. 3. Comparison between the models of the proposed methodology and the baseline. The proposed model showed smaller errors, demonstrating superiority in generalization compared to the baseline.

4 Discussion

The proposed methodology overcomes conventional method limitations by offering precise estimates without needing predefined groups, adapting to specific localities, ages, and periods.

This study enhances understanding of respiratory disease spread, introducing a novel approach to estimate virus proportions in SARS patients. Its findings are practical for public health, providing tools for disease monitoring and supporting prevention and control strategies.

Estimating requires caution, considering uniform testing policies and their stability over time. Moreover, the estimated proportion in SARS cases does not necessarily reflect the general population's proportion, as it is influenced by the severity of virus symptoms.

The PySRAG package includes a detailed web application at https://github.com/joao-1988/PySRAG.

Acknowledgments. Special thanks to the Statistical Modelling Society for the PhD Student Award. J.F.A. Silva gratefully acknowledges financial support from Banco do Brasil. RI was supported through grants 309607/2020-5, 422705/2021-7, 305065/2023-8 Brazilian National Counsel of Technological and Scientific Development (CNPq), and grant 2023/07068-1, São Paulo Research Foundation (FAPESP).

References

1. Brasil, Ministério da Saúde, Secretaria de Vigilância em Saúde: Guia de vigilância epidemiológica: emergência de saúde pública de importância nacional pela doença pelo coronavírus 2019 – covid-19. Ministério da Saúde (2022). https://www.gov.br/saude/pt-br/coronavirus/publicacoes-tecnicas/guias-e-planos/guia-de-vigilancia-epidemiologica-covid-19. ISBN 978-65-5993-025-8
2. Brasil, Ministério da Saúde: Dados Abertos da Saúde (2024). https://opendatasus.saude.gov.br/dataset/srag-2021-a-2024
3. Bastos, L.S., et al.: A modelling approach for correcting reporting delays in disease surveillance data. Stat. Med. **38**, 4363–4377 (2019). https://doi.org/10.1002/sim.8303
4. Hastie, T., Tibshirani, R., Friedman, J.H.: The Elements of Statistical Learning: Data Mining, Inference, and Prediction. Springer, New York (2009)
5. Silva, J.F.A., et al.: Python package PySRAG. https://github.com/joao-1988/PySRAG
6. Brier, G.: Verification of forecasts expressed in terms of probability. Monthly Weather Rev. **78**, 1–3 (1950). https://doi.org/10.1175/1520-0493(1950)078⟨0001:VOFEIT⟩2.0.CO;2

A Computationally Efficient Spatio-Temporal Fusion Model for Reflectance Data

Zhaoyuan Zou(✉), Ruth O'Donnell, Claire Miller, Duncan Lee, and Craig Wilkie

University of Glasgow, Glasgow, UK
z.zou.2@research.gla.ac.uk

Abstract. Fusing remotely-sensed reflectance data from different sources at different spatial and temporal scales is useful to monitor lake water quality. The nonparametric statistical downscaling model (NSD) [5] can account for a change of spatial and temporal support between two remote sensors, but it is computationally demanding for large datasets. This work proposes a method to improve the computational efficiency of the NSD model by endowing it with a Gaussian predictive process. The predictive performance and computational efficiency of both models are compared through simulation and using satellite reflectance data from Lake Garda.

Keywords: Nonparametric statistical downscaling · Gaussian predictive process · reflectance · lake water quality

1 Introduction

Reflectance data are important for monitoring lake water quality, because the water quality parameters such as chlorophyll-a and turbidity can be estimated from these data. This work is motivated by the problem of fusing reflectance data at Lake Garda from two satellite sensors, the Medium Resolution Imaging Spectrometer (MERIS) and the Moderate Resolution Imaging Spectroradiometer (MODIS). MERIS reflectance data are more suitable for lake water than MODIS data, because the MERIS sensor has a finer spatial resolution and key spectral bands to estimate water quality parameters [4]. However, MERIS has fewer observations than MODIS in the temporal dimension. Thus, fusing the reflectance data from these two sensors will maximise the benefits from both. To account for the different spatial and temporal supports of the remote sensors, the nonparametric statistical downscaling model (NSD) was proposed by Wilkie et al. (2019). Since the parameters in the NSD model are estimated by Gibbs sampling, which involves the inversion of a spatial covariance matrix, the computational requirements of the NSD model makes it challenging to apply to large datasets. This work proposes an approximation for the NSD model using the Gaussian predictive process (GPP) [1], which can achieve similar predictive performance to the NSD model but requires less computational time.

J. Einbeck et al. (Eds.): IWSM 2024, CONTRIB.STAT., pp. 81–87, 2024.
https://doi.org/10.1007/978-3-031-65723-8_13

2 Methodology

The NSD model of Wilkie et al. (2019) will be used to fuse the reflectance data from two sensors denoted 1 and 2. Suppose Sensor 2 has more observations in the temporal dimension than Sensor 1, but the reflectance data from Sensor 1 have a finer spatial resolution than those from Sensor 2. The NSD model assumes the reflectance data at each location from each sensor are observations of smooth functions over time, and that the coefficients of these smooth functions are modelled as spatially correlated via a covariance matrix. The vector of reflectance data at location i from Sensors 1 and 2 are presented by $\mathbf{y}_i$ and $\mathbf{x}_i$ for $i = 1, 2, ..., n$. The NSD model is defined as:

$$\begin{aligned} \mathbf{y}_i &\sim N_{q_i}\left(\boldsymbol{\Phi}_i\mathbf{c}_i,\ \frac{1}{p_y}\mathbf{I}_{q_i}\right),\ \mathbf{x}_i \sim N_{p_i}\left(\boldsymbol{\Psi}_i\mathbf{d}_i,\ \frac{1}{p_x}\mathbf{I}_{p_i}\right), \\ c_{ij} &\sim N\left(d_{ij}\beta_{ij} + \alpha_{ij},\ \frac{1}{p_c}\right),\ \mathbf{d}_i \sim N_m\left(\mathbf{0},\ 100 \times \mathbf{I}_m\right), \\ \boldsymbol{\alpha}_j &\sim N_n\left(\mathbf{0},\ \frac{1}{p_\alpha}\exp(-\phi_\alpha\mathbf{D})\right),\ \boldsymbol{\beta}_j \sim N_n\left(\mathbf{1},\ \frac{1}{p_\beta}\exp(-\phi_\beta\mathbf{D})\right), \end{aligned} \tag{1}$$

where $\boldsymbol{\Phi}_i$ and $\boldsymbol{\Psi}_i$ are the basis function matrices with dimension of m. The vectors $\mathbf{c}_i = (c_{i1}, c_{i2}, \cdots, c_{im})$ and $\mathbf{d}_i = (d_{i1}, d_{i2}, \cdots, d_{im})$ are the corresponding coefficients. The coefficients c_{ij} and d_{ij} are related by the intercept α_{ij} and the slope β_{ij} for $j = 1, 2, ..., m$, where m is the number of basis functions. The coefficients $\boldsymbol{\alpha}_j = (\alpha_{1j}, \alpha_{2j}, \cdots, \alpha_{nj})$ and $\boldsymbol{\beta}_j = (\beta_{1j}, \beta_{2j}, \cdots, \beta_{nj})$ follow multivariate normal distributions with precision parameter p_α and p_β, and spatial decay parameters ϕ_α and ϕ_β. The matrix $\mathbf{D}$ is the distance matrix between the n data locations. All parameters are updated via Gibbs sampling steps within a Bayesian MCMC algorithm, except the spatial decay parameters ϕ_α and ϕ_β which do not have closed forms for their posterior distributions, and are hence selected by cross-validation. In each iteration of the Gibbs sampler, the estimation of $\boldsymbol{\alpha}_j$ and $\boldsymbol{\beta}_j$ requires inversion of an $n \times n$ matrix, and this inversion will increase as $O(n^3)$ in the number of locations n. A GPP is one approximation method for representing the spatial process with a lower dimension. Suppose the spatial processes $\boldsymbol{\alpha}_j$ and $\boldsymbol{\beta}_j$ are defined at locations $S = \{s_1, s_2, ..., s_n\}$, the lower-dimensional spatial processes $\boldsymbol{\alpha}_j^*$ and $\boldsymbol{\beta}_j^*$ are defined over a set of knots $S^* = \{s_1^*, s_2^*, ..., s_r^*\}$. The number of knots r is much less than the number of observed data n. The spatial processes $\boldsymbol{\alpha}_j$ and $\boldsymbol{\beta}_j$ are approximated by $\mathbf{Z}\boldsymbol{\alpha}_j^*$ and $\mathbf{V}\boldsymbol{\beta}_j^*$ defined as:

$$\begin{aligned} &\boldsymbol{\alpha}_j^* \sim N_r\left(\mathbf{0},\ \frac{1}{p_\alpha}\exp(-\phi_\alpha\mathbf{D}^*)\right),\ \boldsymbol{\beta}_j^* \sim N_r\left(\mathbf{1},\ \frac{1}{p_\beta}\exp(-\phi_\beta\mathbf{D}^*)\right), \\ &\mathbf{Z} = \exp(-\phi_\alpha\mathbf{D}^\top)(\exp(-\phi_\alpha\mathbf{D}^*))^{-1},\ \mathbf{V} = \exp(-\phi_\beta\mathbf{D}^t op)(\exp(-\phi_\beta\mathbf{D}^*))^{-1}, \end{aligned} \tag{2}$$

where $\mathbf{D}^*$ is the $r \times r$ distance matrix between the selected knots S^*, and $\mathbf{D}^\top$ is the $n \times r$ distance matrix between the observed locations S and the selected knots S^*. The estimation of $\boldsymbol{\alpha}_j^*$ and $\boldsymbol{\beta}_j^*$ requires inverting an $r \times r$ matrix with

$r \ll n$, which reduces the computational time in each iteration of the Gibbs sampling. Then, the nonparametric statistical downscaling model with Gaussian predictive process (NSD-GPP) model is given as a combination of Equations (1) and (2) above. The precision parameters follow the Gamma distribution, $p_y, p_x, p_c, p_\alpha, p_\beta \sim \text{Gamma}(2, 0.01)$.

3 Application to Lake Garda Dataset

The NSD-GPP and the NSD models are applied to the Lake Garda dataset to assess their predictive performance and the computational efficiency. Specifically, the Lake Garda reflectance data [2] for wavelength 412 nm were observed by MERIS and MODIS remote sensors at 211 locations from January 2009 to March 2012. In Equations (1) and (2), MERIS data = $\mathbf{y}$ and MODIS data = $\mathbf{x}$. The 203 locations are randomly divided into ten groups. In each iteration, one group is chosen as the out-of-sample test set and the other nine groups are treated as the training sets. The NSD model is compared to the NSD-GPP model with 25 knots, 49 knots and 100 knots for the Lake Garda dataset respectively, which corresponds to approximately 10%, 25% and 50% of the total locations in Lake Garda. Ten B-splines basis functions, and ϕ_α and ϕ_β equalling 10 are used for both the NSD and NSD-GPP models based on cross-validation. Then, predictions are made for the selected locations in the test set for all months. The root mean squared prediction error (RMSPE) and coverage of the 95% credible intervals over these ten cross-validation iterations are summarised in Table 1. The NSD-GPP model achieves similar RMSPE and coverage as the NSD model for the Lake Garda dataset, but the NSD-GPP model with 25 knots uses about 30% of the computational time of the NSD model. The computational time of the NSD-GPP model increases with the number of knots. Since the reflectance data do not have much spatial variation in each month, a small number of spatial knots in the NSD-GPP model appears suitable to capture the spatial patterns for the Lake Garda dataset. Figure 1 shows the predictions from these models. Both models can appropriately capture the temporal pattern of the MERIS reflectance data at the unobserved locations.

Table 1. Cross-validation results of the NSD-GPP and the NSD models.

Model	RMSPE	Coverage (%)	Time (hour)
NSD-GPP 25 knots	0.0051	97.74	0.35
NSD-GPP 49 knots	0.0050	97.55	0.52
NSD-GPP 100 knots	0.0050	97.25	0.98
NSD	0.0047	97.39	1.12

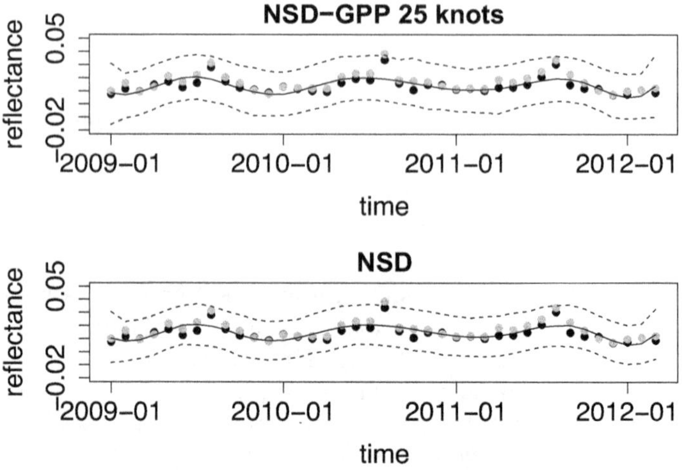

Fig. 1. Prediction of the MERIS reflectance data (black points) at a randomly selected location by the NSD-GPP and the NSD models. Grey points: observed MODIS reflectance, Black solid lines: predictions from the model, Black dashed lines: 95 percent credible intervals of the predictions.

4 Simulation Study

A simulation study was conducted in order to assess the performance of the NSD-GPP model more generally. The data are simulated to mimic the remote-sensing reflectance data at Lake Garda in this study. The data are generated as follows:

$$\begin{aligned} &\mathbf{y}_i \sim N_{q_i}(\alpha_i + \beta_i \mathbf{x}_i, \frac{1}{p_y}\mathbf{I}_{q_i}),\ \mathbf{x}_i \sim N_{p_i}(\boldsymbol{\Psi}_i \mathbf{d}_i, \frac{1}{p_x}\mathbf{I}_{p_i}), \\ &\mathbf{d}_j \sim N_n(\mathbf{0}, \frac{1}{p_d}\exp(-\phi_d \mathbf{D})),\ \boldsymbol{\alpha} \sim N_n(\mathbf{0}, \frac{1}{p_\alpha}\exp(-\phi_\alpha \mathbf{D}), \\ &\boldsymbol{\beta} \sim N_n(\mathbf{1}, \frac{1}{p_\beta}\exp(-\phi_\beta \mathbf{D}),\ p_y = p_x = 100. \end{aligned} \tag{3}$$

In Eq. 3, the matrices $\mathbf{y}_i$ and $\mathbf{x}_i$ are the simulated MERIS and MODIS reflectance data at location i, for $i = 1, 2, \cdots, n$. The matrix $\boldsymbol{\Psi}_i$ represents the Fourier basis functions with dimension three, which aims to generate $\mathbf{x}_i$ with one peak per year. The corresponding coefficients are d_{ij} for the location i and the basis function j, which are represented by the vectors $\mathbf{d}_i = (d_{i1}, d_{i2}, d_{i3})$ and $\mathbf{d}_j = (d_{1j}, d_{2j}, \cdots, d_{nj})$. The vectors $\mathbf{y}_i$ and $\mathbf{x}_i$ are related by the spatially varying intercepts α_i and slopes β_i, where $\boldsymbol{\alpha} = (\alpha_1, \alpha_2, \cdots, \alpha_n)$ and $\boldsymbol{\beta} = (\beta_1, \beta_2, \cdots, \beta_n)$. The spatial decay parameters are ϕ_d, ϕ_α, ϕ_β and the matrix $\mathbf{D}$ represents the distance between the n locations. The precision parameters $p_y = p_x = 100$ are used to simulate the data with relatively large observed error. The data are simulated within a square domain with 225 locations for 39 months, and the distance between two adjacent locations is 0.01. In order to generalise the NSD-GPP model to other reflectance datasets, scenarios based on changing the levels of spatial variation and spatial correlation are investigated and summarised in Table 2. The spatial variation is controlled by the precision parameters $\{p_d, p_\alpha, p_\beta\}$, and a small value of the precision parameter represents a large spatial variation. Since p_y, p_x are fixed to 100 for the simulated datasets, $p_\alpha = p_\beta = p_d = 10$ are used to represent a large spatial variation, and $p_\alpha = p_\beta = p_d = 100$ are to indicate a small spatial variation. The spatial correlation is controlled by the spatial decay parameters ϕ_α, ϕ_β, ϕ_d. The spatial decay parameters are selected based on the effective range of the covariance matrices of $\mathbf{d}_j$, $\boldsymbol{\alpha}_j$, and $\boldsymbol{\beta}_j$ [3]. Then, $\phi_\alpha = \phi_\beta = \phi_d = 15$ represents a strong spatial correlation, and $\phi_\alpha = \phi_\beta = \phi_d = 300$ represents a week spatial correlation. For each scenario, 100 datasets with different random seeds are generated and the output statistics are averaged over these 100 datasets. After generating the data, the NSD-GPP model and the NSD model are applied to these datasets. Ten B-splines basis functions are used because the study of the Lake Garda dataset suggests that ten B-splines basis functions would be enough for one peak per year. The spatial decay parameters ϕ_α and ϕ_β for both the NSD and NSD-GPP models are selected using cross-validation. The results of the average over 100 datasets in each scenario are summarised in Table 3, and the computational time for each model is shown in Table 4. The RMSPE and the coverage have a similar pattern as seen for the Lake Garda dataset, where the RMSPE and the coverage generally decrease with a larger number of knots. Take one dataset in scenario 2 as an example, the prediction at a randomly picked location from the NSD-GPP model and the NSD model are shown in Fig. 2. Both models can appropriately capture the temporal pattern of the simulated data at the unobserved location. This result suggests that the NSD-GPP model with a larger number of knots will achieve a better predictive performance for the datasets with stronger spatial correlation. From these scenarios, the NSD-GPP model with 25 knots and 49 knots approximate the NSD model well, and the NSD-GPP model with 100 knots requires almost the same time as the NSD model with little gain in RMSPE.

Table 2. Scenarios of the simulated data set. ϕ_d, ϕ_α, ϕ_β: spatial decay parameters. p_d, p_α, p_β: precision parameters.

Scenario	$\{\phi_d, \phi_\alpha, \phi_\beta\}$	$\{p_d, p_\alpha, p_\beta\}$
1	15	10
2	15	100
3	300	10
4	300	100

Table 3. Cross-validation results of the NSD-GPP model and the NSD model for the simulation datasets with different scenarios.

Scenario	Model	RMSPE	Coverage
1	NSD-GPP 25 knots	0.181	97.07
	NSD-GPP 49 knots	0.173	96.63
	NSD-GPP 100 knots	0.169	96.10
	NSD	0.163	93.35
2	NSD-GPP 25 knots	0.125	97.065
	NSD-GPP 49 knots	0.123	97.756
	NSD-GPP 100 knots	0.122	97.644
	NSD	0.110	94.769
3	NSD-GPP 25 knots	0.339	88.709
	NSD-GPP 49 knots	0.338	89.203
	NSD-GPP 100 knots	0.338	88.816
	NSD	0.338	88.51
4	NSD-GPP 25 knots	0.147	93.52
	NSD-GPP 49 knots	0.147	93.475
	NSD-GPP 100 knots	0.147	93.469
	NSD	0.146	93.341

Table 4. Computational time of the NSD-GPP model and the NSD-GPP model for the spatial cross-validation of the simulated dataset.

Model	NSD-GPP 25 knots	NSD-GPP 49 knots	NSD-GPP 100 knots	NSD
Time (hour)	0.36	0.55	1.02	1.15

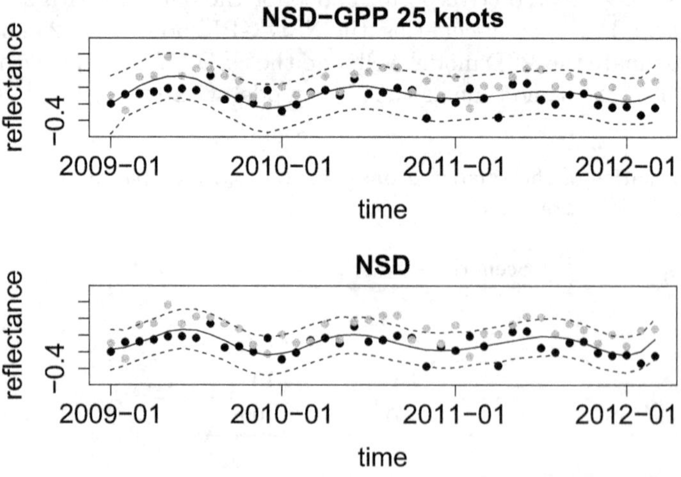

Fig. 2. Prediction of the simulated MERIS reflectance data (black points) at a randomly selected location by the NSD-GPP and the NSD models. Grey points: simulated MODIS reflectance, Black solid lines: predictions from the model, Black dashed lines: 95 percent credible intervals of the predictions.

5 Conclusion

The NSD-GPP model described in this work uses a smaller number of knots compared to the number of observer locations, which reduces the computational time in the Gibbs sampling process in the parameter estimations for the NSD model. Considering the computational time and the improvement of the RMSPE, the NSD-GPP model with the number of knots less than one fourth of the total number of the locations will be considered. In future work, the NSD-GPP model will be extended to allow estimating reflectance data at multiple wavelengths. This could be used to infer water quality parameters.

Acknowledgements. Special thanks to Plymouth Marine Laboratory for data advice. Data are from European Space Agency Lakes Climate Change Initiative project, provided via the Centre for Environment Data Archival (CEDA): https://dx.doi.org/10.5285/a07deacaffb8453e93d57ee214676304.

References

1. Banerjee, S., Gelfand, A.E., Finley, A.O., Sang, H.: Gaussian predictive process models for large spatial data sets. J. R. Stat. Soc. Ser. B Stat. Methodol. **70**(4), 825–848 (2008)
2. Carrea, L., et al.: Satellite-derived multivariate world-wide lake physical variable timeseries for climate studies. Sci. Data **10**(1), 30 (2023)
3. Irvine, K.M., Gitelman, A.I., Hoeting, J.A.: Spatial designs and properties of spatial correlation: effects on covariance estimation. J. Agric. Biol. Environ. Stat. **12**, 450–469 (2007)
4. Palmer, S.C., Kutser, T., Hunter, P.D.: Remote sensing of inland waters: challenges, progress and future directions. Remote Sens. Environ. **157**, 1–8 (2015)
5. Wilkie, C.J., et al.: Nonparametric statistical downscaling for the fusion of data of different spatiotemporal support. Environmetrics **30**(3), e2549 (2019)

Spatial Confounding in Gradient Boosting

Lars Knieper[1(✉)], Thomas Kneib[2], and Elisabeth Bergherr[1]

[1] Chair of Spatial Data Science and Statistical Learning, University of Göttingen, Göttingen, Germany
{lars.knieper,elisabeth.bergherr}@uni-goettingen.de
[2] Chair of Statistics, University of Göttingen, Göttingen, Germany
tkneib@uni-goettingen.de

Abstract. Collinearity between covariates and spatial effects can lead to a bias in the corresponding fixed effects' estimates known as spatial confounding. Recently, the *Spatial+* approach suggests to regress out the spatial effect in the covariate first, before estimating the model of interest. Drastic spatial confounding is observed in gradient boosting due to its step-wise procedure. In this contribution we apply the suggested two-step approach and confirm its ability to correct spatial confounding for gradient boosting as well.

Keywords: gradient boosting · spatial confounding · spatialplus

1 Introduction

Using large data sets from *Inside Airbnb* can help to explain how prices of touristic properties are built. The data hold coordinates as well as several variables about the accommodations. Figure 1 shows a map of Greater Manchester with logarithmised prices per accommodate spread over the city. There is a clear trend to higher prices in the city center of Manchester. Still, it might not be completely the center itself causing higher prices but the proximity to sights and alike next to the amenities the accommodations offer. When complementing *Airbnb* data with variables describing the location, these variables are correlated with the spatial trend of prices.

This collinearity between fixed and spatial effects can lead to the phenomenon of *spatial confounding*. As a result fixed effects' estimates are biased as they get covered by the estimated spatial field instead. A straightforward and powerful two-step approach called *Spatial+* recently showed how unbiased estimates can be achieved again for geo-additive models.

The high number of possible covariates in the *Airbnb* data additionally calls for variable selection as well as regularization, for which gradient boosting will be used. This contribution shows spatial confounding is drastically observed in gradient boosting and further, combines the correction mechanism suggested in *Spatial+* with gradient boosting to overcome this issue.

J. Einbeck et al. (Eds.): IWSM 2024, CONTRIB.STAT., pp. 88–94, 2024.
https://doi.org/10.1007/978-3-031-65723-8_14

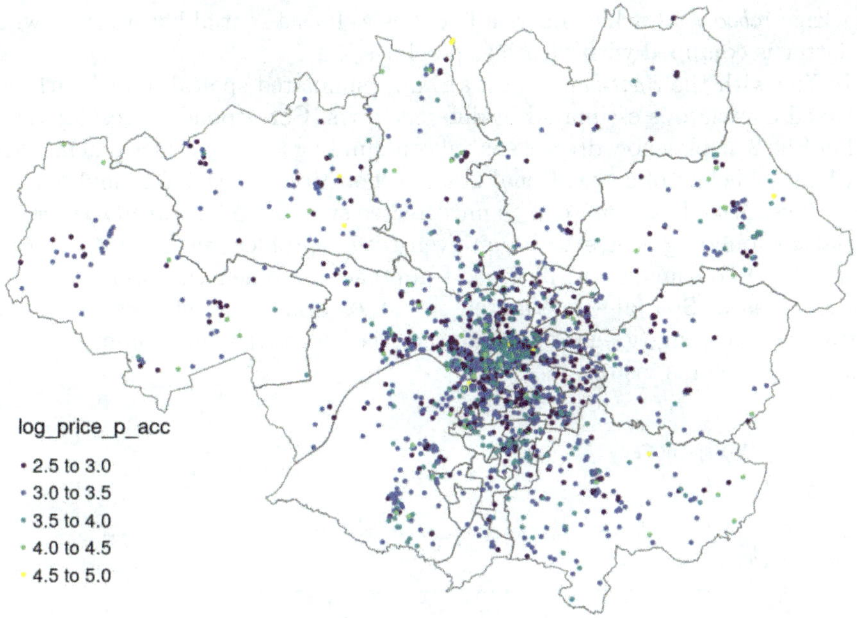

Fig. 1. Log-prices per accommodate for *Airbnbs* in Manchester.

2 Gradient Boosting with Spatial+

In the presence of spatial confounding covariates are correlated with the spatial effect, such that a covariate of this kind can be expressed as

$$x_i^s = f^x(\boldsymbol{z}_i) + \epsilon_i^x, \tag{1}$$

with $\epsilon_i^x \sim \mathcal{N}(0, \sigma_x^2)$. Here, $f^x(\cdot)$ corresponds to a bounded smooth function on a two-dimensional spatial domain, such that $\boldsymbol{z}_i$ represents coordinates of the i-th observation. The crucial first-step of *Spatial+* [2] is to fit the confounded covariate $\boldsymbol{x}^s$ onto the spatial field and retrieve its residuals

$$\boldsymbol{r}^x = (\boldsymbol{I} - \boldsymbol{S}_{\lambda_x})\,\boldsymbol{x}^s. \tag{2}$$

The smoother matrix $\boldsymbol{S}_{\lambda_x}$ is created by two-dimensional thin-plate splines and the smoothing parameter λ is chosen by generalized cross-validation criterion [7]. Afterwards, the obtained residuals $\boldsymbol{r}^x$ are used for the fitting process of a spatial model instead of the original variable $\boldsymbol{x}^s$.

Model-based component-wise gradient boosting [6] is especially helpful for building prediction models on high-dimensional data sets as it incorporates variable selection and regularization. For adapting the Spatial+ procedure, the first and crucial step of *Spatial+* gets applied to all covariates $\boldsymbol{x}_k$ for $k = 1, \ldots, p$. This means all $\boldsymbol{x}_k$ are regressed onto the spatial field and then are replaced by their residuals $\boldsymbol{r}_k^x$ (Eq. 2). Afterwards, the geo-additive model is estimated with

R package *mboost* [3], which offers a linear as well as a spatial baselearner, where the latter is equipped with bivariate p-splines.

In line with the *Spatial+* paper, a simple simulated spatial model with only one fixed covariate is estimated in different ways. Corresponding results visualized in Fig. 2 display how drastic spatial confounding is present in gradient boosting. The coefficient of conventional gradient boosting (*mboost*, red line) does not even converge to the estimate of an uncorrected spatial model (turquoise). Hence, spatial confounding seems to be an even bigger problem in gradient boosting than in common maximum likelihood approaches. When the same correction procedure as in Spatial+ is adapted to the covariate, the well-known picture of gradient boosting (green) converging to the (corrected) maximum likelihood estimate (purple) is visible.

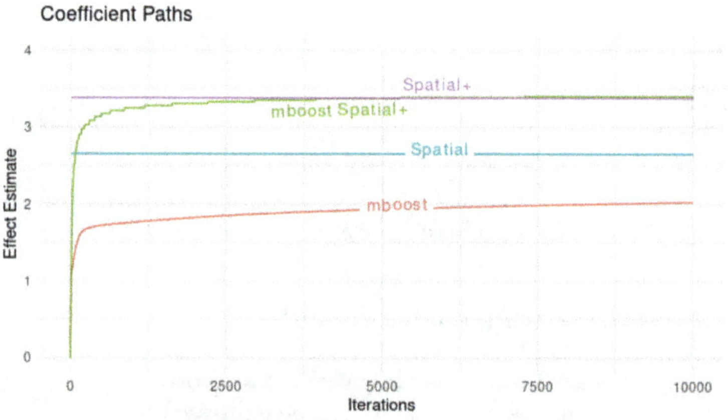

Fig. 2. Coefficient estimates of a spatially confounded fixed effect.

3 Simulation Study

To observe the behaviour of gradient boosting in terms of spatial confounding, a simulation study was conducted for high-dimensional data. Normally distributed response $\boldsymbol{y}$ followed the data generation process of

$$\boldsymbol{y} = 1 - 2\boldsymbol{x}_1^s + 4\boldsymbol{x}_2 - 3\boldsymbol{x}_3^s + 5\boldsymbol{x}_4 - 1\boldsymbol{x}_5 + f(\boldsymbol{z}) + \boldsymbol{\epsilon}^y, \quad \epsilon_i^y \sim \mathcal{N}(0, \sigma_y^2).$$

Hence, spatial confounding might affect covariates $\boldsymbol{x}_1^s$ and $\boldsymbol{x}_3^s$ since they are simulated as described in Eq. 1. Further, $\frac{\sigma_y}{\sigma_x} = 10$ as especially in these cases spatial confounding is expected to arise. To achieve high dimensionality uninformative covariates are added to the simulation, such that $p \in [25, 50, 100]$.

Figure 3 represents fixed effects estimates for informative covariates grouped by usual *mboost* procedure (red boxplots) versus *mboost* with a *Spatial+* correction beforehand (blue boxplots). The observed shrinkage in all estimated effects

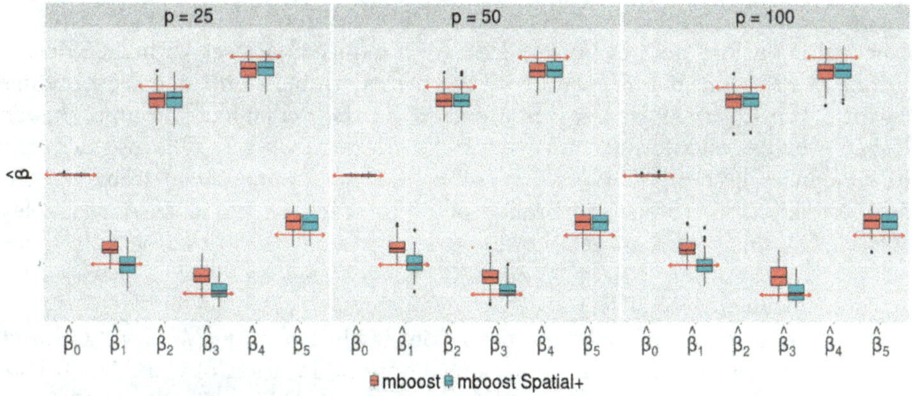

Fig. 3. Coefficient estimates of linear fixed effects.

is indicated by early stopping to prevent overfitting, which is common for gradient boosting.

Even though the correction mechanism is applied to all covariates, the effects of non-confounded covariates ($\hat{\beta}_0, \hat{\beta}_2, \hat{\beta}_4, \hat{\beta}_5$) are very much the same. This is a big advantage as users do not know which covariates are spatially confounded. Hence, the correction can be applied to all covariates without the cost of poorer estimates. For $\hat{\beta}_1$ and $\hat{\beta}_3$ *mboost* shows more shrunk estimates than usual. This corresponds to expected behaviour as it is observed in research concerning spatial confounding. When the correction step of *Spatial+* is implemented these spatially confounded covariate effects are even approaching the true values. Thus, the correction is overcompensating as the desired shrinkage is barely present anymore.

For the shown simulation results thin plate splines are applied for the correction step but bivariate splines implemented in *mboost* are utilised within the gradient boosting procedure. Another simulation study was conducted with an application of bivariate splines via *mboost* also for the correction step, which led to similar results.

Further, it should be mentioned that the degrees of freedom of the spatial base-learners allowed at the beginning of the boosting algorithm heavily influence the number of optimal iterations of the algorithm. More iterations allow for more convergence and therefore larger effect sizes. The degrees of freedom are selected in such a way that the convergence appears comparable to conventional linear models. Thus, for both procedures starting degrees of freedom of 50 are allowed.

4 Data Application

Inside Airbnb [4] offers collections of touristic Airbnb listings from a broad range of cities around the world. For Manchester not only data from the city itself is available but from the area of Greater Manchester, which includes the towns

Wigan, Bolton, Rochdale and Stockport. Data cleaning due to no given prices or accommodations not yet booked leads to a reduced data set with 2295 observations. As the aim is to explain how the prices are built on the corresponding platform the logarithmised prices are used as the dependent variable. *Inside Airbnb* provides all information users of their website can get. This also includes the amenities accommodations are equipped with, which range from general hints as "kitchen" to specific brands of body soap. To group these variables logisticPCA [5] is used to get more general variables that describe accommodations. The resulting variable `gardenPCA` holds amenities like e.g. "backyard", "outdoor furniture" or "BBQ".

Next to information about the properties itself, *OpenStreetMap* via OSMnx [1] is used to retrieve more information about the location of the Airbnb listings. This includes e.g. the number of restaurants and pubs in a radius of one kilometre of each listing. Further, distances to sights and important transport options of Manchester are calculated, like the distance to Albert Square or the Piccadilly station. Additionally, the minimum of these distances is included as a variable as well. These spatially dependent covariates are surely correlated with the spatial field, thus, the method suggested here is necessary for the variable selection process. The spatial dimension is given by the coordinates of each Airbnb accommodation.

The correction step of Spatial+ (Eq. 2) is conducted on all continuous variables of the training data (80/20 split), where these spatial models are then used to apply the correction on test data as well. Hence, 76 potential covariates are given to the boosting algorithms by linear base-learners, which are performed with a 10-fold cross-validation.

Table 1 displays coefficient estimates of selected covariates. Additionally, the third column is the ratio of *mboost*' estimates by *mboost Spatial+* estimates to enable a better comparison. Most of the coefficients are very similar indicated by a ratio close to one. Special attention can to be paid to `garden_PCA` as well as three distance variables (bold variables). The coefficient of `garden_PCA` shows the largest deviation from one in the ratio. This indicates a partial spatial dependence of this variable, which could be related to the less likely existence of garden amenities in the city center.

Distance variables are not chosen by conventional gradient boosting algorithm but in the corrected approach. Still, effect sizes are rather small. This might be due to the fact, that distance variables get very well explained by the correction step in the first place. This is indicated by $R^2 > 0.9$, mostly even almost 1. This corresponds to an (almost) complete spatial dependence of the covariates, which is a known limitation of the Spatial+ approach as in this case it regresses away all variation in the covariate.

However, predictive power on test data increased from an mean squared error of 0.1056 to 0.1015 on log-scale. These predictions are without consideration of the spatial effect, where *mboost Spatial+* still outperforms *mboost* slightly.

Table 1. Boosting estimates of uncorrected (mboost) and spatially corrected variables (mboost Spat+).

covariate	mboost	mboost Spat+	ratio
shared_bathroom	−0.3636	−0.3578	1.02
accommodates	0.2044	0.1912	1.07
bedrooms	0.0820	0.0902	0.91
room_type_Entire.home.apt	0.0563	0.0682	0.83
calculated_host_listings_count	−0.0711	−0.0638	1.11
availability_30	0.0500	0.0483	1.04
host_is_superhost	0.0490	0.047	1.04
Pets_allowed	0.0450	0.0449	1.00
last_review_days	0.0415	0.0404	1.02
reviews_per_month	−0.0317	−0.0344	0.92
Albert_Square_distance	NA	−0.0306	NA
Hair_dryer	0.0294	0.0242	1.21
no_of_bathrooms	0.0254	0.0227	1.12
shower_stuff	0.0225	0.0218	1.03
Streaming_services	0.0234	0.0202	1.16
first_review_days	−0.0188	−0.0198	0.95
Private_entrance	0.0192	0.0177	1.08
number_of_reviews_ltm	−0.0195	−0.0174	1.12
garden_PCA	−0.0109	−0.0147	0.74
Manchester_Piccadilly_distance	NA	−0.0136	NA
review_PCA	−0.0125	−0.011	1.14
National_Football_Museum_distance	NA	−0.0103	NA
instant_bookable	0.0101	0.0096	1.05
availability_365	0.0041	0.0053	0.77
calculated_host_listings_count_entire_homes	−0.0036	−0.0037	0.97
Cleaning_products	NA	−0.002	NA
nearest_distance	NA	−0.0018	NA
host_since_days	−0.0010	−0.0011	0.91
neighbourhood_overview_letter_count	−0.0010	NA	NA

5 Conclusion

This work has shown that gradient boosting is very susceptible to spatial confounding. The approach of Spatial+ works as a correction mechanism very well even though the resulting fixed effects seem to be over-compensated such that shrinkage in terms of regularization vanishes. A major advantage of this correction approach is that the gradient boosting algorithm itself does not need an alteration as the correction happens beforehand. Additionally, correcting also non-confounded covariates does not decrease estimation performance.

The data application showed that by applying the correction predictive performance can be increased. Still, this specific data set of Airbnb accommodations hints that there might be limitations: Spatial+ is not suited for fully spatially confounded covariates as some covariates in this case might be. Therefore, an approach like restricted spatial regression might be more suited but needs an adjustment within the gradient boosting algorithm. This would still be applicable to generalized models, which holds for Spatial+ as well. Hence, this will be dealt with in future steps.

References

1. Boeing, G.: OSMnx: a Python package to work with graph-theoretic OpenStreetMap street networks. J. Open Source Softw. **2**(12), 215 (2017)
2. Dupont, E., Wood, S., Augustin, N.: Spatial+: a novel approach to spatial confounding. Biometrics **78**, 1279–1290 (2022)
3. Hofner, B., Mayr, A., Robinzonov, N., Schmid, M.: Model-based boosting in R: a hands-on tutorial using the R package mboost. Comput. Stat. **29**, 3–35 (2014)
4. Inside Airbnb. https://insideairbnb.com/
5. Landgraf, A.J., Lee, Y.: Dimensionality reduction for binary data through the projection of natural parameters. J. Multivar. Anal. **180**, 104668 (2020)
6. Mayr, A., Binder, H., Gefeller, O., Schmid, M.: The evolution of boosting algorithms. Methods Inf. Med. **53**(6), 419–427 (2014)
7. Wood, S.: Thin-plate regression splines. J. R. Stat. Soc. (B) **65**, 95–114 (2003)

Adaptive Generalized Logistic Lasso and Its Application to Rankings in Sports

Robert Bajons(✉) and Kurt Hornik

Institute of Statistics and Mathematics, Vienna University of Economics and Business, Vienna, Austria
robert.bajons@wu.ac.at

Abstract. The generalized lasso is a popular model for ranking competitors, as it allows for implicit grouping of estimated abilities. In this work, we present an implementation of an adaptive variant of the generalized lasso penalty for logistic regression using conic programming principles. This approach is flexible, robust, and fast, especially in a high-dimensional setting. The methodology is applied to sports data, with the aim of ranking soccer players based on their contribution to possession sequences.

Keywords: Generalized lasso · logistic regression · rankings

1 Introduction

In many fields, e.g. in economics, scientometrics, or sports, there is an innate interest in ranking competitors. However, given the multi-dimensionality and the difficulty of the problem, usually partial rankings, i.e. rankings that allow for groups, are preferred over total rankings. To serve such ranking mentalities and account for potential over-interpretation of insignificant differences between abilities of competitors, Masarotto and Varin (2012) propose the ranking lasso given as the solution of the problem

$$\min_{\boldsymbol{\beta}} \ell\,(Y; X, \boldsymbol{\beta}) + \lambda \sum_{i<j}^{N} w_{ij} |\beta_i - \beta_j|, \tag{1}$$

where w_{ij} are pair-specific weights. The penalty term in Eq. (1) is a variation of the lasso penalty that allows for grouping of the estimated abilities of competitors into several equivalence classes. This problem can be more generally written as

$$\min_{\boldsymbol{\beta}} \ell\,(Y; X, \boldsymbol{\beta}) + \lambda ||D\boldsymbol{\beta}||_1. \tag{2}$$

Here the matrix $D \in \mathbb{R}^{m \times p}$ represents some structural behavior of the coefficients $\boldsymbol{\beta}$. In principle, $\ell(Y; X, \boldsymbol{\beta})$ may represent any convex loss function, however, for our purpose, we consider the (negative) log-likelihood function for the binomial

J. Einbeck et al. (Eds.): IWSM 2024, CONTRIB.STAT., pp. 95–101, 2024.
https://doi.org/10.1007/978-3-031-65723-8_15

response variable Y in the usual logistic regression framework. For squared loss, Eq. (2) is often termed generalized lasso and encompasses various special cases (see Tibshirani and Taylor (2011) for details).

In general, there are many ways to solve the above problem. Masarotto and Varin (2012), e.g., derive an augmented Lagrangian method to solve the problem. However, when incorporating specific ranking-based structures on the coefficients, the dimension of D quickly increases, and consequently such algorithms do not scale reasonably well. In this paper, we present an approach using interior point methods and modern conic programming principles. Such an approach has been proven to be reliable for similar convex problems in Schwendinger et al. (2021) and specifically works well in the context of high-dimensional D. Furthermore, we discuss an application for ranking soccer players, where the matrix D has a particular and high-dimensional structure, which is distinct from the classical ranking lasso case of Eq. (1).

2 Adaptive Generalized Logistic Lasso via Conic Programming

We rewrite Eq. (2) and consider the adaptive generalized logistic lasso (AGLL) problem given as

$$\min_{\boldsymbol{\beta}} -\Big(\sum_{i=1}^{n} y_i \log(h_{\boldsymbol{\beta}}(x_i)) + (1-y_i)\log(1-h_{\boldsymbol{\beta}}(x_i))\Big) + \lambda \sum_{j=1}^{m} w_j |D_j|, \tag{3}$$

with logistic function $h_{\boldsymbol{\beta}}(x) = 1/\big(1+\exp(-\boldsymbol{\beta}^\top x)\big)$. In this case, D_j is the j-th component of $D\boldsymbol{\beta}$, with $D \in \mathbb{R}^{m\times p}$.

In order to use conic programming techniques to solve Problem (3), we first define a conic program (CP) as:

$$\begin{aligned} &\text{minimize } a_0^T x \\ &\quad \text{s.t. } Ax + s = b, \quad s \in \mathcal{K}, \end{aligned} \tag{4}$$

where the set $\mathcal{K}$ is a composition of simple convex cones. Any convex optimization problem can be reformulated into a conic program by expressing it in its equivalent epigraph form. Specifically, Eq. (3) can be reformulated in the following way[1]:

$$\begin{aligned} \min_{(r,\boldsymbol{\beta},\boldsymbol{s},\boldsymbol{t},\boldsymbol{z}_1,\boldsymbol{z}_2)} \; & \sum_{i=1}^{n} t_i + \lambda r \\ \text{s.t. } & (z_{i1}, 1, u_i - t_i) \in K_{\exp}, \\ & (z_{i2}, 1, -t_i) \in K_{\exp}, \\ & z_{i1} + z_{i2} \leq 1, \qquad i = 1,\dots,n, \\ & -s_j \leq D_j \leq s_j, \qquad j = 1,\dots,m, \\ & r - w_1 D_1 - \cdots - w_m D_m \geq 0. \end{aligned} \tag{5}$$

[1] Note that there are other equivalent variants of rewriting the objective function in epigraph form, especially for the likelihood part (see e.g. Schwendinger et al. (2024)).

In the above formulation, the variables $\boldsymbol{r}, \boldsymbol{\beta}, \boldsymbol{s}, \boldsymbol{t}, \boldsymbol{z}_1, \boldsymbol{z}_2$, and $\boldsymbol{u}$ are auxiliary variables. The initial problem (3) is thus rewritten as a conic programming problem as in Eq. (4) on an augmented set of variables $\Theta = (\boldsymbol{r}, \boldsymbol{\beta}, \boldsymbol{s}, \boldsymbol{t}, \boldsymbol{z}_1, \boldsymbol{z}_2)$. Note that the formulation as CP only requires two distinct simple convex cones, namely the exponential cone for the first two lines of Eq. (5) and the linear cone for lines 3–5. These are defined as

$$\begin{aligned} K_{\text{exp}} &= \{x \in \mathbb{R}^3 | x_1 \geq x_2 \exp(x_3/x_2), x_1 > 0, x_2 > 0\}, \quad \text{and} \\ K_{\text{lin}} &= \{x \in \mathbb{R} | x \geq 0\} \end{aligned} \tag{6}$$

respectively. We omit further details on the reformulation procedure in this short paper and refer to Boyd and Vandenberghe (2004) for more information on rewriting convex problems into their epigraph forms.

There are various advantages to using the presented conic approach as opposed to using other methods, such as augmented Lagrangian procedures. First, a wide range of problems can be solved with only a few number of convex cones. For example, many of the most popular models from the GLM family can be modeled with only 3 types of cones: linear, second-order, and exponential cone (Schwendinger et al. (2024)). Furthermore, extensions to penalized versions of GLMs are straightforward by adding cone constraints (e.g. for the lasso penalty, only additional linear cones are required). This makes the conic approach flexible and easily extensible to specific situations. Second, from an algorithmic point of view, the conic solvers do not rely on specific starting values and provide reliable results. That is, when the algorithm signals success in finding an optimal solution, one can be very certain that the found optimum is a global optimum (Schwendinger et al. (2021)). Finally, recent advances in conic programming have led to the development of a variety of solvers, which routinely solve high-dimensional conic problems to proven optimality.

Problem (5) can be solved using a convex optimization solver of choice. The only requirement on the solver is that it can handle the above two types of convex cones. In `R`, there is a range of suitable solvers available via the optimization infrastructure `ROI` (Theußl et al. (2020)). We develop an `R` routine leveraging the flexibility of `ROI`.

Similar to other works (Zou (2006), Masarotto and Varin (2012)), we consider an adaptive variant, where weights w_j are placed on the penalty structure of the components, to avoid inconsistency and reduce bias in the estimation of the effects. We follow Masarotto and Varin (2012) and select the weights to be inversely proportional to the maximum likelihood estimates with a small ridge penalty

$$w_j = \left| D_j \tilde{\boldsymbol{\beta}}_\epsilon \right|^{-1}, \quad \tilde{\boldsymbol{\beta}}_\epsilon = \arg\min_{\boldsymbol{\beta}} \left\{ -\ell(\boldsymbol{\beta}) + \epsilon \sum_i \beta_i^2 \right\}. \tag{7}$$

Therefore, if the structural differences in the effects (represented by the matrix D) are small, a stronger penalization on the structure for these effects is employed. Finally, in order to select the tuning parameter λ, we compute the solution of the AGLL for a sequence of λ-values and minimize an AIC-type criterion of the form

$$\text{AIC}(\lambda) = -2\ell(\boldsymbol{\beta}) + 2\text{enp}(\lambda). \tag{8}$$

This idea follows Tibshirani and Taylor (2011), where enp(λ) is estimated as the number of distinct groups formed by a certain λ.

3 Simulation

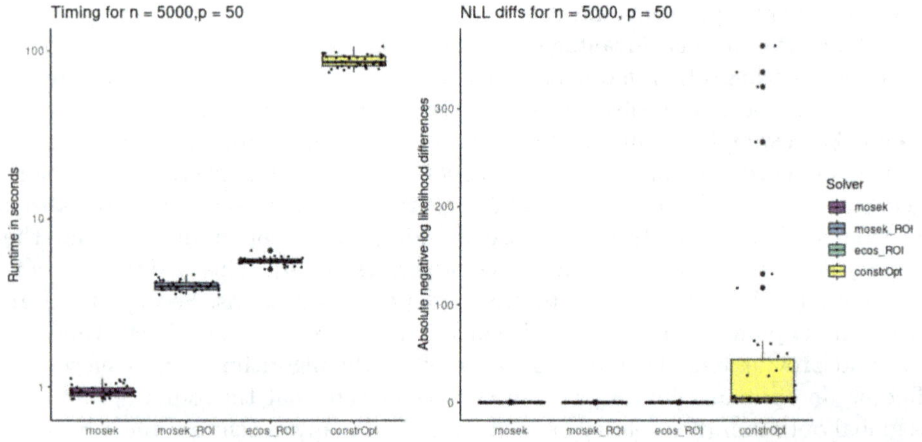

Fig. 1. Left: Comparison of runtime (in seconds) of different solvers. Right: Comparison of differences in negative log-likelihood between the best model and each other model. Displayed are 50 different runs of the simulation setup.

We briefly illustrate the efficiency of our approach in a simulation study. We simulate $n = 5000$ data points from a classical logistic regression model with $p = 50$ covariates. That is, the response variable is drawn from

$$y_i | x_{i1}, \ldots, x_{im} \sim \text{Ber}(\pi_i), \quad m = 1, \ldots, \lfloor \frac{2}{3} p \rfloor, \tag{9}$$

where $\pi_i = 1/(1 + \exp(-\boldsymbol{\beta}^\top x_i))$. The covariate matrix X is drawn from a Gaussian distribution and the coefficients are set such that 4 groups are present, and only 2/3 of the covariates are relevant, i.e. affect the outcome. In total, we compare 4 solvers, 3 of them are conic solvers. First, an implementation of the commercial solver from MOSEK via the `Rmosek`-package (MOSEK Aps (2022)). The other two leverage `ROI`, where we again use MOSEK via `ROI` as well as the open-source solver ECOS (Domahidi et al. (2013)). Finally, to compare the conic solvers to other approaches we use the `constrOpt` function from the alabama-package, which implements an augmented Lagrangian adaptive barrier minimization algorithm (Varadhan (2023)). We evaluate the methods based on runtime, as well as their ability to find the optimal solution for the objective function.

Figure 1 shows the results of our short simulation. It can be seen that the conic solvers are much more efficient in terms of runtime than the augmented Lagrangian solver (left panel of Fig. 1). Using ROI produces a slight overhead, as seen by comparing the usage of the MOSEK solver directly versus via the package. However, the flexibility of ROI allows for easy usage of solvers like ECOS, which is slower than the commercial solver, but only by a small amount. It is important to mention that in our simulation with $p = 50$, the dimension of D is 1275×50. Compared to our application below, this is a rather small problem. Already in this setup, the runtime difference between conic solvers and the augmented Lagrangian method is drastic. In terms of finding the optimal solution (right panel of Fig. 1) the conic solvers also outperform the constrOpt solver, with no notable difference between ECOS and MOSEK.

4 Ranking in Sports

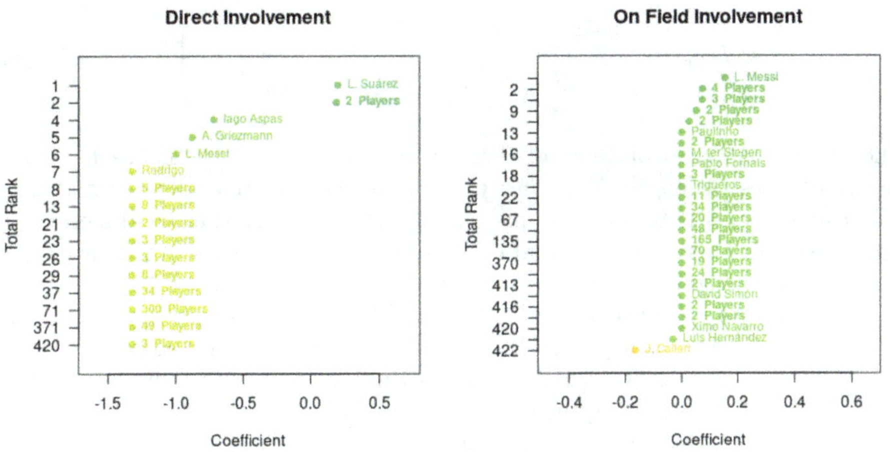

Fig. 2. Strength coefficients for direct (left) and off-ball (right) involvement. Selected groups are displayed with the corresponding group size. Groups of only one player are displayed by the name of the player.

We apply the AGLL to possessions in soccer, with the aim of ranking players based on their contributions to scoring goals. A possession is defined as a sequence of consecutive on-ball events, which ends either by the opponent team gaining possession or by an action of the referee. For each possession, two kinds of information are observed. First, we record which player is actively involved in a possession, and second, we record which player was on the field (offensively and defensively) during a possession, but not directly involved. This data structure allows to separate effects of being part of a possession, from effects of off-ball actions, both of which have substantial impact in soccer. To be more concrete, the units of observation are possessions, where each possession can end in a goal or no goal (binary outcome). The player configuration for each possession is collected in our design matrix X. In our data set, we have 422 players, and therefore 844 total columns of direct and indirect involvements. For ranking players, it then makes sense to differentiate between direct and indirect (off-ball) involvement. That is, we do not want to consider the classical ranking lasso penalty, where effects of direct and indirect involvement would be compared to each other. Instead, the penalty matrix D should account for the fact that we want to compare the direct effects of one player only to the direct ones of the other players and the same for indirect effects. This results in the following form for D:

$$D = \begin{pmatrix} D_{\text{dir}} & \mathbf{0} \\ \mathbf{0} & D_{\text{indir}} \end{pmatrix}. \tag{10}$$

For each of the two components, we are interested in applying a ranking penalty. That is, $D_{\text{dir}} = D_{\text{indir}}$, where

$$D_{\text{dir}} = (A, B, C) = \begin{pmatrix} A_1 & B_1 & C_1 \\ \vdots & \vdots & \vdots \\ A_{N_{\text{dir}}-1} & B_{N_{\text{dir}}-1} & C_{N_{\text{dir}}-1} \end{pmatrix}. \tag{11}$$

The A_i are matrices of zeros of dimension $(N_{\text{dir}} - i) \times (i - 1)$, each B_i is a vector of ones of length N_{dir}, and each C_i is the negative identity matrix of dimension $N_{\text{dir}} - 1$. In our example $N_{\text{dir}} = 422$, and thus the row-dimension of D_{dir} is 88831. Therefore, the total dimension of D is 177662×844. It is evident that an efficient procedure is necessary to solve the AGLL problem, and our conic programming approach works well and fast in such scenarios. The results of our analysis are displayed in Fig. 2. These are in line with the intuition on ranking soccer players. They reflect the difficulty of ranking soccer players while simultaneously emphasizing the necessity of partial rankings, as most players are grouped in similar strength groups, and only a few stand out.

5 Summary

In this work, we consider the generalized lasso penalty for logistic regression. We transform this convex problem into its conic form and develop a framework for solving it using conic programming. The presented approach is flexible and easily extensible and simulations show that it is fast and robust. Finally, we use the methodology to rank soccer players into strength groups.

References

Boyd, S., Vandenberghe, L.: Convex Optimization. Cambridge University Press, Cambridge (2004)

Domahidi, A., Chu, E., Boyd, S.: ECOS: an SOCP solver for embedded systems. In: European Control Conference (ECC), pp. 3071–3076 (2013)

Masarotto, G., Varin, C.: The ranking lasso and its application to sport tournaments. Ann. Appl. Stat. **6**, 1949–1970 (2012)

MOSEK Aps. Rmosek: The R-to-MOSEK optimization interface. R package version 10.0.25 (2022)

Schwendinger, F., Grün, B., Hornik, K.: A comparison of optimization solvers for log binomial regression including conic programming. Comput. Stat. **36**(3), 1721–1754 (2021)

Schwendinger, B., Schwendinger, F., Vana, L.: Holistic generalized linear models. J. Stat. Softw. **108**(7), 1–49 (2024)

Theußl, S., Schwendinger, F., Hornik, K.: ROI: an extensible R optimization infrastructure. J. Stat. Softw. **94**(15), 1–64 (2020)

Tibshirani, R.J., Taylor, J.: The solution path of the generalized lasso. Ann. Stat. **39**(3), 1335–1371 (2011)

Varadhan, R.: alabama: Constrained Nonlinear Optimization. R package version 2023.1.0 (2023)

Zou, H.: The adaptive lasso and its oracle properties. J. Am. Stat. Assoc. **101**, 1418–1429 (2006)

A Biclustering Approach via Mixture of Latent Trait Analyzers for the Analysis of Digital Divide in Italy

Dalila Failli[1(✉)], Bruno Arpino[2], Maria Francesca Marino[1], and Francesca Martella[3]

[1] Dipartimento di Statistica, Informatica, Applicazioni, Università degli Studi di Firenze, viale Morgagni 59, 50134 Firenze, Italy
dalila.failli@unifi.it
[2] Dipartimento di Scienze Statistiche, Università degli Studi di Padova, Via Battisti 241, 35121 Padua, Italy
[3] Dipartimento di Scienze Statistiche, Sapienza Università di Roma, Piazzale Aldo Moro 5, 00185 Rome, Italy

Abstract. We employ an extension of the Mixture of Latent Trait Analyzers (MLTA) model to analyse the digital divide in Italy in a biclustering perspective. In detail, units (individuals) are partitioned into clusters (components) via a finite mixture of latent trait models; in each component, variables (digital skills) are partitioned into clusters (segments) by modifying the linear predictor's specification of the original MLTA model. This allows us to identify homogeneous groups of individuals with respect to subsets of digital skills, also accounting for the influence of demographic features on the probability of being digitally skilled.

Keywords: model-based clustering · co-clustering · finite mixtures · latent variables · EM algorithm

1 Introduction

Biclustering entails the jointly clustering of units (rows) and variables (columns) of a data matrix, especially when relationships between them can be considered symmetrical. In this paper, we employ an extension of the Mixture of Latent Trait Analyzers (MLTA; Gollini and Murphy [5]) proposed by Failli et al. in [4]. This model allows for the identification of parsimonious and interpretable clusters, and for the inclusion of a multi-dimensional latent trait capturing residual heterogeneity between units in terms of observed outcomes.

Our aim is to identify groups of Italian respondents (units) to the European Social Survey round 10 [2] sharing similar subsets of digital skills (variables), also understanding how demographic features influence their propensity to be digitally skilled. In detail, a finite mixture of latent trait models is employed to cluster respondents into subsets called components and, in each of them, variables are partitioned into subsets called segments via a flexible specification

J. Einbeck et al. (Eds.): IWSM 2024, CONTRIB.STAT., pp. 102–108, 2024.
https://doi.org/10.1007/978-3-031-65723-8_16

of the linear predictor. As a result, we are able to obtain both a clustering of individuals based on their digitalisation level and, for each of these clusters, a partitioning of skills based on their diffusion in the population.

2 Data

The ESS includes questions on social behaviour, health, and social inequality. Here, we focus on data entailing digital social contacts in work and family life in Italy, which is still experiencing a wide digital divide. In this framework, units represent individuals, while variables represent the digital skills they master. These identify the ability to use Internet, preference settings, advanced search, and PDFs, as well as the ability to make video calls and send messages to children, parents, or colleagues, and the capacity to share online political posts. Considering only individuals with no missing records, we obtain a data matrix made of 1465 individuals and 7 binary variables. In Table 1 we report the percentage of individuals mastering the different digital technologies. From this table, it is evident that the majority of respondents use the Internet, as well as preference settings, advanced search, PDFs, and messages. With regards to video calls, we may note that only 33% of respondents use this digital technology. Last, only 17% of individuals share online political posts.

Table 1. Percentage of individuals mastering the different digital technologies.

	Skill						
	Internet use	Preference setting	Advanced search	PDF	Video call	Message	Political post
%	75	60	60	57	33	56	17

The data set also contains information on demographic attributes, such as age, education, and health, as well as a variable indicating whether the respondent has children. Table 2 shows the distribution of these variables. From this table, we may note that the sample considered in the analysis includes both young and elderly people, and that the majority of respondents is healthy. In addition, respondents are equally distributed with respect to their gender and to their household's total net income, while the majority of them have a low-to-medium level of education, which also holds for that of the partner. Furthermore, most individuals in the sample have no children and, for those who do have children, these are 12 years old or older. Finally, individuals mainly consist of employed people.

3 The MLTA Model for Biclustering

As detailed by Failli et al. in [4], the original MLTA model (Gollini and Murphy [5]) can be extended to perform a joint clustering of units and variables.

Table 2. Distribution of socio-demographic variables.

Variable	Category	Frequency
Age	<30	0.15
	30–50	0.27
	50–65	0.29
	65–75	0.17
	75+	0.12
Health	Bad	0.04
	Fair	0.25
	Good	0.71
Gender	Male	0.49
	Female	0.51
Education	Low	0.38
	Medium	0.40
	High	0.22
Partner education	Low	0.25
	Medium	0.21
	High	0.11
	No partner	0.43
Household's total net income	Low	0.34
	Medium	0.36
	High	0.30
Children in the household	Children under 12	0.03
	Children over 12	0.21
	No children	0.76
Main activity	Employed	0.48
	Unemployed	0.31
	Retired	0.21

Let Y_{ik} denote a binary random variable and y_{ik} the corresponding observed value for the i-th unit, $i = 1, \ldots, N$, and the k-th variable, $k = 1, \ldots, R$. Focusing on binary outcomes, the model assumes that every unit belongs to one out of G unobserved components identified by a discrete latent variable $\boldsymbol{z}_i = (z_{i1}, \ldots, z_{iG})' \overset{iid}{\sim} \text{Multinomial}(1, (\eta_{i1}, \ldots, \eta_{iG})')$. The generic element of this vector is $z_{ig} = 1$ if unit i belongs to component g, and $z_{ig} = 0$ otherwise. The parameter η_{ig} denotes the probability that unit i belongs to component g, under the constraints that $\sum_{g=1}^{G} \eta_{ig} = 1$ and $\eta_{ig} \geq 0$, for $g = 1, \ldots, G$. Following the proposal by Failli et al. in [3], these probabilities can be modelled via a multinomial logit specification, with parameters $\boldsymbol{\beta}_g$ measuring the impact of covariates $\boldsymbol{x}_i = (x_{i1}, \ldots, x_{iJ})'$ on clustering formation. The model also assumes the existence of a D-dimensional, unit-specific, continuous, latent trait $\boldsymbol{u}_i$, distributed according to a standard D-variate Gaussian density, i.e. $\boldsymbol{u}_i \sim \mathcal{N}_D(\mathbf{0}, \boldsymbol{I})$. This is assumed to capture the heterogeneity between units in terms of observed outcomes.

Conditional on $\boldsymbol{z}_i$ and $\boldsymbol{u}_i$, responses $Y_{i1}, \ldots, Y_{iR}$ are assumed to be independent Bernoulli random variables with probabilities $\pi_{gk}(\boldsymbol{u}_i)$, with $g = 1, \ldots, G$ and $k = 1, \ldots, R$, modelled through the following logistic function:

$$\text{logit}(\pi_{gk}(\boldsymbol{u}_i)) = b_g + \boldsymbol{a}'_{gk}(\boldsymbol{\mu} + \boldsymbol{u}_i). \tag{1}$$

Here, b_g is the component-specific latent effect providing a baseline tendency for units in the g-th component to respond to the different variables, and $\boldsymbol{\mu}$ is a D-dimensional vector of fixed effects which is constant across components. Last, $\boldsymbol{a}_{gk}$ is a D-dimensional row stochastic vector ($D \leq R$) with elements $a_{gkd} = 1$ if, within the g-th component, variable k belongs to segment d, and $a_{gkd} = 0$ otherwise. Thus, vector $\boldsymbol{a}_{gk}$ allows to select a single term only from both $\boldsymbol{\mu}$ and $\boldsymbol{u}_i$.

Maximum likelihood estimates of model parameters can be obtained via an EM algorithm (see Dempster et al. in [1]). Here, a Gauss-Hermite quadrature is employed to approximate integrals not available in closed form.

4 Results

The model is estimated for a number of components, G, and segments, D, ranging from 1 to 4. The optimal specification is selected as the one providing the smallest BIC value, and corresponds to $G = 3$ and $D = 2$, as shown in Table 3.

Table 3. BIC for varying numbers of components G and segments D.

	$D = 1$	$D = 2$	$D = 3$	$D = 4$
$G = 1$	13219.47	11903.23	11779.55	11804.30
$G = 2$	12635.53	9564.11	9381.93	9446.64
$G = 3$	12730.94	**9371.85**	9453.94	9502.80
$G = 4$	12926.99	9483.89	9831.48	9751.54

The corresponding parameter estimates are $\hat{\boldsymbol{b}} = [-2.62, \ -0.03, \ 1.21]$ and $\hat{\boldsymbol{\mu}} = [-1.64, \ 2.28]$. The sign of these estimates reveals three different components of individuals divided according to their level of digital skills, and two segments of digital skills divided according to how widespread they are among individuals in each component. A clearer picture of what has just been pointed out is obtained by looking at the distribution of the estimated probabilities $\hat{\pi}_{gk}(\hat{\boldsymbol{u}}_i)$, for $g = 1, 2, 3$ and $d = 1, 2$, shown in Fig. 1. From here, it is evident that respondents in the first component have a low chance of mastering digital skills classified in segment 1, with a reduced variability around the centre of the distribution. On the other side, for these respondents, the chance of mastering digital skills belonging to segment 2 is medium. Furthermore, heterogeneity between individuals is here more pronounced than in segment 1. As regards respondents classified in the second component, we may note that they have a medium and high chance of mastering digital skills belonging to segment 1 and 2, respectively. As far as the heterogeneity captured by the latent trait, we may see that this has a lower impact on those digital skills belonging to the latter segment. Last, for respondents classified in the third component, the chance of mastering digital skills belonging to segment 1 and 2 is medium-high and high, respectively, with a reduced variability in the second segment.

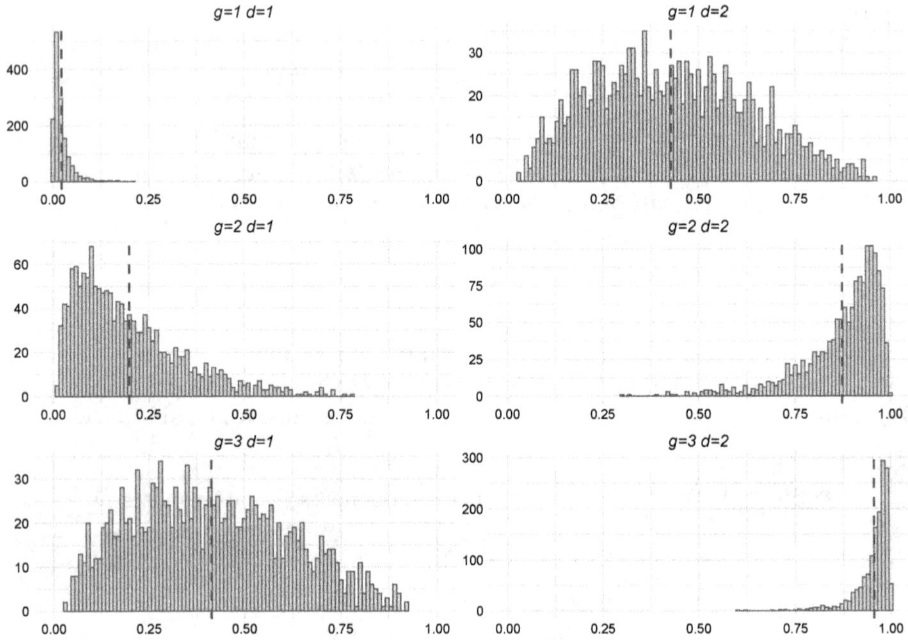

Fig. 1. Distribution of $\hat{\pi}_{gk}(\hat{\boldsymbol{u}}_i)$, $g = 1, 2, 3$, $d = 1, 2$, and corresponding means (in red).

Table 4 shows the classification of digital skills. By looking at this table and at Fig. 1, it is evident that the least prevalent digital skills in the first component (i.e., the least digitalised) are the use of preference settings, advanced search, PDFs, and the sharing of online political posts. In this case, the probability of owning these skills is around 0. In contrast, Internet use, video calls, and online messaging have about 40% chance to be used by the respondents of this component. As far as the second component is concerned, video calls, messaging, and political posting have almost the 20% chance of being used, while Internet, PDFs, preference settings, and advanced search have a higher probability of

Table 4. Classification of digital skills according to $\hat{\boldsymbol{a}}_{gk}$.

Digital skills	$g = 1$	$g = 2$	$g = 3$
Internet	2	2	2
Preference settings	1	2	2
Advanced search	1	2	2
PDFs	1	2	2
Video calls	2	1	1
Messages	2	1	2
Political posts	1	1	1

being used (around 90%). Finally, in the third component, online messaging and video calls are used with a probability of about 0.40, while all the other skills are owned with a probability above 0.90.

The estimated $\boldsymbol{\beta}_g$ coefficients and the corresponding 95% confidence intervals are shown in Table 5. From this table, it is evident that the probability of belonging to the medium digitally active group of individuals (i.e., compo-

Table 5. $\boldsymbol{\beta}$ estimates and 95% confidence intervals. Reference categories are in brackets.

Variable	$\hat{\boldsymbol{\beta}}_2$ (CI)	$\hat{\boldsymbol{\beta}}_3$ (CI)
Intercept	0.03 (0.02, 0.04)	−0.03 (−0.04, −0.02)
Age 30–50 (<30)	−1.28 (−1.84, −0.72)	−2.10 (−2.63, −1.57)
Age 50–65 (<30)	−1.78 (−2.35, −1.21)	−3.44 (−3.99, −2.89)
Age 65–75 (<30)	−3.12 (−3.82, −2.41)	−3.48 (−4.17, −2.78)
Age 75+ (<30)	−3.59 (−4.39, −2.78)	−5.17 (−5.96, −4.38)
Health fair (bad)	−1.52 (−2.22, −0.82)	10.28 (9.54, 11.01)
Health good (bad)	−1.06 (−1.85, −0.27)	10.91 (10.15, 11.67)
Male	0.67 (0.36, 0.98)	0.83 (0.53, 1.14)
Education low (high)	−2.51 (−2.99, −2.04)	−2.91 (−3.38, −2.44)
Education medium (high)	−1.04 (−1.46, −0.62)	−1.18 (−1.58, −0.78)
Partner educ. low (high)	−0.34 (−0.97, 0.28)	−1.33 (−1.93, −0.74)
Partner educ. medium (high)	−0.19 (−0.79, 0.40)	−0.35 (−0.90, 0.20)
No partner (high)	−0.52 (−1.24, 0.21)	−0.80 (−1.49, −0.11)
Income low (high)	−0.99 (−1.40, −0.57)	−1.63 (−2.06, −1.21)
Income medium (high)	−0.68 (−1.06, −0.29)	−1.25 (−1.63, −0.87)
No children (children 12+)	0.26 (−0.20, 0.72)	0.31 (−0.16, 0.77)
Children < 12 (children 12+)	0.68 (−0.23, 1.59)	1.92 (1.03, 2.80)
Retired (employed)	−2.41 (−2.99, −1.82)	−0.19 (−0.72, 0.35)
Unemployed (employed)	−1.21 (−1.62, −0.79)	−0.27 (−0.66, 0.13)

nent 2) is lower for those aged 30–50 years, 50–65 years and over 75 years with respect to those aged less than 30 years. On the other hand, this probability is higher for males compared to females, while it is lower for those who are in good health and for those with a low or medium income level compared to those with a higher income. Furthermore, the likelihood of belonging to the medium digitalised component is lower for those who have a low/medium level of education compared to those who have a higher level of education, and for those who are retired or unemployed compared to those who are employed. Similarly, we may note that the probability of belonging to the most digitalised component (i.e., component 3), compared to the least digitalised one, is higher for those who are healthier, males, and with younger children. In contrast, the probability is lower for those over 30 years of age (and the effect increases with age), for those with a low/medium level of education, a low/medium level of income, and whose partner has a low level of education.

5 Conclusions

In conclusion, the model effectively identifies clusters of individuals with similar digitalisation levels, as well as clusters of digital skills on the basis of how widespread they are among individuals. The analysis also shows that digitalisation in Italy is influenced by age, income and educational level, as well as by partner's educational level and by the presence of young children in the household.

Acknowledgments. Special thanks to the Statistical Modelling Society for the IWSM 2024 PhD student travel award.

References

1. Dempster, A.P., Laird, N.M., Rubin, D.B.: Maximum likelihood from incomplete data via the EM algorithm. J. R. Stat. Soc. Ser. B Methodol. **39**, 1–38 (1977)
2. ESS round 10: Data file edition 3.1. Norwegian Agency for Shared Services in Education and Research (2020). https://doi.org/10.21338/NSD-ESS10-2020
3. Failli, D., Marino, M.F., Martella, F.: Finite mixtures of latent trait analyzers with concomitant variables for bipartite networks: an analysis of COVID-19 data. Multivar. Behav. Res., 1–17 (2024). https://doi.org/10.1080/00273171.2024.2335391
4. Failli, D., Marino, M.F., Martella, F.: Biclustering bipartite networks via extended mixture of latent trait analyzers. arXiv preprint arXiv:2404.09823 (2024)
5. Gollini, I., Murphy, T.B.: Mixture of latent trait analyzers for model-based clustering of categorical data. Stat. Comput. **24**, 569–588 (2014)

Shrinkage in a Bayesian Panel Data Model with Time-Varying Coefficients

Roman Pfeiler(✉) and Helga Wagner

Johannes Kepler University, Linz, Austria
{roman.pfeiler,helga.wagner}@jku.at
https://www.jku.at/institut-fuer-angewandte-statistik/

Abstract. We consider regression models for panel data, where regression effects and within subject dependence are allowed to vary over time. We adopt a Bayesian approach with priors that allow shrinkage to constant and zero effects as well as to simpler dependence structures. The model is evaluated in a simulation study and applied to the analysis of yearly earnings of mothers in Austria who returned to the labour market after maternity leave.

Keywords: Shrinkage prior · Factor model · Random intercept · Income dynamics

1 Introduction

In this paper we consider flexible regression models for panel data from a Bayesian perspective. The flexibility is achieved first by allowing for time-varying effects of covariates, similarly as proposed in [1] for time series data. Secondly, to account for time-varying within subject dependence and between subject heterogeneity we include not just a subject specific intercept, but a subject specific latent variable with weights (i.e. factor loadings) that may also vary over time.

In a Bayesian approach, overspecification of a model with time-varying covariate effects can be prevented by specifying the model appropriately with suitable prior distributions that allow to identify constant or zero effects [2]. We use this specification with shrinkage priors for both regression effects as well as factor loadings and compare the performance to independence priors in a simulation study. Finally, we employ the model to analyse earnings of mothers in Austria who returned to the labour market after maternity leave.

2 Model Specification

2.1 Panel Data Model with Time-Varying Regression Effects

We assume a balanced panel where data on $i = 1, \ldots, n$ subjects at time points $t = 1, \ldots, T$ are available. We denote by y_{it} the response for subject i at time

J. Einbeck et al. (Eds.): IWSM 2024, CONTRIB.STAT., pp. 109–115, 2024.
https://doi.org/10.1007/978-3-031-65723-8_17

t and by $\mathbf{x}_{it}$ the $d \times 1$ vector of covariate values (including an intercept). The regression model with time-varying effects is then given as

$$y_{it} = \mathbf{x}_{it}^\top \boldsymbol{\beta}_t + \epsilon_{it},$$

where $\boldsymbol{\beta}_t$ is the $d \times 1$ vector of regression effects at time point t and ϵ_{it} is the error term. Smoothing of the regression effects over time is accomplished by a random walk prior

$$\boldsymbol{\beta}_t = \boldsymbol{\beta}_{t-1} + \boldsymbol{\omega}_t, \quad \boldsymbol{\omega}_t \sim \mathcal{N}(\mathbf{0}, \mathbf{Q}),$$

where the covariance matrix of the increments is diagonal, $\mathbf{Q} = \text{diag}(\theta_1^2, \dots, \theta_d^2)$. The prior on the initial values $\boldsymbol{\beta}_0$ is specified as $\boldsymbol{\beta}_0 \sim \mathcal{N}(\boldsymbol{\beta}, c\mathbf{Q})$.

To allow shrinkage of the time-varying effects $\boldsymbol{\beta}_t$ to constant or zero effects we use the non-centered parameterization proposed in [2]

$$\begin{aligned}
\boldsymbol{\beta}_t &= \boldsymbol{\beta} + \boldsymbol{\Theta}\tilde{\boldsymbol{\beta}}_t, \\
\tilde{\boldsymbol{\beta}}_t &= \tilde{\boldsymbol{\beta}}_{t-1} + \tilde{\boldsymbol{\omega}}_t, \quad \tilde{\boldsymbol{\omega}}_t \sim \mathcal{N}(\mathbf{0}, \mathbf{I}),
\end{aligned}$$

where $\boldsymbol{\Theta} = \text{diag}(\theta_1, \dots, \theta_d)$ with $\theta_j = \sqrt{\theta_j^2}$ and the initial values $\tilde{\boldsymbol{\beta}}_0$ follow a multivariate standard Normal distribution $\tilde{\boldsymbol{\beta}}_0 \sim \mathcal{N}(\mathbf{0}, c\mathbf{I})$. The observation equation can then be written as

$$y_{it} = \mathbf{x}_{it}^\top \boldsymbol{\beta} + \mathbf{x}_{it}^\top \boldsymbol{\Theta}\tilde{\boldsymbol{\beta}}_t + \epsilon_{it}.$$

We place independent shrinkage priors on the elements of both the process standard deviations $\boldsymbol{\theta} = (\theta_1, \dots, \theta_d)^\top$ as well as the constant effects $\boldsymbol{\beta} = (\beta_1, \dots, \beta_d)^\top$, which are specified hierarchically as

$$\begin{aligned}
\theta_j|\xi_j^2 &\sim \mathcal{N}(0, \xi_j^2), \quad \xi_j^2|a^\xi, \kappa^\xi \sim \mathcal{G}\left(a^\xi, \frac{a^\xi \kappa^\xi}{2}\right), \\
\beta_j|\tau_j^2 &\sim \mathcal{N}(0, \tau_j^2), \quad \tau_j^2|a^\tau, \kappa^\tau \sim \mathcal{G}\left(a^\tau, \frac{a^\tau \kappa^\tau}{2}\right),
\end{aligned}$$

where $a^\xi, \kappa^\xi, a^\tau, \kappa^\tau$ are additional hyperparameters.

2.2 Latent Variable Model

To model dependence of the observations of one subject we model ϵ_{it} using a subject specific latent factor $f_i \sim \mathcal{N}(0, 1)$ as

$$\epsilon_{it} = \lambda_t f_i + \zeta_{it}, \qquad \zeta_{it} \sim \mathcal{N}(0, \sigma^2). \tag{1}$$

With $\boldsymbol{\lambda} = (\lambda_1, \dots, \lambda_T)^\top$ the covariance matrix of the error vector $\boldsymbol{\epsilon}_i = (\epsilon_{i1}, \dots, \epsilon_{iT})^\top$ is $\boldsymbol{\Omega} = \boldsymbol{\lambda}\boldsymbol{\lambda}^\top + \sigma^2 \mathbf{I}$ with time-varying within subject dependence of the response. If $\lambda_t = \lambda$ for all $t \in \{1, \dots, T\}$, $\boldsymbol{\Omega}$ is of compound-symmetry structure. To allow for smoothing of the loadings over time and shrinkage to a compound-symmetry structure or to zero, similarly as for the regression effects we use a random walk prior on the factor loadings in non-centered representation

$$\lambda_t = \lambda + \psi \tilde{\lambda}_t, \quad t = 2, \dots, T,$$
$$\tilde{\lambda}_t = \tilde{\lambda}_{t-1} + \tilde{\nu}_t, \quad \tilde{\nu}_t \sim \mathcal{N}(0, 1),$$

with initial loading $\tilde{\lambda}_1 \sim \mathcal{N}(0, c_\lambda)$. Independent shrinkage priors on ψ and λ are specified as for the regression effects in Subsect. 2.1.

2.3 Posterior Inference

Inference on the model parameters can be accomplished by MCMC methods iterating over the following three steps:

1. Step R: Sample the time-varying effects $\boldsymbol{\beta}_1, \dots, \boldsymbol{\beta}_T$, the process standard deviations $\theta_1, \dots, \theta_d$ and associated hyperparameters from the posterior of the linear regression model

$$y_{it} - \lambda_t f_i = \mathbf{x}_{it}^\top \boldsymbol{\beta} + \mathbf{x}_{it}^\top \boldsymbol{\Theta} \tilde{\boldsymbol{\beta}}_t + \zeta_{it}, \quad \zeta_{it} \sim \mathcal{N}(0, \sigma^2).$$

2. Step F: Sample the latent factors f_i for all $i \in \{1, \dots, n\}$, the time-varying factor loadings $\lambda_1, \dots, \lambda_T$, the process standard deviation ψ and associated hyperparameters from the posterior of the linear regression model

$$y_{it} - \mathbf{x}_{it}^\top \boldsymbol{\beta}_t = \lambda f_i + \psi f_i \tilde{\lambda}_t + \zeta_{it}, \quad \zeta_{it} \sim \mathcal{N}(0, \sigma^2).$$

3. Step V: Sample the homoscedastic error variance σ^2.

In most sampling steps direct sampling from the full conditionals is feasible.

3 Simulation Study

To assess the performance of the approach for rather short panels we simulate $nsim = 100$ data sets of $n = 10,000$ subjects at $T = 8$ different time points. We use $d = 4$ regressors including the constant for the intercept and simulate the other 3 regressors independently from a standard Normal distribution.

We specify the initial values of the regression effects as $\boldsymbol{\beta} \equiv (\beta_1, \beta_2, \beta_3, \beta_4)^\top = (4, 0, 1, 1)^\top$ and the process standard deviations as $\boldsymbol{\theta} \equiv (\theta_1, \theta_2, \theta_3, \theta_4)^\top = (1, 0, 0.2, 0)^\top$. The time-varying regression effects are generated from the model for each data set and hence will differ across the data sets. For the error term, we assume the factor model specified in Eq. (1) with $\lambda_t = 0.6$ for all $t \in \{1, \dots, 8\}$ in all data sets. Figure 1 compares the distribution of the squared error for the regression effects and factor loadings under shrinkage and independence priors.

For effects that are constant over time the shrinkage prior performs much better, whereas results are similar under both priors for time-varying effects. Also for the factor loadings, which are constant (or time-invariant) in this simulation scenario, the shrinkage prior yields smaller squared errors.

To assess the performance for time-varying factor loadings we simulate data in the same setup as before but now consider time-varying factor loadings with prespecified values $\boldsymbol{\lambda} = (0.50, 0.55, 0.60, 0.65, 0.62, 0.59, 0.56, 0.53)^\top$. Figure 2 shows estimation results for the factor loadings and the posterior of the signed process standard deviation ψ in one of the simulated data sets as well as the squared error of the factor loadings for all $nsim = 100$ data sets. As for the regression effects, results are similar under shrinkage and independence priors, if factor loadings are actually time-varying.

To investigate the performance for a smaller data set, we repeated the simulations for data sets with $n = 100$ subjects (not shown). As expected squared errors are higher than for $n = 10,000$, but also in these smaller samples shrinkage is effective when appropriate and squared errors are smaller than under the independence prior for constant or zero effects and loadings whereas results are similar if they vary over time.

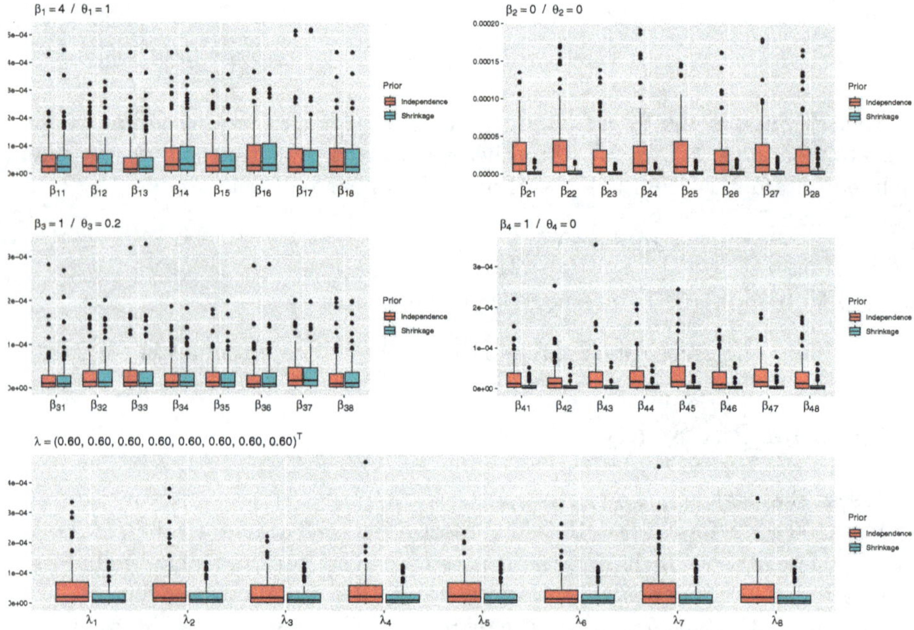

Fig. 1. Squared error of effects and **time-invariant** loadings ($n = 10,000$)

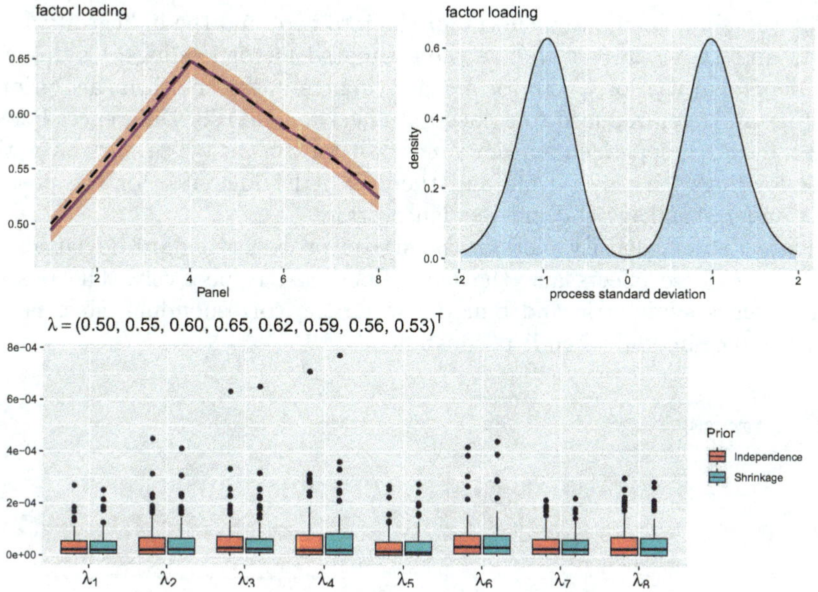

Fig. 2. Posterior means [black line: shrinkage prior; blue line: independence prior; dashed line: true values of data generating process; coral area: 95% HPD interval based on estimation with shrinkage prior], signed process standard deviations and squared error of **time-varying** loadings ($n = 10,000$)

4 Case Study: Mother's Yearly Income

We analyse yearly earnings of mothers in Austria after their return to the labour market after maternity leave. The data set consists of $n = 8,887$ mothers with earnings observed in $T = 8$ consecutive years.

To analyse the data we apply our model, which allows for effects and within subject dependence that can vary over time but encourages shrinkage to simpler models to avoid overspecification.

We model the yearly log-income of mothers in terms of indicator variables for two (`child2`), three or more children (`child3`), return to the same employer (`same.emp`), duration of maternity leave longer than 24 months (`leave.dur`) and blue-collar worker (`blue.c`) as well as job experience in years (`experience`) and base income before birth of child (`lbasec`).

Figure 3 shows estimated effects for the intercept and the indicator variables `child3` and `leave.dur` as well as the estimated factor loadings. Compared to the independence prior, posterior mean estimates under the shrinkage prior are smoother and even reduced to a constant effect for `child3`. Differences between shrinkage and independence prior are small for effects which vary over time. Factor loadings vary over time and there is little difference for the posterior means under shrinkage and independence prior.

Figure 4 shows density plots of the signed process standard deviations $\pm\theta_j$ and $\pm\psi$ for these effects and the factor loadings, respectively. The posterior distribution is symmetric and bimodal when the corresponding effect is time-varying and unimodal when it is constant.

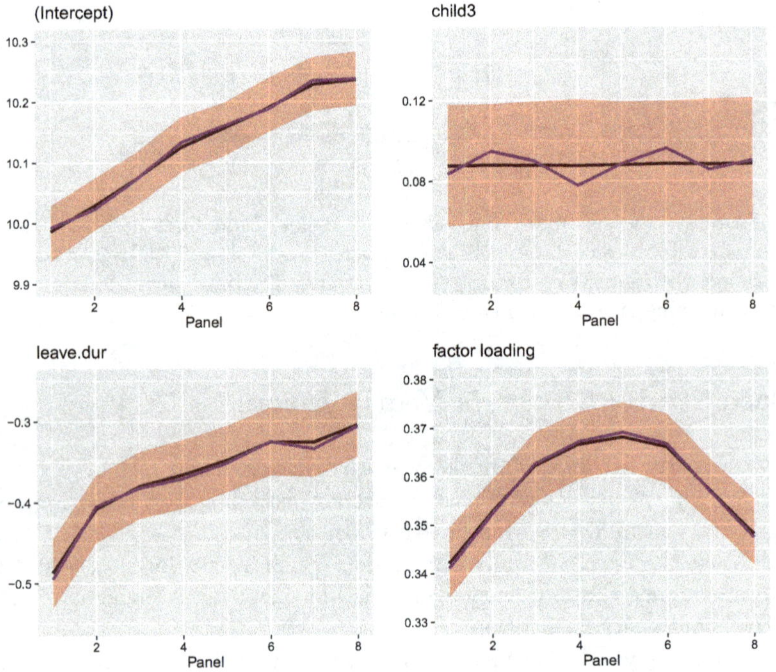

Fig. 3. Posterior means of selected covariates and factor loadings (black lines: shrinkage prior [with 95% HPD interval in coral]; blue lines: independence prior)

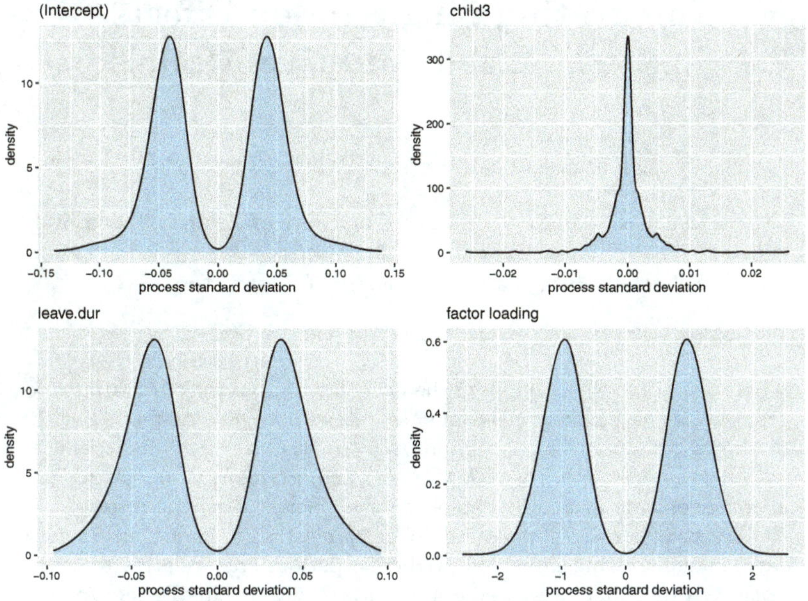

Fig. 4. Signed process standard deviations of selected covariates and factor loadings

5 Conclusion

We propose a flexible Bayesian panel data model where within subject dependence is captured by a latent factor and regression effects as well as factor loadings may vary over time. To avoid overspecification, we use priors that encourage shrinkage of time-varying effects and loadings to constant or zero effects. Posterior mean estimates are similar to those under an independence prior for time-varying effects and loadings but have lower squared error when effects and loadings are constant or zero.

References

1. Bitto, A., Frühwirth-Schnatter, S.: Achieving shrinkage in a time-varying parameter model framework. J. Econom. **210**, 75–97 (2019). https://doi.org/10.1016/j.jeconom.2018.11.006
2. Frühwirth-Schnatter, S., Wagner, H.: Stochastic model specification search for Gaussian and partially Non-Gaussian state space models. J. Econom. **154**, 85–100 (2010). https://doi.org/10.1016/j.jeconom.2009.07.003

Integrating Single Index Effects in Generalized Additive Models

Claudia Collarin[1(✉)] and Matteo Fasiolo[2]

[1] Department of Statistical Sciences, University of Padova, Padua, Italy
claudia.collarin@phd.unipd.it
[2] School of Mathematics, University of Bristol, Bristol, UK

Abstract. Linearly combining the elements of a vector of covariates to get a scalar-valued feature is common practice in regression modelling. In this work, we propose a novel approach to integrate single index effects in Generalised Additive Models (GAMs). In particular, model fitting and inference are performed by exploiting the efficient methods proposed in [7]. We consider an application to daily electricity load consumption data, demonstrating improved predictive performance relative to traditional GAMs. This integrated approach provides a valuable tool to capture complex relationships in real-world applications, while preserving interpretability.

Keywords: Generalised Additive Models · Single Index Models · Projection Pursuit Regression

1 Introduction

Generalised Additive Models (GAM; [4]) are a class of models that offer an attractive balance between flexibility and interpretability. Specifically, by developing non-linear effects through linear combinations of basis functions, they facilitate the modelling of complex relationships between the response variable and the predictors. However, this flexibility has a downside, because each smooth component contains regression coefficients that must be estimated. Hence, the number of smooth effects contained in a GAM must be limited, which poses a challenge in the presence of many covariates. In some cases, the number of covariates can be reduced by combining them to get a smaller set of features. As an example, here we consider a model for the regional electricity load at time t, L_t, which takes into account the outdoor temperature measured at 25 weather stations. The most obvious way to integrate these measurements into a GAM is to first summarise them through a linear combination $\mathbf{T}_t\alpha$. In practice, α is often chosen on the basis of expert knowledge or via a cross-validation routine, which requires refitting the model multiple times.

The objective of this work is to prevent refitting and to estimate α simultaneously with all other model parameters. This is achieved by adopting the efficient fitting framework proposed in [7], which is applied to fit generalised

J. Einbeck et al. (Eds.): IWSM 2024, CONTRIB.STAT., pp. 116–120, 2024.
https://doi.org/10.1007/978-3-031-65723-8_18

additive models that include smooth transformations of covariates' linear combinations. Throughout this paper, we will denote this class of smoothers as *single index* effects. Note that estimating all parameters together provides inferential as well as computational advantages. Specifically, using a single objective function, namely the penalised log-likelihood, for parameter estimation leads to a parameters vector distribution that captures all components of variability.

Projection Pursuit Regression (PPR; [6]) and Generalised Partially Linear Single Index Models (GPLSIM; [1]) are two model classes that are related to our proposal. Specifically, PPR is designed to build the regression surface by summing up M single index effects of the covariate vector $\mathbf{x}$, expressed as $E[Y] = \sum_{m=1}^{M} s_m(\mathbf{x}^\top \alpha_m)$. The main differences relative to our method are PPR's restriction to only one single index effect, $s_1(\cdot)$ and the requirement that $s_1(\cdot)$ be a function whose argument is a linear combination of all covariates. GPLSIM incorporates a single index smooth effect within the Generalised Linear Model (GLM) framework, expressing the linear predictor η as a sum of a linear combination of covariates and a single index of a subset of covariates $\mathbf{z}$, that is, $\eta = X^\top \beta + s(\mathbf{z}^\top \alpha)$. Over the past two decades, researchers have focused on developing a stable fitting algorithm for this class of models using P-splines ([8,9], and [10]). The model we propose can be seen as an extension of GPLSIM to the GAM framework.

2 Incorporating Single Index Effects into Generalised Additive Models

Define the vector of the response variables as $\mathbf{y} = (y_1, \ldots, y_n)^\top$ and let $\mathbf{x}_1, \ldots, \mathbf{x}_n$ represent the associated d-dimensional covariates. Assume that each y_i follows an exponential family distribution with a linear predictor μ that is modelled by linear, standard smooth, and single index components. Let $f_k(\cdot)$ represent the K standard smooths and $s_p(\cdot)$ denote the P single index effects. The proposed model is expressed as

$$\mu_i = g^{-1}\left(\mathbf{Z}_i^\top \gamma + \sum_{k=1}^{K} f_k\left(\mathbf{X}_i^{S_k}\right) + \sum_{p=1}^{P} s_p\left(\mathbf{X}_i^{S_p} \alpha_p\right)\right), \tag{1}$$

where g is a monotonic link function, $\mathbf{Z}_i^\top$, $\mathbf{X}_i^{S_k}$, and $\mathbf{X}_i^{S_p}$ are subsets (which may overlap) of the i-th row of the design matrix, γ is the vector of linear regression coefficients and α_p is the weight vector in the linear combination of the single index effect s_p. $S_k, S_p \subseteq \{1, \ldots, d\}$ are a subset of indexes that indicate which covariates should be considered for a particular effect. For example, if $S_k = \{1, 3\}$, then $\mathbf{x}_i^{S_k} = (x_1, x_3)$ is a two-dimensional vector formed by the first and third elements of $\mathbf{x}_i$. All functions f_k's and s_p's are assumed to be fourth order differentiable and are estimated via P-spline bases $\left\{h_1^j, \ldots, h_{L_j}^j\right\}$ [2]

$$f_k(\mathbf{x}^{S_k}) = \sum_{l=1}^{L_k} h_l^k(\mathbf{x}^{S_k}) b_l^k \qquad\qquad s_p(\mathbf{x}^{S_p}) = \sum_{l=1}^{L_p} h_l^p(\mathbf{x}^{S_p}) \beta_l^p, \tag{2}$$

where b_l^k and β_l^p are regression coefficients. Omitting the final term on the right-hand side of (1) results in a standard GAM model, while excluding the penultimate term yields a GPLSIM with several single index components.

Although the model of this section belongs to the GAM class, it is important to recognise that the linear predictors non-linearly depend on the single index inner parameters, α_p. The efficient framework described in [7] allows for such non-linearities. In particular, the single-index coefficients are jointly estimated with the other parameters that appear in (1) using a penalised maximum likelihood approach. Additionally, the selection of smoothing parameters is achieved by optimising a Laplace approximation to the marginal likelihood. Joint fitting permits uncertainty quantification and inference via an asymptotic Gaussian approximation to the Bayesian posterior distribution of both the regression and single index coefficients.

3 GefCom2014 Data Application

Applications for the model class described in the previous section include scenarios in which the response shows a non-linear relationship with a subset of covariates and, simultaneously, there is a need to aggregate these variables to keep the model simple and interpretable. An example of such data is that used in the electricity load forecasting track of the 2014 Global Energy Forecasting Competition (GefCom2014, [5]). Here, we analyse daily records of the hourly load from 12:00 p.m. to 1:00 p.m. (L_t), spanning from 8 January 2005 to 30 November 2011.

We fit a GAM to data collected from January 8, 2005 to December 31, 2009, and use the remaining data to validate the results. Data include a cyclic variable that indicates position within the year (S_t), a factor variable indicating the day of the week (D_t), a counter representing time (t), the electricity loaded the day before ($L_{t-24}, \ldots, L_{t-47}$) and the previous week at 12:00 ($L_{t-48}, L_{t-72}, \ldots, L_{t-168}$), and predicted temperatures ($\mathbf{T}_t$) at noon at 25 weather stations.

We model the load via a Gaussian Generalised Additive Model where the mean is modelled by

$$L_t = \sum_{j=1}^{7} \delta_{jD_t} \gamma_j + f_1(t) + f_2(S_t) + s_1(\mathbf{T}_t \alpha_t) + s_2(\mathbf{L}_t \alpha_l), \tag{3}$$

where δ_{jD_t} is the Kronecker delta, used to denote dummy variables of the day of the week, and $\mathbf{L}_t$ is a row vector of lagged loads. For comparison, we consider a naïve model where α_t is set to $\frac{1}{25}(1, \ldots, 1)$ and $s_2(\mathbf{L}_t \alpha_l)$ is substituted by $f_3(L_{t-24}) + L_{t-48}\gamma_8 + \cdots + L_{t-168}\gamma_{14}$. Hence, this model uses standard smooth effects for the average temperature across stations and for L_{t-24}, and linear effects for $L_{t-48}, \ldots, L_{t-168}$.

The resulting fitted effects and the inner coefficients of the single index are illustrated in Figs. 1 and 2, respectively. It should be noted that $\mathbf{T}_t \alpha_1$ can be

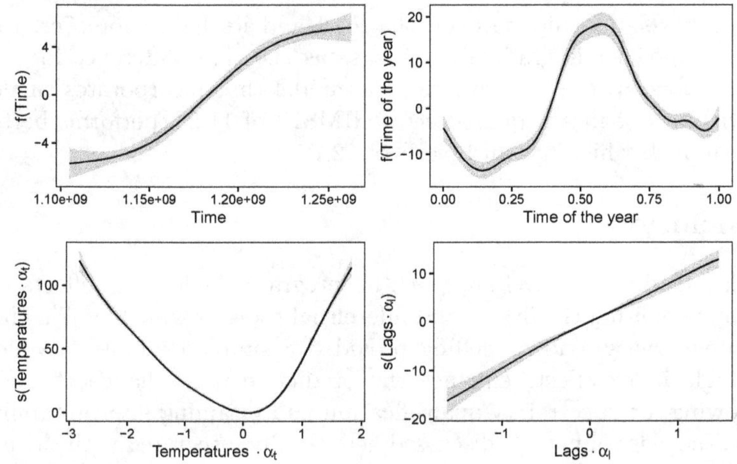

Fig. 1. Fitted smooth effects with 95% credible bands of time, time of the year, linear combination of temperatures and of lagged load values.

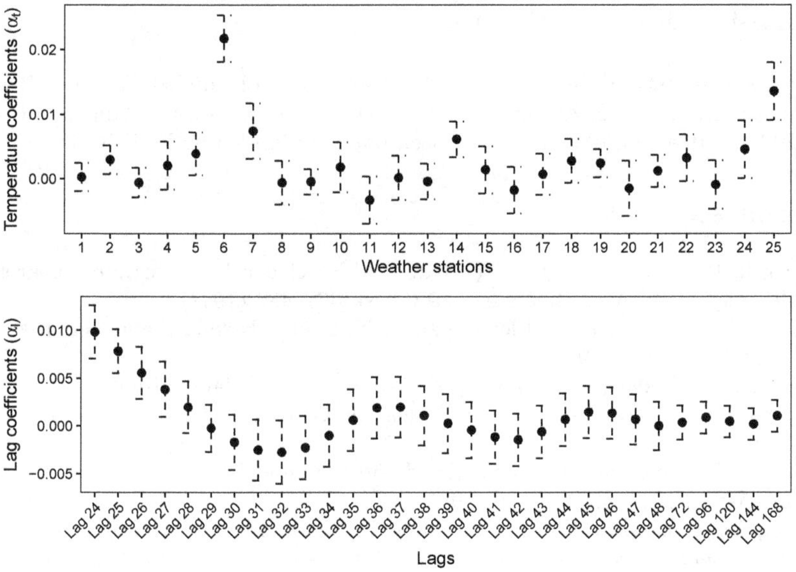

Fig. 2. Inner single index coefficients with 95% credible intervals.

seen as a weighted average of temperatures, with only a few stations making substantial contributions to the average, while others play a less important role. As expected, there is an increase in the load occurring as the average temperature deviates from the mean. The exact locations of these stations remain unknown; otherwise, it would have been interesting to explore their geographical relationships with the consumption centres. In terms of lagged values, we observe an almost linear relationship between the load and its lags. Moreover, the coefficients of lagged loads gradually decrease as the time difference increases. In terms of performance in the test set, the model that incorporates single index effects, with a root mean squared error (RMSE) of 11.56, performs better than the naïve model, which has an RMSE of 12.77.

4 Conclusions

Our work introduces a novel approach to integrate single index effects in GAM models, by exploiting the fitting and inferential tools provided by [7]. The application to electricity load modelling provided a simple example in which integrated single index effects enhance the predictive performance of the model, while allowing for uncertainty quantification and retaining interpretability. Furthermore, the class of models discussed here is fully integrated with the packages `mgcv` [7] and `mgcViz` [3], which allows users to take advantage of the efficiency and stability of the fitting algorithms provided by the former and to adopt the rich visualisation framework made available by the latter. The code and data to reproduce the results and the graphs are available at https://github.com/ccollarin/single_index_IWSM2024.git.

Acknowledgments. Claudia Collarin PhD scholarship is funded by PON "Research and Innovation" 2014 - 2020 Action IV.5 "PhDs on Green issues." - Ministerial Decree 1061/2021. Matteo Fasiolo's work has been partially funded by EDF R&D.

References

1. Carroll, R.J., Fan, J., Gijbels, I., Wand, M.P.: Generalized partially linear single-index models. J. Am. Stat. Assoc. **92**(438), 477–489 (1997)
2. Eilers, P.H., Marx, B.D.: Flexible smoothing with B-splines and penalties. Stat. Sci. **11**(2), 89–121 (1996)
3. Fasiolo, M., Nedellec, R., Goude, Y., Wood, S.N.: Scalable visualization methods for modern generalized additive models. J. Comput. Graph. Stat. **29**(1), 78–86 (2020)
4. Hastie, T., Tibshirani, R.: Generalized additive models: some applications. J. Am. Stat. Assoc. **82**(398), 371–386 (1987)
5. Hong, T., Pinson, P., Fan, S., Zareipour, H., Troccoli, A., Hyndman, R.J.: Probabilistic energy forecasting: global energy forecasting competition 2014 and beyond. Int. J. Forecast. **32**(3), 896–913 (2016)
6. Friedman, J.H., Stuetzle, W.: Projection pursuit regression. J. Am. Stat. Assoc. **76**(376), 817–823 (1981)
7. Wood, S.N., Pya, N., Säfken, B.: Smoothing parameter and model selection for general smooth models. J. Am. Stat. Assoc. **111**, 1548–1563 (2016)
8. Yu, Y., Ruppert, D.: Penalized spline estimation for partially linear single-index models. J. Am. Stat. Assoc. **97**, 1042–1054 (2002)
9. Yu, Y., Wu, C., Zhang, Y.: Penalised spline estimation for generalised partially linear single-index models. Stat. Comput. **27**, 571–582 (2017)
10. Zu, T., Yu, Y.: Gplsim: an R package for generalized partially linear single-index models. R J. **15**(1) (2023)

An Underrated Prior Distribution for Proportions. The Logistic–Normal for Dynamical Football Predictions

Rui Martins[1,2](✉)

[1] Faculdade de Ciências da Universidade de Lisboa (FCUL), Lisbon, Portugal
rmmartins@fc.ul.pt

[2] Centro de Estatística e Aplicações da Universidade de Lisboa (CEAUL), Lisbon, Portugal

Abstract. The result of a football match in terms of Home–Win, Draw or Away–Win can be modelled by considering the observed outcome as a realization of a Multinomial random variable with three mutually exclusive events over a single trial. Most applications consider the Dirichlet distribution to represent the prior uncertainty about the Multinomial's proportion parameters, mainly because of conjugacy and the reduced number of parameters. As alternative we propose to use the Logistic–Normal, a multivariate prior distribution for proportions but to which little attention has been paid. This approach was motivated by the question – Are women's and men's football leagues equally predictable? The models developed are applied to the main Portuguese women's and men's football leagues over seven seasons, starting from 2016–2017 up to 2022–2023. The work also provides estimates of latent team-specific strengths and addresses the variability between and within seasons, along with insights of each team's home advantage.

Keywords: Compositional data · Dynamic models · Football prediction · Logistic-Normal prior · Sports comparison

1 Introduction

The beginning of the 21st century witnessed an acceleration in women's football popularity and consequently of practitioners and fans worldwide. Historically, the focus of analytics has been confined to men's leagues, hindering the establishment of robust comparisons with women's league.

The outcomes of a football game are generally analysed following two distinct perspectives: (i) goal-based approach where the number of goals scored by each team are modelled with a suitable model for counts, e.g. Poisson [1–3]; (ii) outcome-based approach where the final result in terms of Home–Win, Draw or Away–Win, is considered a realization of a Multinomial random variable with three mutually exclusive events over a single trial [4,5]. It will be this last perspective that will be followed in the remainder of this work.

J. Einbeck et al. (Eds.): IWSM 2024, CONTRIB.STAT., pp. 121–127, 2024.
https://doi.org/10.1007/978-3-031-65723-8_19

Despite being mathematically simple, the dependence variates in a Dirichlet distribution are always negatively correlated, which may not represent adequate prior beliefs for the parameters of a Multinomial distribution. One of the most attractive alternatives is the Logistic–Normal prior, because methods involving such distribution can be easily formulated as transformations of some Multivariate–Normal model where the richness of its covariance structure is at researcher's disposal [6].

This work provides a model that enables the estimates of latent characteristics related to team-specific strengths and assesses the competitiveness across women's and men's leagues, both within- and between-seasons.

2 Data

We analysed a series of 7 seasons of football match results from the main Portuguese women's and men's football leagues, starting from 2016–17 up to 2022–23. During a season each of the 12 clubs in the women's league plays the others twice (double round–robin system), once at the home field and once away, for 22 rounds. Teams receive three points for a win and one point for a draw. No points are awarded for a loss. Teams are ranked by total points. The same rules apply to the men's league, simply the number of teams increases to 18 and the number of rounds per season to 34. At the end of each season, the last 2 or 3 teams (depending on the years) are relegated to the lower league.

2.1 Methodology

Let us consider a particular match outcome, $z_{qsr,ij}$, consisting of the observed 3-dimensional vector result for the game opposing team i playing at home against team j playing away: $z_{qsr,ij} = (1, 0, 0)$, home-win; $z_{qsr,ij} = (0, 1, 0)$, draw; $z_{qsr,ij} = (0, 0, 1)$, away-win. Here $i, j = 1, \ldots, t_{qs} \wedge i \neq j$ and t_{qs} represents the number of teams in season s for league $q \in \{w, m\}$, depending on whether it is the women's or men's league. Additionally, the analysed number of seasons, S_q, and rounds per season, R_{qs}, can vary between leagues, i.e. $s \in \{1, \ldots, S_q\}$ and $r \in \{1, \ldots, R_{qs}\}$. In fact, s should be written in the form, e.g. 2016–17, but to keep the notation simple we will consider that the subscript s varies between 1 and number of analysed seasons, which is 7 in this case. In a double round–robin system the total number of games per season is $G_{qs} = \binom{t_{qs}}{2} \times 2 = t_{qs}(t_{qs} - 1)$.

It is natural to assume that $Z_{qsr,ij} = (z_{qsr,ij1}, z_{qsr,ij2}, z_{qsr,ij3})$ follows a multinomial distribution, $\mathcal{M}(.;.)$, with $\sum_{l=1}^{3} z_{qsr,ijl} = 1$ and vector of probabilities $\theta_{qsr,ij} = (\theta_{qsr,ij1}, \theta_{qsr,ij2}, \theta_{qsr,ij3})$, being $0 < \theta_{qsr,ijl} < 1$, $l = 1, 2, 3$, and $\sum_{l=1}^{3} \theta_{qsr,ijl} = 1$. We purposely assume no probabilities of 0 or 1 associated to the different outcomes of a game. Within this framework we consider:

$$Z_{qsr,ij} \mid \theta_{qsr,ij} \sim \mathcal{M}(1;\ \theta_{qsr,ij}) \tag{1}$$

$$\theta_{qsr,ij} \sim f(\iota_{qsr,ij}), \tag{2}$$

where $f(\iota_{qsr,ij})$ represents a stochastic process possibly time-dependent with parameters ι. To represent the prior distribution for the vector $\theta_{qsr,ij}$, as already mentioned above, we consider the Logistic–Normal for $f(.)$.

The appeal of this little-used distribution has it roots in the relationship with the Multivariate–Normal. Logistic–Normal models can be framed as a transformation of adequate Multivariate–Normal models.

Suppose that $\phi(\cdot)$ represents the additive log–ratio (alr) transformation [6] of a 3-dimensional vector in the 2-Simplex, $\theta_{qsr,ij} = (\theta_{qsr,ij1}, \theta_{qsr,ij2}, \theta_{qsr,ij3}) \in \mathbb{S}^2$ into a 2-dimensional vector in the 2-dimensional Euclidean space, $w_{qsr,ij} = (w_{qsr,ij1}, w_{qsr,ij2}) \in \mathbb{R}^2$:

$$\phi(\theta_{qsr,ij}) = w_{qsr,ij} = \left[\log\left(\frac{\theta_{qsr,ij1}}{\theta_{qsr,ij2}}\right), \log\left(\frac{\theta_{qsr,ij3}}{\theta_{qsr,ij2}}\right)\right]. \tag{3}$$

With the inverse transformation below we get the so-called alr–coordinates:

$$\begin{aligned}\theta_{qsr,ij} &= \phi^{-1}(w_{qsr,ij})\\ &= \left(\frac{e^{w_{qsr,ij1}}}{1+\sum_{l=1}^{2} e^{w_{qsr,ijl}}}, \frac{1}{1+\sum_{l=1}^{2} e^{w_{qsr,ijl}}}, \frac{e^{w_{qsr,ij2}}}{1+\sum_{l=1}^{2} e^{w_{qsr,ijl}}}\right).\end{aligned}$$

The 3-dimensional vector, $\theta_{qsr,ij}$, is said to have a Logistic–Normal distribution, $\mathcal{LN}(\mu, \mathbf{\Sigma})$, on $\mathbb{S}^2$ if any of its vector of log-ratio coordinates has a joint 2–variate normal distribution, $\mathcal{N}(\mu, \mathbf{\Sigma})$ on $\mathbb{R}^2$. In (3) $\theta_{qsr,ij2}$ seems to be treated differently to the other θ. However, the Logistic–Normal distribution is permutation invariant, i.e. regardless the ordering of the elements in $\theta_{qsr,ij}$ its associated density function is invariant.

A major benefit of this approach is that the modelling possibilities of the Multivariate–Normal covariance structure can be transfer to the Logistic–Normal, which allows many assumptions for the correlation between the elements of $\theta_{qsr,ij}$.

2.2 Model Specification

Given the above and (1)–(2) we can write the Multinomial–Logistic–Normal (MLN) model as a Multinomial–Multivariate–Normal (MMN) model:

$$\begin{aligned} Z_{qsr,ij} \mid \theta_{qsr,ij} &\sim \mathcal{M}(1;\ \theta_{qsr,ij})\\ \theta_{qsr,ij} &= \phi^{-1}(w_{qsr,ij})\\ w_{qsr,ij} \mid \mu_{qsr,ij}, \mathbf{\Sigma}_q &\sim \mathcal{N}(\mu_{qsr,ij}, \mathbf{\Sigma}_q).\end{aligned}$$

The team's and game's properties associated to the probability of a home–win, draw or away–win, will enter the model through the location parameter vector μ in the following way:

$$\log\left(\frac{\theta_{qsr,ij1}}{\theta_{qsr,ij2}}\right) = \mu_{qsr,ij1} = \beta_{10} + \zeta_{qsr,i} - \zeta_{qsr,j} + \psi_{q,i}, \tag{4}$$

$$\log\left(\frac{\theta_{qsr,ij3}}{\theta_{qsr,ij2}}\right) = \mu_{qsr,ij2} = \beta_{20} + \zeta_{qsr,j} - \zeta_{qsr,i}. \tag{5}$$

Equation (4) represents the log-odds of a home–win relatively to a draw. Whereas (5) represents the log-odds of an away–win relatively to a draw. Parameters β_{10} and β_{20} are the intercepts roughly describing an empirical mean. Parameters $\zeta_{.,i}$ and $\zeta_{.,j}$ are, respectively, the team's i and j strengths that we will model dynamically from season–to–season and round–to–round. Finally, $\psi_{q,i}$ is the home effect for team i in league q. For the (2×2) prior covariance matrix $\mathbf{\Sigma}_q$, it is assumed an adequate prior covariance structure which may depend on the team, round or season, but for now it will be only a function of the league, q:

$$\mathbf{\Sigma}_q = \begin{bmatrix} \sigma_{q1}^2 & \rho_q \cdot \sigma_{q1} \cdot \sigma_{q2} \\ \rho_q \cdot \sigma_{q1} \cdot \sigma_{q2} & \sigma_{q2}^2 \end{bmatrix} \tag{6}$$

where $0 < \sigma_{q1}, \sigma_{q2} < \infty$ and $-1 < \rho_q < 1$. This defines the correlation between $w_{q1,.}$ and $w_{q2,.}$ equal to ρ. All the remaining parameters are modelled with appropriate prior distributions of traditional forms.

For identifiability purposes it is required that $\sum_{i=1}^{t_{qs}} \zeta_{qsr,i} = 0$ holds for all the rounds, r, within each season, s. The strength parameters, $\zeta_{qsr,i}$, therefore represent the strength, relatively to an average team with a strength of 0.

2.3 Teams Merits

Teams merits or team strengths will be specified as a dynamic model. The evolution component of our formulation will describe the stochastic behaviour of the time-dependent parameters, ζ.

Below we present the structure for the home team i, omitting the specification for the visiting team j, which can be written in a similar way, only substituting the subscript i with j. These strength parameters are meant to vary autoregressively from season–to–season and round–to–round, i.e.:

$$\zeta_{q,(s+1),1,i} | \zeta_{qsR_{qs},i} \sim \mathcal{N}(\gamma_q^{(szn)}\, \zeta_{qsR_{qs},i}, \sigma_q^{2(szn)}); \; s = 1, \ldots, S_q - 1 \tag{7}$$

$$\zeta_{q,s,(r+1),i} | \zeta_{qsr,i} \sim \mathcal{N}(\gamma_q^{(rnd)}\, \zeta_{qsr,i}, \sigma_q^{2(rnd)}); s = 1, ..., S_q; r = 1, ..., R_{qs} - 1 \tag{8}$$

$$\zeta_{q,1,1,i} \sim \mathcal{N}(0,\; \sigma_q^{2(szn)}) \tag{9}$$

Equation (7) encapsulates the evolution of strength between the last round of season s and the first round of season $s+1$, while the short-term changes within a season, i.e. from round-to-round, are considered in (8). A consequence from this definition is that recent matches are more important to estimate current merits than matches played longer ago. The variance parameters $\sigma_q^{2(rnd)}$ and $\sigma_q^{2(szn)}$ represent the "evolution variance" between rounds and seasons, respectively. $\gamma_q^{(rnd)}$ and $\gamma_q^{(szn)}$ are auto-regressive coefficients. If stationarity is a requirement we would limit the process using $|\gamma_q^{(rnd)}| < 1$ and $|\gamma_q^{(szn)}| < 1$ and in that case team merits are prevented from "exploding" both within and between seasons. The case where $\gamma_{\alpha,.} = \gamma_{\beta,.} = 1$ means that we assume a random-walk and the succession of team properties is unpredictable. The case that we chose admits a certain degree of rapid improvement of team merits, e.g., when a new coach arrives, and in that case both $\gamma_{\alpha,.}$ and $\gamma_{\beta,.}$ are not restricted. Although some care is needed in defining its prior distributions. More complicated, dynamic structures can be considered as in [2] where the authors consider Brownian motion to tie together two time points.

Some references argue that there is no particular reason to believe that the home field advantages for each team are quite different. Although in our formulation we consider a team-specific home advantage, $\psi_{qsr,i} \equiv \psi_{q,i}$. We define its prior distribution as

$$\psi_{q,i} \mid \sigma^2_{q,\psi} \sim \mathcal{N}(0,\ \sigma^2_{q,\psi}); \quad i = 1, \ldots, t_{qs}. \tag{10}$$

Finally, we assume the following half-Cauchy prior distributions for the standard deviations above:

$$\sigma_q^{(szn)}, \sigma_q^{(rnd)} \sim \mathcal{C}^+(0, \tau_1); \quad \sigma_{q,\psi} \sim \mathcal{C}^+(0, \tau_2).$$

and for the between- and within-season regression parameters we define

$$\gamma_q^{(szn)} \sim \mathcal{N}(0.99, 1); \quad \gamma_q^{(rnd)} \sim \mathcal{N}(0.98, 1)$$

because we expect small changes from season-to-season for each team and even smaller changes from round-to-round.

3 Results

The MLN model here presented for modelling a three-way game result is an alternative to the traditional cumulative link model and to the Bradley–Terry model extension that allows for ties. For the datasets analysed here, the proposed Logistic–Normal prior outperformed the Dirichlet prior and the dynamic approach for estimating the team strengths improved the results when compared to the static form of the model. Further work is planned to use the Logistic–Normal prior for quantifying specialist's opinions about each probability enrolled in the 3-dimensional Multinomial model here considered.

Table 1. Summary of average week-level team strength parameters, average of autoregressive parameters and variance taken on the log-odds scale.

League	ζ						γ		σ	
	min	$Q_{2.5}$	Q_{25}	Q_{75}	$Q_{97.5}$	max	$\gamma^{(rnd)}$	$\gamma^{(szn)}$	$\sigma^{(rnd)}$	$\sigma^{(szn)}$
Women	−17.6	−12.2	−5.4	3.8	17.9	20.7	0.996	0.98	0.895	4.66
Men	−1.4	−1.2	−0.4	0.4	3.2	3.8	0.995	0.97	0.035	0.92

The first columns of Table 1 (from min to max) show a summary for the posterior merits of each team for all rounds across the seasons for both leagues.

Overall, there is a larger variability in the strength in women's league. A 95% credibility interval (CI) for the median is $(-12.2, 17.9)$ (on the log-odds scale). As a curiosity a difference between two team–strengths of $+0.5$ on the log-odds scale, in favor of the first team, implies a chance of its win of $\exp\{0.5\} = 1.65$ relatively to a draw in a game played at a neutral site. And a chance of $\exp\{-0.5\} = 0.607$ of a win of the second team relatively to a draw in the same game.

The last columns of Table 1 show the posterior mean along with the standard deviation of the autoregressive parameteres and the evolution variance for the rounds and for the seasons. The posterior mean of $\gamma^{(szn)}$ are 0.98 and 0.97, which implies that relatively to each league, we expect almost the same amount of shrinkage from one season to the next. Although, this corresponds to larger reversions in season-level strengths for women, because there are larger gaps in their team–specific strengths.

All the evolution standard deviations for the men's league are small, so we don't expect to much changes in team strengths within and between seasons. Although the standard deviation for the women's league is substantially large, which means that some teams might improve or decrease a lot from one season to the next.

The 95% CI for the correlation parameter (not shown in the table) of the men's league, ρ_m, is $(0.15, 0.42)$, whereas for the women's league we get $(-0.4, 0.01)$. This means that for each game the log-odds of a win *vs* a draw in the men's league defined in (3), regardless it is from the home or the away team, tends to be the most likely outcome. While for women that relation is not present and those log-odds may be deemed independent.

We found no evidence of home advantage in the women's league for any team but one – Fiães SC. The team participated only in the 2021–2022 season with only one victory, and curiously, away. In the men's championship, 6 teams stand out for having a positive home effect: S.L. Benfica, V. Guimarães, Marítimo, F.C. Porto, Sp. Braga and Sporting CP. No team has a negative effect from playing at home. Except for the Marítimo, the remaining 5 teams are consistently the top 5 in the league. In fact, it is curious that Marítimo is identified with the advantage of playing at home, as it is the only team from Madeira Island and has not been performing very well, having been relegated at the end of the 2022/23 season. We suspect this may be related to the long distance to mainland Portugal and the consequent air travel!

Now to answer our main question – Are women's and men's football leagues equally predictable? – as in [7] we consider the posterior distribution of the probabilities that given a pair of teams randomly chosen the better team wins the game. The better team is defined to be the one *a priori* with the highest strength. Figure 1 shows the empirical cumulative distribution functions (ECDF) for the posterior predicted probabilities of the "theoretically" best team to win the game for 10 000 simulated games over the 7 seasons of each league. Without considering a home-advantage the median probabilities are 0.56 for men and 0.83 for women. Considering the home-effect the medians are, respectively, 0.72 and 0.70. When playing at home the best team in a game of the men's league is favored to win the game 72% of the times. While for the women's league the scenario is that on a neutral field, without home-advantage, the best team wins in 83% of the occasions. It is interesting to note that when considering the home-advantage for women's league the median decreases. This might be related to the absence of a clear home-effect in this league and with the situation where one team has in fact a negative home-effect.

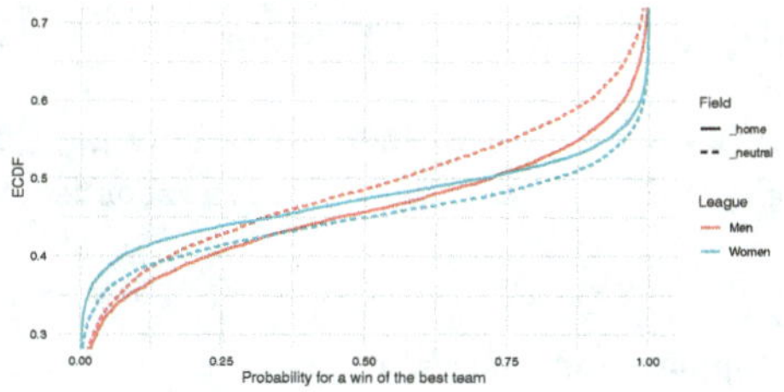

Fig. 1. Empirical Cumulative Density Function for 10 000 simulated games. Probability for a win of the best team.

4 Discussion

The standard approach involving the conjugate prior distribution (Dirichlet) has been here replaced by the less conventional approach of a logistic transformation followed by the employing of a multivariate normal distribution to the transformed parameters. This allowed a more flexible approach readily allowing for prior covariance structures between the parameters, permitting a meaningful hierarchical model. Clearly, in contrast to the men's league, the Portuguese women's league is more predictable in the sense that the team considered *a priori* as the best tends to win game more frequently.

References

1. Maher, M.J.: Modelling association football scores. Stat. Neerl. **3**(36), 109–118 (1982)
2. Rue, H., Salvesen, O.: Prediction and retrospective analysis of soccer matches in a league. J. R. Stat. Soc. Ser. D (Stat.) **3**(49), 399–418 (2000)
3. Egidi, L., Pauli, F., Torelli, N.: Combining historical data and bookmakers' odds in modelling football scores. Stat. Model. **18**(5–6), 436–459 (2018)
4. Tsokos, A., Narayanan, S., Kosmidis, I., Baio, G., et al.: Modelling outcomes of soccer matches. Mach. Learn. **108**, 77–95 (2019)
5. Egidi, L., Torelli, N.: Comparing goal-based and result-based approaches in modelling football outcomes. Soc. Indic. Res. **2**, 801–813 (2021)
6. Aitchison, J.: The Statistical Analysis of Compositional Data. Chapman & Hall, New York (1986)
7. Lopez, M.J., Matthews, G.J., Baumer, B.S.: How often does the best team win? A unified approach to understanding randomness in North American sport. Ann. Appl. Stat. **12**(4), 2483–2516 (2018)

A Comparison of Extreme Gradient and Gaussian Process Boosting for a Spatial Logistic Regression on Satellite Data

Michael Renfrew and Bruce J. Worton(✉)

School of Mathematics, The University of Edinburgh, Edinburgh, UK
M.A.Renfrew@sms.ed.ac.uk, bruce.worton@ed.ac.uk

Abstract. A popular and successful method of obtaining regression models using decision tree learners is XGBoost. However, the method implicitly assumes conditional independence of the predictions given the data and is not statistically efficient for autocorrelated data, as arises in spatial statistics. GPBoost incorporates a Gaussian process in a mixed effects model, and is demonstrated for our remote sensing model to reduce the generalisation error dramatically.

Keywords: Gaussian processes · gradient boosting · logistic regression · machine learning · spatial regression

1 Extreme Gradient Boosting

A popular and successful algorithm in machine learning regression is extreme gradient boosting (XGBoost), introduced by Chen and Guestrin [3]. It combines iterative improvement of weak learners, in this case decision trees, in a process termed *boosting*, with the regularised objective function

$$L = \sum_{i=1}^{N} \ell(y_i, F(\mathbf{x}_i)) + \sum_{m=1}^{M} \Omega(h_m) , \qquad \Omega(h) = \gamma T + \tfrac{1}{2}\lambda \|\mathbf{w}\|^2 ,$$

where ℓ is a loss function suitable for the task, i.e. sum of squares or binary cross-entropy, T is the number of leaves of each tree, and $\mathbf{w}$ is a weight vector corresponding to the leaves. The parameters γ and λ are thus hyperparameters used to control tree complexity. A second-order Taylor series approximation of L increases the practical efficiency of the algorithm.

This algorithm therefore inherits the assumptions of decision-tree based regression analysis, including the conditional independence of predictions given the regressors. However, in practice this assumption fails to hold, in many applications, for spatial modelling.

The statistical properties of boosting, and regression and classification trees, have been reviewed by Bühlmann and Hothorn [2].

J. Einbeck et al. (Eds.): IWSM 2024, CONTRIB.STAT., pp. 128–133, 2024.
https://doi.org/10.1007/978-3-031-65723-8_20

2 Gaussian Process Boosting

A novel technique called Gaussian process boosting (GPBoost) is proposed by Sigrist [5] which relaxes the usual zero-mean assumption of Gaussian processes, defined by letting $\mathbf{b} = (b(s_1), \ldots, b(s_m))^T$ be multivariate Gaussian with $\mathrm{Cov}(b(s), b(s')) = c(s, s')$.

The form of the covariance function $c(s, s')$ is a hyperparameter to be optimised and depends on the application. Some usual choices are a Matérn kernel, exponential (special case of Matérn where $\nu = \frac{1}{2}$) or squared exponential ($\nu \to \infty$).

This Gaussian-process derived random effect $\mathbf{b}$ is combined with the application of a decision tree-boosting algorithm to yield $F(\cdot)$ for the form of a geostatistical mixed-effects model as given by Cressie and Wikle [4],

$$\mathbf{y} = F(X) + Z\mathbf{b} + \epsilon \ , \ \ \mathbf{b} \sim \mathrm{N}(\mathbf{0}, \Sigma) \ , \ \ \epsilon \sim \mathrm{N}(\mathbf{0}, \sigma^2 I_n) \ .$$

The base learner used for the decision tree-boosting algorithm may take several forms, however the most appropriate is the form of a regression tree as introduced by Breiman et al. [1].

This combines the flexibility and accuracy of tree and boosting algorithms with the lack of conditional independence introduced by the spatially autocorrelative nature of such models, and is comparable to techniques such as integrated nested Laplacian approximation with stochastic partial differential equations (INLA-SPDE) or fixed-rank kriging (FRK).

3 Model Specification and Experimental Design

To compare the algorithms of Sects. 1 and 2, a model was constructed as follows. A total of 119,967 tiles of Google Static Maps API satellite imagery at zoom level 18, each representing approximately 0.147 km^2, were sampled for Samburu County, Kenya (Fig. 1). The presence of a boma, a temporary overnight livestock enclosure employed by East African nomadic pastoralists, was ascertained with the use of an artificial intelligence object detection model trained to recognise these structures. For each cell, if any of the 100 model detections had a detection confidence score of 0.7 or greater, the cell was deemed to contain a boma.

Then, 20 squares of 27×27 tiles in dimension containing at least 20 positive tiles were selected uniformly at random from the Samburu County layer. For each square, each of six train/test splits were obtained at random, with the constraint that each group contain at least one positive tile. Spatial logistic regressions were then constructed with the spatial predictor variables in Table 1 using both XGBoost and GPBoost.

The XGBoost models at each train/test split and sample square pair were obtained using the default hyperparameters of the Python package and a binary logistic objective function.

For the GPBoost models, the learning rate was set to 0.1, the maximum tree depth to 3, and maximum boosting rounds to 50. The covariance function was set to the default *exponential*.

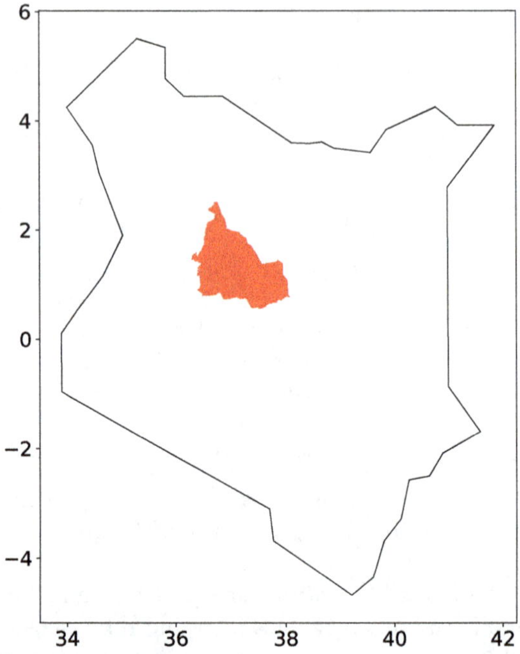

Fig. 1. Location of Samburu County study site (*red region*), overlaid on outline of Kenya

Table 1. Datasets giving rise to variables comprising the model matrix (FAO: Food and Agriculture Organization, ESA: European Space Agency, USGS: United States Geological Survey)

Dataset	No. variables	Source of the dataset
Gridded Livestock of the World (2010 & 2015)	16	FAO
Land Use and Land Cover 2016	55	ESA
Global Soil Organic Carbon v1.5	1	FAO
Shuttle Radar Topography Mission	8	USGS
Koppen-Geiger climatology	31	GloH2O
Total	111	

4 Results

Table 2 shows means and standard deviations (in parentheses) for the following canonical logistic regression evaluation measures across training splits.

- **Area under the curve (AUC):** representing the area under the receiver operating characteristic curve as the classification threshold is varied over [0,1]. Ranges from 0% (worst) to 100% (best classification performance overall).

- **F1 score:** defined as the harmonic mean of *precision* and *recall.* The classification threshold was chosen so as to maximise the F1 in the training sets, and this was reported. The F1 score at that threshold was then evaluated in the test set.

The AUC for XGBoost was superior to that of GPBoost for all but two train splits (50% and 5%), for which the standard deviations in the GPBoost observations were 0% points, suggesting an artefact. This is typical of the ability of XGBoost to tightly fit the data. Note that as the training proportion decreases there is a general downward trend in the AUC for XGBoost but no noticeable trend for GPBoost.

The F1 score obtained on the training data for XGBoost is also in general better and less variable than that of GPBoost, although there is a noticeable decline in performance when the available training data is shrunk from 25% to 5%. Also, the noticeable increase in standard deviation of the XGBoost performance over this range (from 9% points to 18% points and nearly a factor of 5 times worse than with 95% training data) suggests some critical threshold of training data proportion beyond which the algorithm breaks down more rapidly.

The F1 score obtained on the test data is an indicator of how well the models obtained by each individual algorithm generalise. The general machine learning paradigm is to select the best performing model (usually by varying hyperparameters) according to appropriate metrics on the training data set or averaged across k-folds of validation data for a cross-validation (not performed here) and evaluate these same metrics on unseen data (the test data).

In this case, hyperparameters included the covariance function, the learning rate, tree depth, among others, as well as the binary decision threshold. At the given threshold, and at each proportion of training data across variates, the model of each algorithm was generalised to the test data and an F1 score produced.

For both XGBoost and GPBoost, the test F1 scores are lower than the train. This is to be expected, as most machine learning algorithms involve some degree of overfit, whereby the model more accurately describes the given data than the true process. However, note that generalisation performance is much better for GPBoost at every level of incorporated training data, and does not appear to degrade as strongly as XGBoost when the proportion of training data is decreased.

Figure 2 demonstrates an example of the ground truth boma-containing tile locations on a 27×27 grid, along with the models fitted by XGBoost and GPBoost on the whole data.

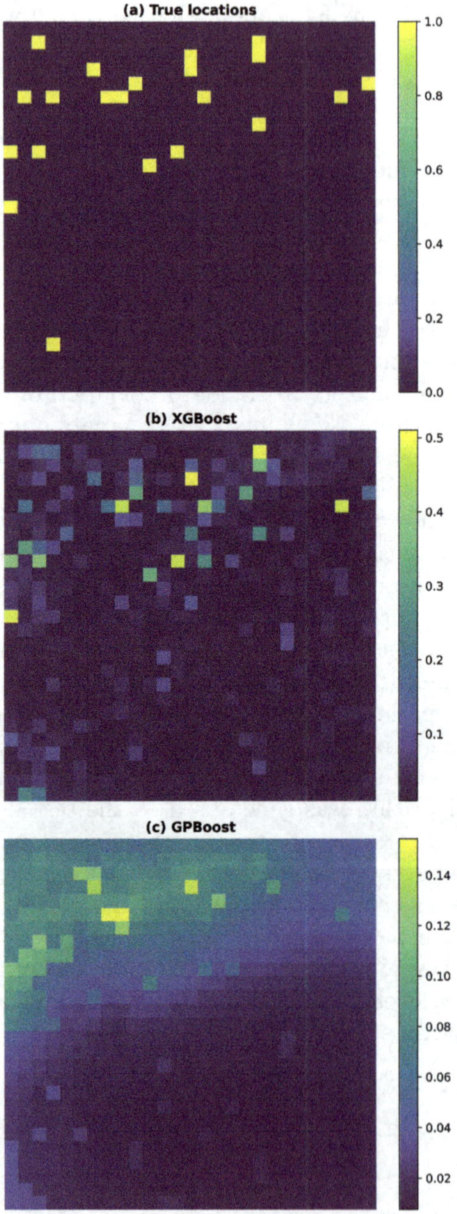

Fig. 2. Illustration of models obtained on a 27×27 square. **a** locations actually containing bomas, as determined by object detection. **b** XGBoost fitted probabilities. **c** GPBoost fitted probabilities

Table 2. Algorithm performance evaluation metrics (%). Standard deviations are shown in parentheses (percentage points)

Train (%)	Train AUC		Train F1		Test F1	
	XGBoost	GPBoost	XGBoost	GPBoost	XGBoost	GPBoost
95	99.0 (0.8)	90.0 (20)	88.3 (4)	81.2 (38)	15.0 (21)	69.5 (39)
90	99.1 (0.7)	92.5 (18)	87.4 (4)	85.9 (34)	15.4 (18)	68.1 (41)
80	99.3 (0.7)	92.5 (18)	89.4 (5)	85.9 (34)	12.0 (14)	77.1 (32)
50	99.7 (0.2)	100.0 (0)	92.4 (5)	100.0 (0)	11.6 (8)	80.8 (18)
25	99.6 (0.9)	95.0 (22)	93.1 (9)	95.1 (21)	12.5 (8)	69.0 (27)
5	98.3 (2.0)	100.0 (0)	83.5 (18)	100.0 (0)	7.0 (7)	98.9 (5)

5 Discussion

On inspection of Fig. 2, it is apparent that GPBoost has discerned a smoother, more graduated pattern than XGBoost, suggesting a significant contribution of the Gaussian process random effects to the overall model. Table 2 shows that the obtained fit generalises to the test data much more successfully for GPBoost, even at very low proportions of incorporated training data, although there is more variability in its performance.

Acknowledgements. The authors would like to thank the anonymous referees for their extremely valuable comments and suggestions on an earlier version of this paper. Michael Renfrew is supported by the Natural Environment Research Council of the United Kingdom (NERC) through a SENSE CDT studentship (grant no. NE/T00939X/1).

References

1. Breiman, L., Friedman, J., Stone, C.J., Olshen, R.A.: Classification and Regression Trees. Chapman and Hall/CRC, New York (1984)
2. Bühlmann, P., Hothorn, T.: Boosting algorithms: regularization, prediction and model fitting. Stat. Sci. **22**, 477–505 (2007)
3. Chen, T., Guestrin, C.: XGboost: a scalable tree boosting system. In: Krishnapuram, B., et al. (eds.) Proceedings 22nd ACM SIGKDD International Conference on Knowledge Discovery and Data Mining, San Francisco, pp. 785–794 (2016)
4. Cressie, N., Wikle, C.K.: Statistics for Spatio-Temporal Data. Wiley, Hoboken (2011)
5. Sigrist, F.: Gaussian process boosting. J. Mach. Learn. Res. **23**, 1–46 (2022)

Gene Coexpression Analysis with Dirichlet Mixture Model: Accelerating Model Evaluation Through Closed-Form KL Divergence Approximation Using Variational Techniques

Samyajoy Pal(✉) and Christian Heumann

LMU Munich, Ludwigstr. 33, 80539 Munich, Germany
Samyajoy.Pal@stat.uni-muenchen.de

Abstract. Gene coexpression analysis poses unique challenges, particularly in clustering normalized gene profiles where dedicated algorithms are lacking. Compositional in nature, normalized gene profiles find a fitting solution in the Dirichlet Mixture Model (DMM). This study pioneers the application of DMM for clustering normalized gene profiles, recognizing the necessity for efficient model evaluation. Central to this evaluation is the Kullback-Leibler (KL) Divergence, a critical metric for DMMs. In addressing the computational challenges associated with KL Divergence in DMMs, we introduce a novel variational approach. This method provides a closed-form solution, markedly improving computational efficiency for rapid model comparisons and robust estimation evaluations. Through validation on real and simulated data, our approach demonstrates superior efficiency and accuracy compared to traditional Monte Carlo-based methods. This innovation opens new frontiers for expeditious exploration of diverse DMM models, propelling advancements in the statistical analysis of compositional gene expression data.

Keywords: Gene Coexpression · Dirichlet Mixture Model (DMM) · Normalized Gene Profiles · Kullback-Leibler Divergence · Variational Approach

1 Introduction

RNA-sequence (RNA-seq) data often come with read counts or pseudo-counts, representing the number of reads aligned to specific genes or genomic regions. When using normalized expression profiles, which indicate the proportion of normalized counts for each feature, the data become compositional. Dirichlet Mixture Model (DMM) has proven to be more effective than other clustering algorithms for compositional data [1]. The Kullback-Leibler (KL) Divergence [2]

J. Einbeck et al. (Eds.): IWSM 2024, CONTRIB.STAT., pp. 134–141, 2024.
https://doi.org/10.1007/978-3-031-65723-8_21

stands as a fundamental measure in statistics, quantifying the statistical distance between probability distributions. The Kullback-Leibler (KL) divergence (also recognized as relative entropy) between two probability density functions $f(x)$ and $g(x)$ is defined by the integral expression:

$$D(f\|g) \stackrel{\text{def}}{=} \int f(x) \log\left(\frac{f(x)}{g(x)}\right) \mathrm{dx} \,. \tag{1}$$

It operates as a measure of the dissimilarity between the probability distributions encoded by $f(x)$ and $g(x)$. In statistical inference, generally $f(x)$ is the distribution with true parameter values and $g(x)$ is the distribution with estimated parameter values. The KL divergence exhibits fundamental properties known as divergence properties: self-similarity, self-identification, and positivity. These properties underscore the significance of KL divergence in capturing the nuances of distributional disparities, making it a cornerstone in statistical analyses. While closed-form solutions for KL Divergence exist for the Dirichlet distribution, there is no analytically tractable solution available for DMM. This study addresses these challenges by proposing a variational approach to approximate KL Divergence in DMMs. Unlike other methods such as Monte Carlo based approximation [3], our approach provides a closed-form solution, substantially enhancing computational efficiency. Validation using real and simulated data demonstrates its superiority in efficiency and accuracy over traditional Monte Carlo-based approaches. The results underscore the potential of our variational approximation to accelerate the estimation process while improving the quality of estimates.

2 Methods

Let $\boldsymbol{X}_1, \boldsymbol{X}_2, \ldots, \boldsymbol{X}_N$ denote a random sample of size N, where $\boldsymbol{X}_i$ is a p dimensional random vector with probability density function $f(\boldsymbol{x}_i)$ on $\mathbb{R}^p$.

The Dirichlet density is given by

$$f(\boldsymbol{x}_i) = \frac{\Gamma(\sum_{m=1}^{p} \alpha_m)}{\prod_{m=1}^{p} \Gamma(\alpha_m)} \prod_{m=1}^{p} x_{im}^{\alpha_m - 1} \,, \tag{2}$$

where $\sum_{m=1}^{p} x_{im} = 1, x_{im}\text{'s} > 0\,, \alpha_{jm}\text{'s} > 0$ and $\Gamma(\cdot)$ denotes a gamma function. The density of a mixture model with k mixture components for one observation $\boldsymbol{x}_i$ is given by the mixture density

$$p(\boldsymbol{x}_i) = \sum_{j=1}^{k} \pi_j f(\boldsymbol{x}_i \mid \boldsymbol{\alpha}_j) \,, \tag{3}$$

where $\boldsymbol{\pi} = (\pi_1, \ldots, \pi_k)$ contains the corresponding mixture proportions with $\sum_{j=1}^{k} \pi_j = 1,\ 0 < \pi_j < 1$. The density component of mixture j is given by $f(\boldsymbol{x}_i \mid \boldsymbol{\alpha}_j)$ and $\boldsymbol{\alpha}_j$, $j = 1, 2, ..., k$ is the vector of component specific parameters for each density. Then $\boldsymbol{\alpha} = (\boldsymbol{\alpha}_1, \ldots, \boldsymbol{\alpha}_k)$ denotes the vector of all parameters of the model.

The parameters of Dirichlet mixture model, can be estimated using an Expectation-Maximization (EM) algorithm [4]. In our previous work [1] we presented a Hard version [5] of the EM algorithm to estimate the parameters. The log likelihood of the model for a sample of size N is then given by

$$\log p(\boldsymbol{x}_1, \ldots, \boldsymbol{x}_N | \boldsymbol{\alpha}, \pi) = \sum_{i=1}^{N} \log \left[\sum_{j=1}^{k} \pi_j f(\boldsymbol{x}_i | \boldsymbol{\alpha}_j) \right] . \tag{4}$$

Latent variables Z_i's are introduced, which are categorical variables taking on values $1, \ldots, k$ with probabilities $\pi_1, \ldots, \pi_k$ such that $Pr(\boldsymbol{X}_i | Z_i = j) = f(\boldsymbol{x}_i \mid \boldsymbol{\alpha}_j)$, $j = 1, \ldots, k$. The cluster membership probabilities of data point i for cluster j can be obtained by γ_{ij}, where,

$$\gamma_{ij}(x_i) = Pr(Z_i = j | \boldsymbol{x}_i, \boldsymbol{\alpha}_j) = \frac{\pi_j f(\boldsymbol{x}_i | \boldsymbol{\alpha}_j)}{\sum_{j=1}^{k} \pi_j f(\boldsymbol{x}_i | \boldsymbol{\alpha}_j)} . \tag{5}$$

Hard EM maximizes the classification log likelihood; it applies a delta function approximation to the posterior probabilities $Pr(Z_i = j | \boldsymbol{X} = \boldsymbol{x}, \boldsymbol{\alpha})$, where $Z_i, i = 1, \ldots, N$ are the latent variables representing class labels. The approximation changes the E step as follows,

$$Pr(Z_i = j | \boldsymbol{x}_i, \boldsymbol{\alpha}_j) \approx \mathbb{I}(j = z_i^*), \tag{6}$$

where, $z_i^* = \underset{j}{\operatorname{argmax}}\, \gamma_{ij}$. γ_{ij}'s are nothing but the responsibilities (probabilities) for each data point that belongs to different clusters. In other words, it introduces a classification step, where all the data points are classified into different clusters based on the posterior probability. Let N_j be the number of data points in cluster j. Then, the ML estimates of π_j is obtained as $\dfrac{N_j}{N}$. And estimates of $\boldsymbol{\alpha}_j$'s are obtained by finding the MLE using N_j data points in cluster j. However, as the solution is not analytically tractable, some numerical methods need to be used. It is generally done by fixed-point iteration. The iterative equation that needs to be solved is given by

$$\Psi(\alpha_{jm}^{new}) = \Psi(\sum_{m=1}^{p} \alpha_{jm}^{old}) + \frac{1}{N_j} \sum_{i=1}^{N_j} \log(x_{im}) , \tag{7}$$

where, Ψ is the digamma function. The inverse of diggama function is used to get the estimates of α_{jm}. Now, let's explore various approximations to compute the KL distance for DMM.

2.1 KL Divergence: Monte Carlo Approach

Monte Carlo sampling is frequently employed by researchers to compute KL divergence. Let f_a and g_b be two DMMs (see Eq. 3). The approach involves drawing a sample $\boldsymbol{x}_i$ from the probability density function f_a such that,

$$E_{f_a}[\log f_a(\boldsymbol{x}_i)/g_b(\boldsymbol{x}_i)] = D(f_a \| g_b) .$$

Utilizing N independent and identically distributed samples $\{\boldsymbol{x}_i\}_{i=1}^N$, the estimation is expressed as follows:

$$D_{\mathrm{MC}}(f_a \| g_b) = \frac{1}{N} \sum_{i=1}^{N} \log f_a(x_i)/g_b(x_i) \rightarrow D(f_a \| g_b) , \tag{8}$$

as $N \rightarrow \infty$. The variance of the estimation error is $\frac{1}{N}\mathrm{Var}_{f_a}[\log f_a/g_b]$. To compute $D_{\mathrm{MC}}(f \| g)$, it is necessary to generate the independent and identically distributed samples $\{\boldsymbol{x}_i\}_{i=1}^N$ from f_a. Drawing a sample $\boldsymbol{x}_i$ from the DMM f_a involves initially drawing a discrete sample a_i according to the probabilities π_a. Subsequently, a continuous sample $\boldsymbol{x}_i$ is drawn from the resulting Dirichlet component $f_{a_i}(\boldsymbol{x})$. The Monte Carlo method satisfies the similarity property; however, the positivity property does not hold. The identification property is likely to fail only under highly artificial circumstances and with very low probability.

2.2 KL Divergence: Variational Approach

Let us denote $\langle . \rangle$ as the inner product. In our context $\langle . \rangle_x$ means expectation with respect to $\mathbf{x}$.

Theorem 1. *Let $\boldsymbol{X}$ be an $p \times 1$ random vector. Assume two Dirichlet distributions u and v specifying the probability distribution of $\boldsymbol{X}$ as,*

$$u : \boldsymbol{X} \sim \mathrm{Dir}(\alpha_{11}, \ldots, \alpha_{1p})$$
$$v : \boldsymbol{X} \sim \mathrm{Dir}(\alpha_{21}, \ldots, \alpha_{2p}) .$$

Then, the Kullback-Leibler divergence of u from v is given by,

$$\begin{aligned} \mathrm{D}(u \,||\, v) = & \log \frac{\Gamma\left(\sum_{i=1}^{p} \alpha_{1i}\right)}{\Gamma\left(\sum_{i=1}^{p} \alpha_{2i}\right)} + \sum_{i=1}^{p} \log \frac{\Gamma(\alpha_{2i})}{\Gamma(\alpha_{1i})} \\ & + \sum_{i=1}^{p} (\alpha_{1i} - \alpha_{2i}) \left[\psi(\alpha_{1i}) - \psi\left(\sum_{i=1}^{p} \alpha_{1i} \right) \right] . \end{aligned} \tag{9}$$

Proof. For Dirichlet distributions KL divergence is,

$$\begin{aligned} \mathrm{D}(u \,||\, v) &= \int_{\boldsymbol{X}^p} \mathrm{Dir}(\boldsymbol{x}; \alpha_{11}, \ldots, \alpha_{1p}) \log \frac{\mathrm{Dir}(\boldsymbol{x}; \alpha_{11}, \ldots, \alpha_{1p})}{\mathrm{Dir}(\boldsymbol{x}; \alpha_{21}, \ldots, \alpha_{2p})} \, \mathrm{d}\boldsymbol{x} \\ &= \left\langle \log \frac{\mathrm{Dir}(x; \alpha_{11}, \ldots, \alpha_{1p})}{\mathrm{Dir}(x; \alpha_{21}, \ldots, \alpha_{2p})} \right\rangle_{u(\boldsymbol{x})} \end{aligned} \tag{10}$$

We can do some algebraic manipulations using the probability density function of the Dirichlet distribution to get,

$$\begin{aligned}
\mathrm{D}(u\,||\,v) &= \left\langle \log \frac{\frac{\Gamma(\sum_{i=1}^{p}\alpha_{1i})}{\prod_{i=1}^{p}\Gamma(\alpha_{1i})} \prod_{i=1}^{p} {x_i}^{\alpha_{1i}-1}}{\frac{\Gamma(\sum_{i=1}^{p}\alpha_{2i})}{\prod_{i=1}^{p}\Gamma(\alpha_{2i})} \prod_{i=1}^{p} {x_i}^{\alpha_{2i}-1}} \right\rangle_{u(\boldsymbol{x})} \\
&= \log \frac{\Gamma\left(\sum_{i=1}^{p}\alpha_{1i}\right)}{\Gamma\left(\sum_{i=1}^{p}\alpha_{2i}\right)} + \sum_{i=1}^{p} \log \frac{\Gamma(\alpha_{2i})}{\Gamma(\alpha_{1i})} + \sum_{i=1}^{p} (\alpha_{1i} - \alpha_{2i}) \cdot \langle \log x_i \rangle_{u(\boldsymbol{x})} \ .
\end{aligned}$$

Moreover,

$$\langle \log \boldsymbol{x}_i \rangle = \psi(\alpha_i) - \psi\left(\sum_{i=1}^{p}\alpha_i\right) .$$

Thus the Kullback-Leibler divergence of u from v becomes:

$$\mathrm{D}(u\,||\,v) = \log \frac{\Gamma\left(\sum_{i=1}^{p}\alpha_{1i}\right)}{\Gamma\left(\sum_{i=1}^{p}\alpha_{2i}\right)} + \sum_{i=1}^{p} \log \frac{\Gamma(\alpha_{2i})}{\Gamma(\alpha_{1i})} + \sum_{i=1}^{p} (\alpha_{1i} - \alpha_{2i}) \left[\psi(\alpha_{1i}) - \psi\left(\sum_{i=1}^{p}\alpha_{1i}\right)\right] .$$

Proposition 1. *Let f_a and g_b be two DMMs such that,*

$$f_a = f(x) = \sum_a \pi_a Dir(\boldsymbol{x}; \boldsymbol{\alpha}_a)$$

$$g_b = g(x) = \sum_b \omega_b Dir(\boldsymbol{x}; \boldsymbol{\alpha}_b)$$

Then using a variational approach, an approximated KL divergence can be expressed as,

$$D_{\text{variational}}(f||g) = \sum_a \pi_a \log \frac{\sum_{a'} \pi_{a'} e^{-D(f_a||f_{a'})}}{\sum_b \omega_b e^{-D(f_a||g_b)}} . \tag{11}$$

Proof. [6] has provided a similar proof for Gaussian Mixture Models. That approach can be adopted for DMMs as well. We can define the log-likelihood,$L_f(g)$ as, $L_f(g) = \langle[\log g(\boldsymbol{x})]\rangle_{f(\boldsymbol{x})}$. Then KL divergence can be written in terms of log-likelihood in the following way.

$$D(f||g) = L_f(f) - L_f(g) \ . \tag{12}$$

We define variational parameters,$\phi_{b|a} > 0$ such that $\Sigma_b \phi_{b|a} = 1$. Using Jensen's inequality we can show,

$$\begin{aligned} L_f(g) &\stackrel{\text{def}}{=} \langle \log g(x) \rangle_{f(x)} \\ &= \left\langle \log \sum_b \omega_b g_b(x) \right\rangle_{f(x)} \\ &= \left\langle \log \sum_b \phi_{b|a} \frac{\omega_b g_b(x)}{\phi_{b|a}} \right\rangle_{f(x)} \\ &\geq \left\langle \sum_b \phi_{b|a} \log \frac{\omega_b g_b(x)}{\phi_{b|a}} \right\rangle_{f(x)} \\ &\stackrel{\text{def}}{=} \mathcal{L}_f(g, \phi) . \end{aligned} \tag{13}$$

The above is a lower bound on $L_f(g)$. We can get the best bound by maximizing $\mathcal{L}_f(g, \phi)$ with respect to ϕ. The maximum value is obtained with:

$$\hat{\phi}_{b|a} = \frac{\omega_b e^{-D(f_a \| g_b)}}{\sum_b' \pi_b' e^{-D(f_a \| g_{b'})}} . \tag{14}$$

Likewise, we define ,

$$\mathcal{L}_f(f, \psi) \stackrel{\text{def}}{=} \left\langle \sum_{a'} \psi_{a'|a} \log \frac{\pi_{a'} f_{a'}(x)}{\psi_{a'|a}} \right\rangle_{f(x)} . \tag{15}$$

The optimal $\psi_{a'|a}$ is given by,

$$\hat{\psi}_{a'|a} = \frac{\pi_{a'} e^{-D(f_a \| f_{a'})}}{\sum_{\hat{a}} \pi_{\hat{a}} e^{-D(f_a \| f_{\hat{a}})}} \tag{16}$$

Now, like Eq. 12, we can define $D_{\text{variational}}(f \| g) = \mathcal{L}_f(f, \hat{\psi}) - \mathcal{L}_f(g, \hat{\phi})$. After substituting $\hat{\phi}_{b|a}$ and $\hat{\psi}_{a'|a}$, we finally get,

$$D_{\text{variational}}(f \| g) = \sum_a \pi_a \log \frac{\sum_{a'} \pi_{a'} e^{-D(f_a \| f_{a'})}}{\sum_b \omega_b e^{-D(f_a \| g_b)}} .$$

$D_{\text{variational}}(f \| g)$ satisfies the self similarity and self identification property. However, it may not always satisfy the positivity property. In that case we may use the absolute value of the divergence.

3 Results

We conducted extensive experiments using both simulated and real data sets, including three simulated data sets (Data Set 1, Data Set 2, Data Set 3) drawn from different Dirichlet distributions and a real gene expression data set (Modencodefly Data [7]). Data Set 3 and Modencodefly Data are highdimensional in nature. The Modencodefly Data has been pre-processed and top 75 genes were chosen based on variation. Each experiment was conducted only once. The primary metrics for comparison were the Kullback-Leibler (KL) Divergence and the time taken for each approach.

Table 1. Comparison of KL Divergence and Time Taken for Different Data Sets

Data Set	(N, p, k)	Metric	Variational	Monte Carlo $n = 10000$	Monte Carlo $n = 100000$	Monte Carlo $n = 1000000$
Data Set 1	(4200, 3,3)	KL Div	0.0017	0.0024	0.0021	0.0017
		Time	**0.0004**	1.7	17.3391	181.3682
Data Set 2	(4200, 3,3)	KL Div	0.0022	0.0024	0.0024	0.0022
		Time	**0.0005**	1.7283	17.4883	180.9482
Data Set 3	(230, 75,6)	KL Div	6.2723	6.1737	6.1815	6.1824
		Time	**0.0014**	3.6702	37.4568	384.2183
Modencodefly	(147, 75,6)	KL Div	34.7652	33.5581	33.5471	33.5579
		Time	**0.0014**	3.6353	36.0671	375.7836

From Table 1, it is evident that our proposed variational approach consistently provided faster solutions for all data sets. Notably, the Monte Carlo method yielded KL Divergence values closer to the variational method as we increase the number of samples, which increases the execution time to a great extent. When $N \to \infty$ Monte Carlo technique offers accurate KL divergence, as the variance of the estimation error becomes zero. From our results we see that with increasing N, the KL divergence obtained using Monte Carlo technique approaches that of variational technique, implying that variational technique offers more accurate results than Monte Carlo technique for moderate N with much less execution time, indicating that our solution is more robust and applicable for practical applications.

4 Conclusion

This study addresses the efficient estimation of Kullback-Leibler (KL) Divergence in Dirichlet Mixture Models (DMM). Despite the analytical tractability of KL Divergence for Dirichlet distributions, extending it to DMMs has been challenging, leading past research to rely on computationally intensive Monte Carlo methods. In response, we propose a novel variational approach, providing a closed-form solution that significantly enhances computational efficiency. The method is validated using both simulated and real-world datasets, demonstrating superior efficiency and accuracy over traditional Monte Carlo-based methods. Notably, our approach exhibits robustness by providing accurate solutions which can be achieved only by a very large number of samples using Monte Carlo based methods. This transformative solution opens avenues for rapid exploration of diverse DMM models, advancing statistical analyses of RNA-seq data in gene co-expression analysis.

References

1. Pal, S., Heumann, C.: Clustering compositional data using Dirichlet mixture model. Plos One **17**(5), e0268,438 (2022)
2. Csiszár, I.: I-divergence geometry of probability distributions and minimization problems. Ann. Probabil. 146–158 (1975)
3. Ma, Z., Rana, P.K., Taghia, J., Flierl, M., Leijon, A.: Bayesian estimation of Dirichlet mixture model with variational inference. Pattern Recogn. **47**(9), 3143–3157 (2014)
4. Dempster, A.P., Laird, N.M., Rubin, D.B.: Maximum likelihood from incomplete data via the EM algorithm. J. Roy. Stat. Soc.: Ser. B (Methodol.) **39**(1), 1–22 (1977)
5. Celeux, G., Govaert, G.: A classification EM algorithm for clustering and two stochastic versions. Comput. Stat. Data Anal. **14**(3), 315–332 (1992)
6. Hershey, J.R., Olsen, P.A.: Approximating the kullback leibler divergence between gaussian mixture models. In: 2007 IEEE International Conference on Acoustics, Speech and Signal Processing-ICASSP 2007, vol. 4, pp. IV–317. IEEE (2007)
7. Graveley, B.R., et al.: The developmental transcriptome of drosophila melanogaster. Nature **471**(7339), 473–479 (2011)

Optimizing Variable Selection in Multi-Omics Datasets: A Focus on Exclusive Lasso

Dayasri Ravi(✉) and Andreas Groll

Department of Statistics, TU Dortmund University, Vogelpothsweg 78, 44227 Dortmund, Germany
{ravi,groll}@statistik.tu-dortmund.de

Abstract. Multi-omics datasets pose significant challenges due to their structured nature, where highly correlated variables are grouped within a complex, high-dimensional framework. Traditional Lasso methods encounter limitations in handling correlated features within these groups effectively. To address this issue, we propose using Exclusive Lasso, focusing on inducing sparsity at the intra-group level. Additionally, we introduce an efficient algorithm for solving the related optimization problem. By prioritizing feature selection robustness within correlated group structures, our proposed methodology offers a promising solution to the challenges inherent in analyzing biological datasets. This advancement enhances our ability to extract meaningful insights from multi-omics data, thus facilitating deeper understanding and exploration of complex biological systems.

Keywords: Variable selection · Composite penalty · Exclusive Lasso

1 Introduction

Effectively utilizing multi-omics data, encompassing genomics, epigenomics, transcriptomics, proteomics, metabolomics, and microbiomics, presents a considerable challenge. The critical characteristic of multi-omics data lies in the extensive dimensionality of the datasets. This poses specific requirements for constructing prediction models, as they must handle datasets where the number of variables significantly surpasses the number of observations. Another challenge in working with multi-omics data is its structured nature, where variables are grouped into non overlapping categories. This structural organization should be considered when constructing prediction models. A crucial aspect of multi-omics data is the high dimensionality within each omic group of datasets. In such scenarios, incorporating the group structure during model building or prioritizing clinical variables becomes beneficial. Otherwise, clinical variables which are very few in number may be overshadowed by the vast amount of omics data. It is widely recognized that a substantial portion of omics data lacks informativeness for prediction due to redundancy or irrelevance [1,2]. The importance of feature

J. Einbeck et al. (Eds.): IWSM 2024, CONTRIB.STAT., pp. 142–147, 2024.
https://doi.org/10.1007/978-3-031-65723-8_22

selection is indisputable, often requiring sparse and interpretable models that include only a limited number of variables.

Various group regularizers, including the well-known Group Lasso [3], have been extensively explored to address this challenge. Group Lasso employs $L_{2,1}$-norm regularization to promote sparsity between groups. This means that features within the same group, such as genomics or proteomics, are either selected or excluded together. However, genomics data are typically grouped together due to their high correlation. Incorporating inter-group sparsity could lead to overlooking this interdependence among groups. We propose the Exclusive Lasso [4], incorporating an $L_{1,2}$-norm regularization term to address this challenge. This term promotes sparsity within groups while allowing for a relaxation of sparsity between groups, ensuring that at least one variable from each group is selected. We introduce the *Newton Method-$L_{1,2}$ Sparsity Algorithm* (*NM-$L_{1,2}$ Sparsity Algorithm*) as an alternative estimation approach for the Exclusive Lasso, employing a quadratic approximation of the $L_{1,2}$-norm.

The paper is organized as follows. Section 2 introduces the Exclusive Lasso technique and the new estimation procedure. Results from simulation studies and real-data applications are presented in Sect. 3 and Sect. 4 concludes.

2 Methods

For $\boldsymbol{\beta} = (\beta_1, \ldots, \beta_p)^\top$, we consider the problem of the form

$$\min_{\boldsymbol{\beta}} f(\boldsymbol{\beta}) = L(\boldsymbol{\beta}) + \frac{\lambda}{2} \sum_{g \subset \mathcal{G}} \left(\sum_{k \in g} |\beta_k| \right)^2, \tag{1}$$

where $L(\boldsymbol{\beta})$ is a loss function, $\lambda \geq 0$ is the penalty parameter and $\mathcal{G}$ is a collection of non-overlapping predefined groups of indices g such that $\bigcup_{g \subset \mathcal{G}} = \{1, \ldots, p\}$.

Following [5], we use a quadratic approximation for the transformation of the L_1 norm into a differentiable function given by $|x| \approx \sqrt{x^2 + c}$. Here, c is a small positive number. With this approximation, the penalty term from Eq. (1) can be rewritten as

$$P(\boldsymbol{\beta}) = \frac{1}{2} \sum_{g \subset \mathcal{G}} \left(\sum_{k \in g} \sqrt{\beta_k^2 + c} \right)^2. \tag{2}$$

Let $S = \{1, \ldots, p\}$ be the set of indices corresponding to the entries of $\boldsymbol{\beta}$. We construct square matrices $\mathbf{M}_g$ with dimensions $|S \cap g|$ such that

$$\mathbf{M}_{g_{ij}} = \begin{cases} 1, & \text{if } i = 1, \\ 0, & \text{if } i > 1. \end{cases}$$

Let $\mathbf{B} \in \mathbb{R}^{p \times 1}$ represent the vector $\left(\sqrt{(\beta_1^2 + c)}, \ldots, \sqrt{(\beta_p^2 + c)} \right)^\top$, then

$$\frac{\partial \mathbf{B}}{\partial \beta_k} = \frac{\beta_k}{\sqrt{(\beta_k^2 + c)}} \quad \& \quad \frac{\partial^2 \mathbf{B}}{\partial \beta_k^2} = \frac{c}{(\beta_k^2 + c)^{\frac{3}{2}}}.$$

We rewrite the penalty term as $0.5 \cdot (\mathbf{GB})^{\mathbf{T}}\mathbf{GB}$, where $\mathbf{G} \in \mathbb{R}^{p \times p}$ is a block diagonal matrix with matrices $\mathbf{M}_g$. Using matrix and vector differentiation rules, the gradient and Hessian of the penalty term $P(\boldsymbol{\beta})$ can be derived as

$$\frac{\partial}{\partial \beta_k} P(\boldsymbol{\beta}) = \mathbf{B}^{\mathbf{T}}(\mathbf{C} + \mathbf{C}^{\mathbf{T}}) \frac{\partial \mathbf{B}}{\partial \beta_k}$$

where $\mathbf{C} \in \mathbb{R}^{p \times p} = \mathbf{G}^{\mathbf{T}}\mathbf{G}$. With $\mathbf{D} \in \mathbb{R}^{p \times p} = \mathbf{C} + \mathbf{C}^{\mathbf{T}}$, we obtain

$$\frac{\partial^2}{\partial \beta_k^2} P(\boldsymbol{\beta}) = \left[\frac{\partial \mathbf{B}}{\partial \beta_k} \mathbf{D}^T \frac{\partial \mathbf{B}}{\partial \beta_k} + \mathbf{B}^T \mathbf{D} \frac{\partial^2 \mathbf{B}}{\partial \beta_k^2} \right].$$

We perform Newton iterations of the form $\boldsymbol{\beta}^{(l+1)} := \boldsymbol{\beta}^{(l)} - t(\nabla^2 g(\boldsymbol{\beta}^{(l)}))^{-1} \nabla g(\boldsymbol{\beta}^{(l)})$, where $g(\boldsymbol{\beta})$ is a continuous and twice-differentiable approximation function of $f(\boldsymbol{\beta})$. Following [6], we choose step size t using a back-tracking line search satisfying the Armijo condition.

3 Results

We evaluate our algorithm by comparing it with the standard Lasso [7] using simulated data and a real-world multi-omics dataset.

3.1 Simulation Studies

Following [4], we simulate two examples with $n = 100$ observations and $p = 100$ variables. In the first example, the variables are divided into four equal groups, with the true parameter being non-zero in the first index of each group. The data is simulated from a multivariate normal distribution with a Toeplitz covariance matrix with entries $\Sigma_{i,j} = a^{|i-j|}$ for variables in the same group, and $\Sigma_{i,j} = b^{|i-j|}$ for variables in different groups. For the first covariance matrix, we opt for a strong correlation of $a = b = 0.9$, simulating high correlation both within and between groups. For the second scenario, we use a moderate correlation of $a = 0.9$ and $b = 0.6$, resulting in high correlation within and medium correlation between group. Finally, for the third scenario, both within- and between-group correlations are set at a moderate level of $a = b = 0.6$. We repeat the same set of scenarios for the second example. Here, the variables are divided into the same four equal groups, with the true parameter being non-zero in more than one index of each group. In all the above scenarios, the data is simulated using the model $\boldsymbol{y} = \boldsymbol{X}\boldsymbol{\beta} + \boldsymbol{\varepsilon}$ where $\boldsymbol{\varepsilon} \sim \mathcal{N}(0, 1)$ and $\lambda = \max_i |\boldsymbol{X}_i^T \boldsymbol{y}|$. We report the results in terms of average variable selection accuracy, standard error (SE), and root mean square error (RMSE) on external test data for 50 simulations in Table 1 and 2 (Figs. 1 and 2).

Table 1. Example 1: Comparison of variable selection methods

		NM-$L_{1,2}$	Lasso
Scenario 1	Accuracy (SE)	**0.74** (0.015)	0.31 (0.015)
	RMSE	**1.35**	2.349
Scenario 2	Accuracy (SE)	**0.86** (0.022)	0.33 (0.017)
	RMSE	**1.37**	2.178
Scenario 3	Accuracy (SE)	**0.95** (0.015)	0.36 (0.018)
	RMSE	**1.65**	2.208

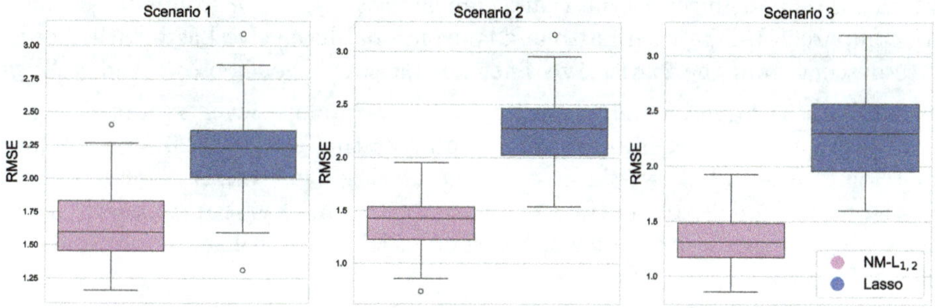

Fig. 1. Example 1: Root Mean Square Error (RMSE) for Two Models

Table 2. Example 2: Comparison of variable selection methods

		NM-$L_{1,2}$	Lasso
Scenario 1	Accuracy (SE)	**0.84** (0.024)	0.29 (0.015)
	RMSE	**2.07**	4.15
Scenario 2	Accuracy (SE)	**0.91** (0.017)	0.31 (0.015)
	RMSE	**2.22**	3.89
Scenario 3	Accuracy (SE)	**0.95** (0.011)	0.30 (0.014)
	RMSE	**2.52**	3.66

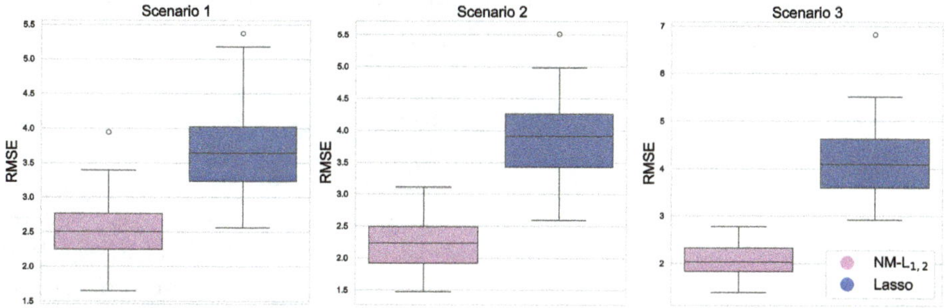

Fig. 2. Example 2: Root Mean Square Error (RMSE) for Two Models

3.2 Down Syndrome Analysis

We validate the effectiveness of the proposed variable selection algorithm using multi-omics data to predict Down Syndrome. Down Syndrome (DS) is attributed to the presence of either a complete or partial extra copy of human chromosome 21 (HSA21) [8]. It is the most common genetic condition in humans, occurring in about 1 in 700 live births. Our data comprises of 29 individuals with DS, along with their mothers and unaffected siblings. The family-centric approach is preferred as it allows for a comprehensive examination of potential influences on DNA methylation patterns, encompassing both genetic and environmental (lifestyle) factors within familial contexts. There are two molecular data types (methylation and glycomics data) and clinical data, i.e., three groups of variables. We compare *NM-*$L_{1,2}$ with Lasso and conventional Exclusive Lasso with coordinate descent from the `Exclusive Lasso` R package. We choose $\lambda = \max_i |\boldsymbol{X}_i^T \boldsymbol{y}|$ such that it is large enough to estimate one variable in each group. We randomly split the dataset into a training and a testing set, with 20% of the data for testing. Figure 3 shows the Receiver Operating Characteristic (ROC) curve for the three models. In contrast to the other two models, our approach showcases superior predictive performance, emphasizing the utilization of optimally chosen features.

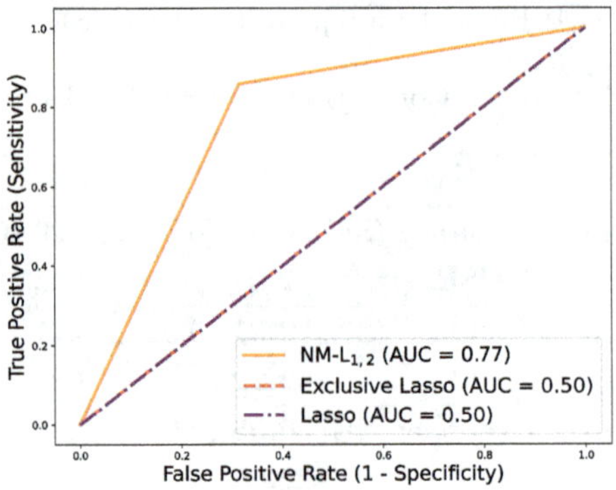

Fig. 3. Receiver Operating Characteristic (ROC) Curve for Three Models

4 Conclusion

In this work, we develop a novel algorithm to solve the Exclusive Lasso problem. Our findings demonstrate superior performance, surpassing that of standard Lasso, particularly in scenarios with highly correlated features. We propose the use of Exclusive Lasso for within-group variable selection, frequently encountered in biological datasets, especially in the context of multi-omics studies.

Acknowledgments. This work has been supported by the Research Training Group "Biostatistical Methods for High-Dimensional Data in Toxicology" (RTG 2624, Project R2) funded by the Deutsche Forschungsgemeinschaft (DFG, German Research Foundation-Project Number 427806116).

References

1. Libralon, G.L., de Carvalho, A.C.P.D.L.F., Lorena, A.C.: Pre-processing for noise detection in gene expression classification data. J. Braz. Comput. Soc. **15**, 3–11 (2009)
2. Li, Y., Mansmann, U., Du, S., Hornung, R.: Benchmark study of feature selection strategies for multi-omics data. BMC Bioinf. **23**(1), 412 (2022)
3. Yuan, M., Lin, Y.: Model selection and estimation in regression with grouped variables. J. R. Stat. Soc. Ser. B Stat Methodol. **68**(1), 49–67 (2006)
4. Campbell, F., Allen, G.I.: Within group variable selection through the exclusive lasso (2017)
5. Oelker, M.R., Tutz, G.: A uniform framework for the combination of penalties in generalized structured models. Adv. Data Anal. Classif. **11**(1), 97–120 (2017)
6. Schmidt, M., Fung, G., Rosales, R.: Fast optimization methods for L1 regularization: a comparative study and two new approaches. In: Kok, J.N., Koronacki, J., Mantaras, R.L., Matwin, S., Mladenič, D., Skowron, A. (eds.) ECML 2007. LNCS (LNAI), vol. 4701, pp. 286–297. Springer, Heidelberg (2007). https://doi.org/10.1007/978-3-540-74958-5_28
7. Tibshirani, R.: Regression shrinkage and selection via the lasso. J. R. Stat. Soc. Ser. B Stat Methodol. **58**(1), 267–288 (1996)
8. Bacalini, M.G., et al.: Identification of a DNA methylation signature in blood cells from persons with down syndrome. Aging (Albany NY) **7**(2), 82 (2015)

Non-parametric Frailty Model for the Natural History of Prostate Cancer; Using Data from a Screening Trial

Ilse Cuevas Andrade[1](✉), Ardo van den Hout[1], and Nora Pashayan[2]

[1] University College London, Gower Street, London WC1E 6BT, UK
{ilse.andrade.21,ardo.vandenhout}@ucl.ac.uk
[2] University of Cambridge, Trinity Lane, Cambridge, England CB2 1TN, UK

Abstract. Mixed-effects models for survival, known as frailty models, can be used to capture individual or cluster-specific unobserved heterogeneity. A common choice is assuming the random effects follow a parametric distribution, e.g. a normal distribution. However, computing the marginal likelihood can be computationally expensive and infeasible in a high-dimension setting. Alternatively, a non-parametric approach avoids the normality assumption for random effects and can be less computationally demanding. The data used are from the Prostate, Lung, Colorectal, and Ovarian (PLCO) Cancer Screening Trial. The aim is to model prostate cancer progression to evaluate screening strategies, considering the PSA longitudinal biomarker, accounting for unobserved heterogeneity, interval-censored, left-truncation, and right-censored data.

Keywords: Continuous-time Markov model · Latent-class model · Cancer screening

1 Introduction

Prostate cancer is the second most commonly diagnosed cancer in men. The prostate-specific antigen (PSA) test measures the PSA levels in the blood. A PSA level above 3.0 or 4.0 ng/mL can be considered abnormal. However, different factors can cause the PSA level to fluctuate. The PSA levels can be used to assess if further clinical investigation is required, i.e. imaging or biopsy studies.

Different models have been proposed to include PSA when modelling disease progression. Following a multi-state framework, a mixed-effects model for survival can be fitted, known as the frailty model. The frailty term, as a random effect, can be specified for an individual or can be cluster-specific. One way to specify this type of model is by assuming a parametric frailty distribution, e.g. log-normal or gamma frailty. The former is a common choice, followed by using the Gauss-Hermite quadrature to estimate the marginal likelihood. An optimisation that includes integration can be computationally expensive and can become infeasible in a high-dimension setting.

J. Einbeck et al. (Eds.): IWSM 2024, CONTRIB.STAT., pp. 148–152, 2024.
https://doi.org/10.1007/978-3-031-65723-8_23

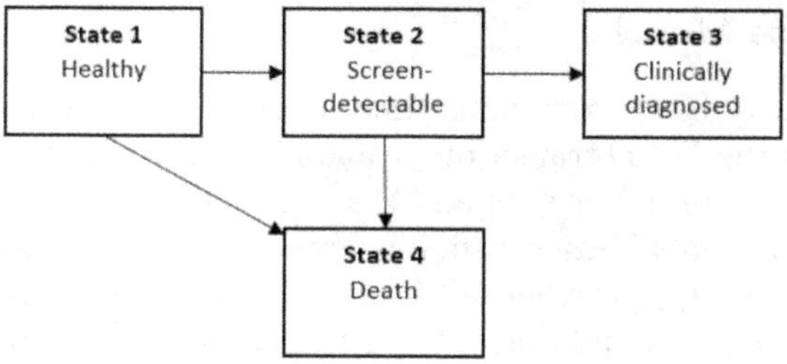

Fig. 1. Four-state progressive model for prostate cancer.

Conversely, a non-parametric frailty approach removes the assumption of normality for the random effects, and there is no need to estimate the marginal likelihood.

In this study, we consider panel data from the (PLCO) Cancer Screening Trial. The trial included 76,685 men who were randomised and split into a screening and control group. The screening group received an annual PSA test for six years. The men were aged 55 to 74 and followed up for a median of 13 years.

We aim to extend the four-state natural history model developed by Bhatt et al. [2] to account for unobserved heterogeneity; see Fig. 1. We propose a multi-state non-parametric frailty model to consider unobserved heterogeneity linking the biomarker trajectories with the transition probability from a healthy to a screen-detectable state. This model can inform screening frequency before transitioning to a clinically diagnosed state.

2 Methods

The model contains K latent classes, each representing a subpopulation. We conduct the maximum likelihood estimation on the K classes. Logistic regression models the probability of a subject belonging to a latent class. The longitudinal submodel, multi-state model, and likelihood function are described in the following sections.

2.1 Longitudinal Submodel

Denoting z_{ij} as a repeated PSA measurement for subject i at time jth, the longitudinal model for z_{ij} is

$$\mu_{ij.k}(t) = \log(z_{ij} + 1) = \gamma_{1.k} + \gamma_{2.k} t_{ij} + \epsilon_{ij} , \quad (1)$$

where $\epsilon_{ij} \overset{\text{iid}}{\sim} N(0, \sigma)$, and $k \in \{1, 2\}$. The PSA values increase exponentially in some prostate cancer cases. The natural logarithm of the PSA values was used as the dependent variable in the longitudinal submodel.

2.2 Multi-state Model

Let $\{Y_t \mid t \in [0, \infty)\}$ be a continuous-time Markov chain on the state space S, and let $P(t, u)$ be the $D \times D$ transition probability matrix with entries $p_{rs}(t, u) = P(Y_u = s \mid Y_t = r)$, for $0 \leq t \leq u$, and $r, s = 1 \ldots D$.

The transition probabilities can be derived from the transition hazards, $P(t, u) = \exp((u - t)Q(t))$, where Q is the $D \times D$ generator matrix with off-diagonal (r, s) entries q_{rs} and diagonal entries $q_{rr} = -\sum_{s \neq r} q_{rs}$.

The transition-specific hazards can be defined by combining a baseline hazard with a log-linear regression $q_{rs}(t \mid x) = q_{rs.0}(t) \exp\left(\beta_{rs}^{\top} x\right)$, where $\beta_{rs} = (\beta_{rs.1}, \ldots, \beta_{rs.p})^{\top}$ is a parameter vector, and $x = (x_1 \ldots x_p)^{\top}$ is the covariate vector.

Defining the natural history of prostate cancer as presented in Fig. 1, the transition hazards for the multi-state model are defined by

$$\begin{aligned} q_{12.k}(t) &= \exp\left(\beta_{12} + \alpha_{12.k}\mu_{ij.k}(t)\right) \\ q_{14.k} &= \exp\left(\beta_{14}\right) = q_{24.k} \\ q_{23.k} &= \exp\left(\beta_{23}\right) \end{aligned} \tag{2}$$

,

where $\mu_{ij.k}(t)$ is defined by (1), and $k \in \{1, 2\}$. Following the model assumptions defined by Bhatt et al. [2], the parameter constraints for this model are such that $q_{14.k} = q_{24.k}$.

2.3 Likelihood Function

We adapt the non-parametric maximum likelihood estimation of mixed models by Aitkin [1] to our multi-state framework. Assuming $\mathbf{y} = (y_1, \ldots, y_J)$ are the observed states of individual i, and considering the presence of classes $C_k, k = 1, \ldots, K$. with probability of class-membership $P(i \in C_k)$. The likelihood function contribution of individual i can be written as

$$\begin{aligned} L_i(\boldsymbol{\theta} \mid \mathbf{y}, \mathbf{x}) &= P\left(Y_J = y_J, \ldots, Y_2 = y_2 \mid Y_1 = y_1, \boldsymbol{\theta}, \mathbf{x}\right) \\ &= \sum_{k=1}^{K} P\left(Y_J = y_J, \ldots, Y_2 = y_2 \mid Y_1 = y_1, \boldsymbol{\theta}, \mathbf{x}, i \in C_k\right) P\left(i \in C_k\right), \end{aligned} \tag{3}$$

where K is the number of classes.

Let $\pi_k = P(i \in C_k), k = 1, \ldots, K$, be defined as the *masses*. The estimation of the masses, π_k, are subject to the restriction $\sum_{k=1}^{K} \pi_k = 1$. This can be conducted using a logit transformation. Let $K = 2$, then the masses can be estimated by $\pi_1 = \frac{1}{1+\exp(\psi_1)}$, and $\pi_2 = 1 - \pi_1$, with $\psi_1 \in \mathbb{R}$. Then, the likelihood function $L = \prod_{i=1}^{N} L_i(\boldsymbol{\theta} \mid \mathbf{y}, \mathbf{x})$, for all N individuals can be optimised using a general-purpose optimiser, e.g. `optim` in R.

3 Application

The PLCO trial included 76,685 men who were randomised into the screening and control groups. The screening group received an annual PSA test for six years. The observed transitions from the screening group can only be from healthy to screen-detectable, right-censored, or dead, whereas the control group can only be observed transitioning from a healthy state to clinically diagnosed, right-censored, or dead. Given the study design, identifiability can be a challenge.

For this exploratory research, we sampled 7000 individuals randomly, considering 3500 individuals per group. We fitted the frailty multi-state model defined in Sect. 2, considering the four-state model illustrated in Fig. 1. The general-purpose optimiser `optim` in R was used to maximise the likelihood function. The delta method was applied to derive the standard errors for the masses π_k. The estimates and standard errors are shown in Table 1.

Table 1. Estimated parameters for the four-state mover/stayer non-parametric maximum likelihood Model with $K = 2$. S.E. stands for standard errors.

Parameters	Estimates	SE	Class C_1 parameters		
β_{12}	−7.363	0.446	Parameters	Estimates	SE
$\alpha_{12.1}$	4.107	0.643	b_1	−1.765	0.045
$\alpha_{12.2}$	2.106	0.294	π_1	0.854	0.006
β_{23}	−0.810	0.106			
β_D	−4.355	0.030			
$\gamma_{1.1}$	−0.032	0.042			
$\gamma_{1.2}$	0.111	0.006			
$\gamma_{2.1}$	0.129	0.083			
$\gamma_{2.2}$	0.212	0.013			
$\sigma = \exp(\theta)$	$\exp(-1.146) = 0.318$	0.002			

The probability of belonging to C_1 is estimated to be 0.854 with a standard error of 0.006, as shown in Table 1. The estimates and standard errors are in Table 1. The association parameter for both classes is positive, meaning a higher PSA value increases the transition hazard from a healthy state to a screen-detectable state. Table 1 shows that individuals in class C_1 (movers) are more likely to move to the next living state than individuals in class C_2 (stayers). This is given by the class-specific association parameter $\alpha_{12.k}$; class C_1 has a higher coefficient.

The extension of this model will be explored by fitting more flexible forms for the longitudinal submodel, allowing time-varying hazards for the transition to death and accounting for left-truncation data.

Acknowledgements. Research reported in this publication was supported by the National Cancer Institute (NCI) of the National Institutes of Health under Award Number U01CA253915. The authors thank the National Cancer Institute for access to

NCI's data collected by the Prostate, Lung, Colorectal and Ovarian (PLCO) Cancer Screening Trial. The statements contained herein are solely those of the authors and do not represent or imply concurrence or endorsement by NCI.

References

1. Aitkin, M.: A general maximum likelihood analysis of variance components in generalized linear models. Biometrics **55**, 117–128 (1999)
2. Bhatt, R., van den Hout, A., Pashayan, N.: A multistate survival model of the natural history of cancer using data from screened and unscreened populations. Stat. Med. **40**, 3791–3807 (2021)

Parametric and Non-parametric Bayesian Imputation for Right Censored Survival Data

Shirin Moghaddam[1(✉)], John Newell[2], and John Hinde[2]

[1] Department of Mathematics and Statistics (MACSI), University of Limerick, Limerick, Ireland
shirin.moghaddam@ul.ie

[2] School of Mathematical and Statistical Sciences, University of Galway, Galway, Ireland
{john.newell,john.hinde}@universityofgalway.ie

Abstract. A common feature of much survival data is censoring due to incompletely observed lifetimes. Survival analysis methods have been designed to take account of this and provide appropriate relevant summaries, such as the Kaplan-Meier plot and the median is easily read off this plot. However, a single summary is not really a relevant quantity for communication to an individual patient, as it conveys no notion of variability and uncertainty. The aim of this paper is to consider censored data as a form of missing data and impute them using Bayesian methods. We introduce two novel parametric and non-parametric Bayesian approaches for imputing right censored observations to be used as a complement to formal inferential methods and to allow more interpretable displays to be made for physicians and patients.

Keywords: Survival Analysis · Bayesian Methods · Imputation Methods · Dirichlet process · Censored Observation

1 Introduction

The main interest in survival analyses is studying the time to an event (usually death, recurrence or remission). In survival analysis subjects are followed until the event of interest has happened. Subjects who do not experience the event are referred to as censored. Due to censoring, methods of plotting individual survival times such as the histogram or the density plot are invalid. Therefore, graphical displays of time-to-event data usually take the form of a Kaplan-Meier survival plot, and the median is easily read off this plot. However, a density plot of the data is perhaps more informative than a single summary statistic, Gould (1985). By imputing values for the censored observations and combining original complete and imputed data, it is possible to plot the histogram or density of the complete data to complement the information given by Kaplan-Meier plots.

J. Einbeck et al. (Eds.): IWSM 2024, CONTRIB.STAT., pp. 153–158, 2024.
https://doi.org/10.1007/978-3-031-65723-8_24

2 Methods

For a flexible approach to impute censored observations using predictive distributions we review the previously published parametric framework (Moghaddam et al., 2022) and present a new non-parametric Bayesian approach.

2.1 Parametric Bayesian Approach

In the parametric approach to impute censored observations in a Bayesian framework, a specific distribution needs to be considered for the survival times. To represent the imputation method, we consider a general parametric model for the data that depends on a parameter θ, say $f(t|\theta)$. Also $p(\theta)$ is assumed as a prior distribution for θ, which is independent of any observed data. By using Bayes theorem, the prior distribution $p(\theta)$ is updated to a posterior distribution $p(\theta|D) \propto p(D|\theta)p(\theta)$, where D denotes the observed data. The density for the survival time conditional on a (right) censoring time is:

$$f(t \mid T \geq c, \theta) = \frac{f(t \mid \theta)}{S(c \mid \theta)}, \quad t \geq c \tag{1}$$

where $S(c|\theta) = P(T \geq c \mid \theta)$.

For the imputation approach, individual sample values from the predictive distribution, conditional on the observed censoring time, can be generated using the following density:

$$f(t \mid T \geq c, D) = \int f(t \mid T \geq c, \theta)p(\theta \mid D)d\theta \tag{2}$$

Suppose we have a posterior density $p(\theta|D)$ and that we can generate a random sample from this distribution, say $\theta^{(1)}, \theta^{(2)}, ..., \theta^{(s)}$ where $\theta^{(s)}$ is the s-th component of the sample. Then to sample $t^{(k)}$, observations from the predictive conditional distribution, first of all, $\theta^{(k)}$ are sampled from the posterior density $p(\theta \mid D)$, then $t^{(k)}$ are generated from the density $f(t \mid T \geq c, \theta^{(k)})$. The sampled $t^{(k)}$ is a draw from the predictive distribution conditional on the observed censoring time. This can be done repeatedly to obtain a Monte Carlo sample $\{t^{(k)} : k = 1, ..., s\}$. The mean of the predictive distribution can be approximated numerically by $\sum_{k=1}^{s} t^{(k)}/s$, and the median of the predictive distribution by the median of the sample.

2.2 Non-parametric Bayesian Approach

A common motivation in using non-parametric Bayesian methods is to account for model uncertainty about the choice of a parametric distribution. Under the non-parametric Bayesian paradigm, the unknown distribution of the model is treated as a random parameter with stochastic non-parametric priors, such as the Dirichlet process, Ferguson (1973). Assume $t_1, ..., t_n$ are n independent survival times, where t_i is the survival time for individual i, δ_i is the associated censoring indicator, and x_i a p-dimensional vector of categorical and continuous covariates. Let $f(.|\mu,\sigma^2)$ denote arbitrary location-scale parametric densities. For each individual i, conditional on the observed covariates x_i a Dirichlet process mixture model for the data is defined as:

$$\begin{aligned} f_{x_i=x}(t_i;G) &= \int f(t_i|\mu,\sigma^2)G(d\mu\sigma^2) \\ G &\sim DP(\alpha G_0) \end{aligned} \tag{3}$$

For right-censored observartions, Individual sample values are generated from the predictive distribution, conditional on the observed censoring time, $p(t_{new}|T \geq c, D)$.

The `LDDPsurvival` function in the `DPpackage` in R, Jara et al. (2011), can be used to impute these censored observations in a non-parametric way.

3 Simulation

One hundred datasets are generated from a $Weibull(1,4)$ with different sample sizes. Potential censoring times were also generated from anexponential distribution. Specific percentages (p) of censoring are then applied and these censored observations are imputed using both parametric and non-parametric Bayesian methods. In the parametric Bayesian approach, the distribution of the data needs to be pre-specified so a Weibull distribution is assumed for the data together with lognormal and Gamma distributions as priors for the shape and scale parameters of the Weibull distribution, respectively. Consequently, as a visual measure to see how well the model is working, these 100 completed datasets are also compared to the range and interquartile range of the Kaplan-Meier estimates. The steps for plotting the bound and interquartile ranges are as follows:

- A total of 100 sets of data with the desired sample size are simulated from the specific Weibull distribution with no censoring.
- The survivor curve of each dataset is estimated using a Kaplan-Meier estimator.
- The Kaplan-Meier estimated value for each of the 100 simulation sets is subtracted from the true value of the Weibull distribution survivor function at specific time points.
- The maximum, minimum and quartiles of these differences are used to define a bound range and interquartile range over the time period of interest.

From Fig. 1 and Fig. 2, in both parametric and non-parametric Bayesian methods, as the sample size increased the imputed values became closer to the true values. Also, for the same sample size by increasing the percentage of censoring the imputed values became less accurate. Furthermore, for most of the time, the imputation values are within the Kaplan-Meier estimates, especially in the cases of low or medium percentages of censoring. However, with a high percentage of censoring, p = 50%, the parametric Bayesian approach works quite well as the boxplots are symmetric around zero line and all the medians are nearly zero. This is not unexpected as we assume the correct distribution in the parametric Bayesian approach.

4 Application

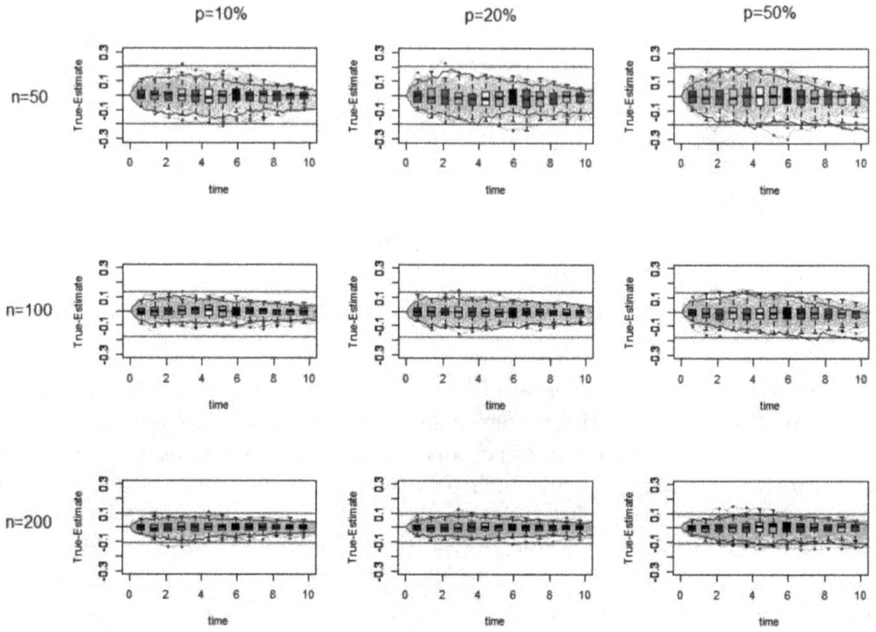

Fig. 1. The difference between the true values and the estimated ones (True-Estimate) (grey lines) using parametric Bayesian approach for 100 datasets is presented for different sample sizes (n = 50, 100, 200) and different percentages of censoring (p = 10%, 20%, 50%). Survival times are generated from $Weibull(1, 4)$ using exponential censoring. In each individual panel, the red bound and the blue bound are the bound and interquartile range for the Kaplan-Meier estimates, respectively. Over the range of different time points, the boxplots of True-Estimate values are also plotted. (Color figure online)

The 6-MP dataset, Gehan (1965), is the duration of remission in weeks for 42 leukaemia patients where 21 patients were allocated to a drug treatment group and the rest of them to a control group. There is no censoring in the control group while there are 12 censored observations in the intervention group. Figure 3 shows the boxplot for intervention and control group where the censored observations in the intervention group were imputed using parametric Bayesian and non-parametric Bayesian approaches which shows the effectiveness of the treatment in comparison to the control group.

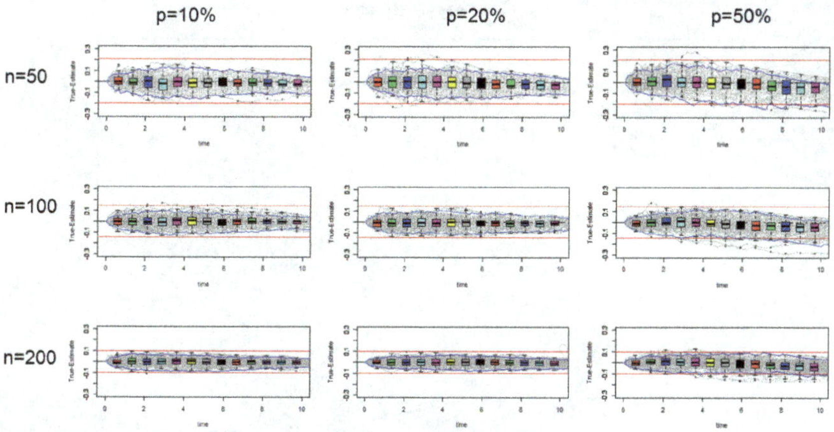

Fig. 2. The difference between the true values and the estimated ones (True-Estimate) (grey lines) using non-parametric Bayesian approach for 100 datasets is presented. Survival times are generated from $Weibull(1, 4)$ using exponential censoring for different sample size and different percentage of censoring. In each individual panel, the red bound and the blue bound are the bound and interquartile range for the Kaplan-Meier estimates, respectively. Over the range of different time points, the boxplots of True-Estimate values are also plotted. (Color figure online)

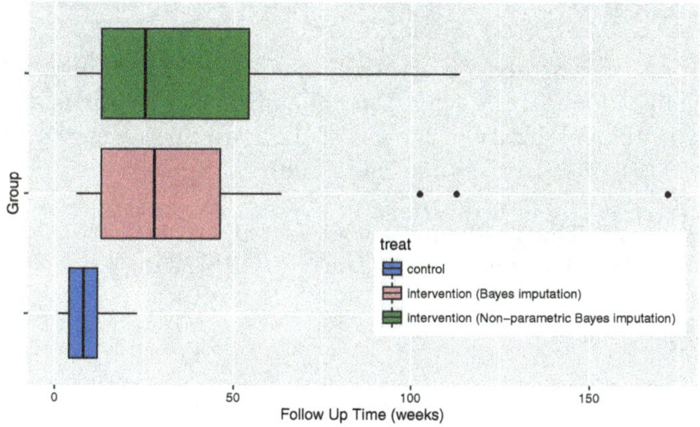

Fig. 3. Box plot for control and intervention group in 6-MP data by imputing censored observations using parametric Bayes and non-parametric Bayesian approaches.

As a 'complete' dataset is available upon imputation a plot of the estimated density function can be made using the `logspline` function, Kooperberg et al. (2023). The plots, using the two imputation approaches, are given in Fig. 4. There is little to choose between the imputation methods when comparing the plots for the treatment group (i.e. where censoring was present) so there is no substantial evidence against using a parametric assumption for the response distribution.

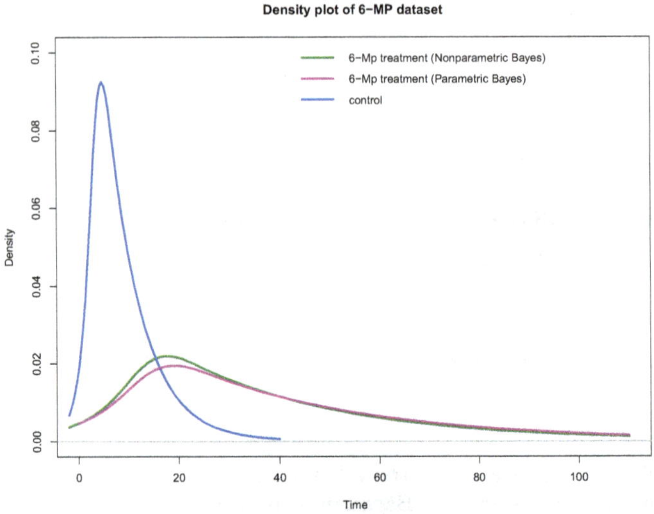

Fig. 4. Comparing the density plot of control and treatment group using parametric and non-parametric Bayesian approaches to impute censored observations in treatment group.

5 Conclusion

The imputation of censored observations not only allows more interpretable graphics to be produced for a wider general audience (physicians and patients), but it opens up the possibility of the use of standard formal methods of analysis for continuous responses, Royston et al. (2008).

Acknowledgments. This research was funded by the Irish Research Council (IRC) Government of Ireland Postgraduate Scholarship GOIPG/2013/1314.

References

Ferguson, T.S.: A Bayesian analysis of some non-parametric problems. Ann. Stat. 209–230 (1973)

Gehan, E.A.: A generalized Wilcoxon test for comparing arbitrarily singly-censored samples. Biometrika **52**, 203–224 (1965)

Gould, S.J.: The median is not the message. Discover **6**, 40–42 (1985)

Jara, A., Hanson, T., Quintana, P., Rosner, G.: DPpackage: bayesian semi- and non-parametric modeling in R. J. Stat. Softw. **40**, 1–30 (2011)

Kooperberg, C., Moler, C., Dongarra, J.: logspline: routines for logspline density estimation. R Pack. Vers. **2**(1), 21 (2023)

Moghaddam, S., Newell, J., Hinde, J.: A bayesian approach for imputation of censored survival data. Stats **5**, 89–107 (2022)

Royston, P., Parmar, M.K., Altman, D.G.: Visualizing length of survival in time-to-event studies: a complement to Kaplan-Meier plots. J. Natl. Cancer Inst. **100**, 92–97 (2008)

An Updated Wilcoxon–Mann–Whitney Test

Paul Wilson(✉)

University of Wolverhampton, Wolverhampton, UK
pauljwilson@wlv.ac.uk
https://researchers.wlv.ac.uk/PaulJWilson

Abstract. The Wilcoxon–Mann–Whitney test, also known as the Wilcoxon rank–sum test and the Mann-Whitney U test, is a non-parametric method used to compare differences between two independent variables when the dependent variable is either ordinal or continuous. The associated test statistic follows a discrete distribution, the quantiles and corresponding p-values of which are traditionally determined using "traditional" definitions. We show that the utilisation of the mid-quantiles and mid p-values leads to a test with improved attainment rates and power.

Keywords: Mann-Whitney-Wilcoxon test · mid p-values · discrete test statistics

1 Introduction

The Mann-Whitney-Wilcoxon test, also known as the Wilcoxon rank-sum test (Wilcoxon 1945), or the Mann-Whitney U test (Mann and Whitney 1947) is used to compare two independent samples and determine whether their underlying population distributions differ significantly. It is a non-parametric test that does not assume normality of data. Instead, it relies on ranks of observations. The distribution of the test statistic of the Mann-Whitney-Wilcoxon test is discrete on the non-negative integers. The distribution may be approximated by a normal distribution, this approximation is commonly employed for sample sizes greater than 20, in this paper however we use the exact distribution of the test statistic throughout. The "traditional" definition of a p-value as the "probability of observing a test statistic at least as extreme as that observed" is well suited to the case where the distribution of the test statistic is continuous, but not so when it is discrete. (See Wilson and Einbeck (2023)). For example, Wilson and Einbeck (2018) show that the test of zero-modification introduced in that paper has much improved attainment and power when mid, as opposed to traditional, p-values are employed.

J. Einbeck et al. (Eds.): IWSM 2024, CONTRIB.STAT., pp. 159–165, 2024.
https://doi.org/10.1007/978-3-031-65723-8_25

2 Mid–quantiles and Mid p-Values

For discrete distributions, Franck (1986) strongly advocates the use of the mid p-value. Mid p-values are defined by:

$$p_{\text{mid}} = P(X < x) + \tfrac{1}{2}P(X = x). \qquad (1)$$

Mid–quantiles are defined analogously. Let X be a discrete random variable with distinct values $v_1 < v_2 < \cdots < v_d$. Let $P(X = v_i) = p_i$ and $\pi_j = \sum_{i=0}^{j-1} p_i + \frac{1}{2}p_j$.

$$\xi_{\text{mid}}(p) = \begin{cases} v_1 & \text{if } p < p_1/2 \\ v_k & \text{if } p = \pi_k,\ k = 1, \ldots, d \\ \lambda v_k + (1-\lambda)v_{k+1} & \text{if } p = \lambda\pi_k + (1-\lambda)\pi_{k+1} \\ & 0 < \lambda < 1,\ \ k = 1, \ldots, d-1 \\ v_d & \text{if } p > \pi_d \end{cases} \qquad (2)$$

In essence, mid–quantiles and mid p-values align for values at which the mid p-values exist, and are obtained by linear interpolation at values in between. See Fig. 1. (For a more detailed account of mid–quantiles see Ma et al. (2011) or Wilson and Einbeck (2017)).

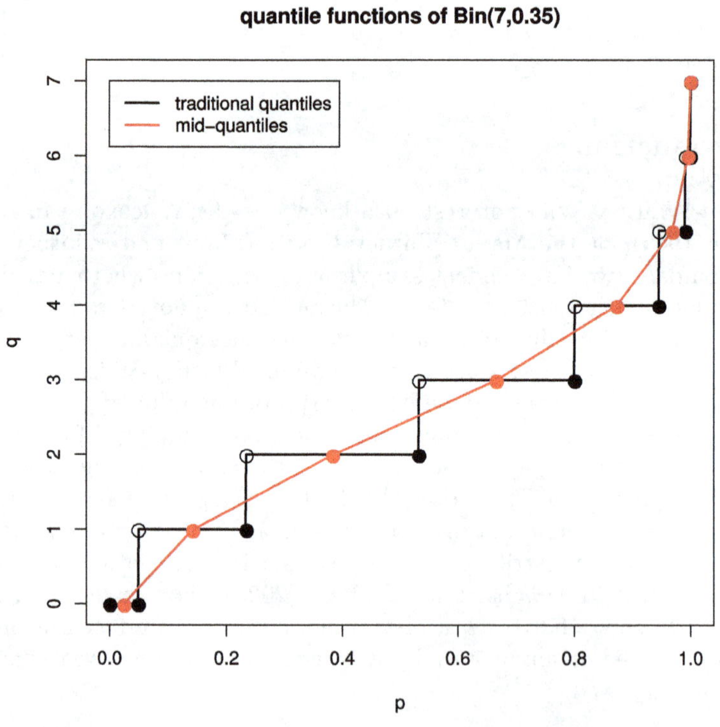

Fig. 1. Attainment: Traditional and mid-quantiles

The employment of mid p-values and mid-quantiles has many advantages: under the null hypothesis the expected values of mid$-p$ values for discrete test statistics and traditional p-values for continuous test statistics are equal, and their variances are approximately equal. Wilson and Einbeck (2023) point out that for continuous distributions the definitions of traditional and mid p-values are equivalent and propose that the definition of the mid p-value should be used for *all* p-values.

3 Application to the Wilcoxon-Mann-Whitney Test

Table 1 displays the critical values of the distribution of the Wilcoxon-Mann-Whitney test statistic at a significance level of $\alpha = 0.025$ (one tailed)/$\alpha = 0.05$ (two tailed), where these values have been determined using mid-quantile techniques. Criticial values based upon mid-quantiles will either coincide with those based upon traditional values, or be one greater. Entries in bold font indicate those values which are one greater.

3.1 Attainment Rates

Figure 2 illustrates the attainment (type-one error) rates obtained under both traditional- and mid-quantile methods when Wilcoxon-Mann-Whitney tests are performed on two equally sized samples. It is apparent that attainment achieved when mid-quantile techniques are employed is either equal or superior to that achieved under traditional techniques.

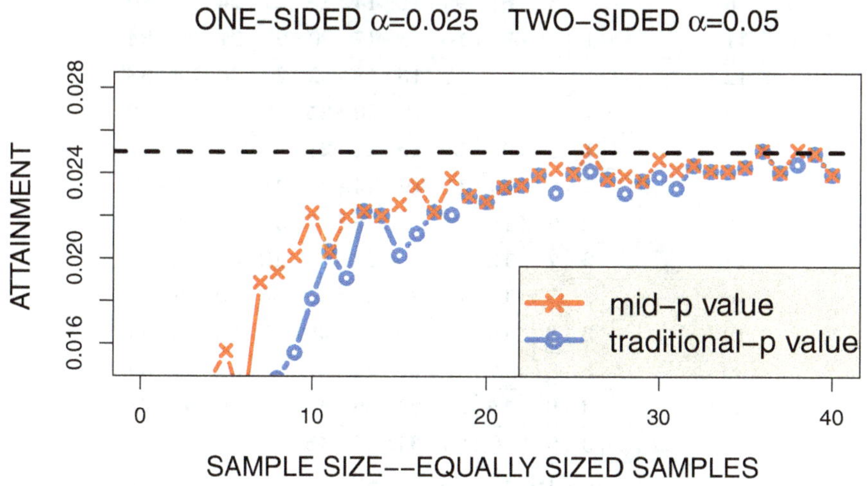

Fig. 2. Attainment: Wilcoxon-Mann-Whitney test, two equally sized samples

Figure 3 illustrates the attainment rates obtained under both traditional- and mid-quantile methods when Wilcoxon-Mann-Whitney tests, are performed on two samples, one of size 8, and the size of the other ranging from 3 to 40. Figure 4 illustrates the attainment rates obtained under both traditional- and mid-quantile methods when Wilcoxon-Mann-Whitney tests, are performed on two samples, where the larger sample is of size ten greater then the smaller, the size of the smaller varying from three to forty. It is clear that in both cases attainment achieved when mid-quantile techniques are employed is either equal or superior to that achieved under traditional techniques

Table 1. Critical Values of the Mann-Whitney-Wilcoxon test based upon mid-quantiles. Entries in normal font correspond to those using traditional quantiles. Entries in bold font are one greater than those derived from traditional quantiles.

$n_1 \downarrow$ | $n_2 \rightarrow$	1	2	3	4	5	6	7	8	9	10	11	12
1	–	–	–	–	–	–	–	–	–	–	–	–
2	–	–	–	–	–	–	–	–	–	1	1	1
3	–	–	–	–	–	1	**2**	2	**3**	3	**4**	4
4	–	–	–	**1**	**2**	2	3	4	**5**	**6**	**7**	**8**
5	–	–	–	**2**	3	**4**	5	6	7	**9**	**10**	11
6	–	–	1	2	**4**	5	**7**	8	10	**12**	13	**15**
7	–	–	**2**	3	5	**7**	**9**	**11**	**13**	15	17	18
8	–	–	2	4	6	8	**11**	13	15	**18**	**20**	22
9	–	–	**3**	**5**	7	10	**13**	15	**18**	**21**	23	26
10	–	–	3	**6**	**9**	11	14	**18**	**21**	**24**	**27**	**30**
11	–	1	4	7	**10**	13	17	20	23	**27**	30	**34**
12	–	1	4	**8**	11	**15**	18	22	26	**30**	**34**	**38**
13	–	1	4	8	12	16	20	**25**	**29**	33	37	**42**
14	–	1	5	9	13	**18**	22	**27**	**32**	36	**41**	**46**
15	–	**2**	**6**	10	**15**	19	24	29	34	39	44	49
16	–	**2**	6	11	**16**	21	26	**32**	37	42	**48**	53
17	–	2	**7**	**12**	17	**23**	28	34	**40**	**46**	**52**	57
18	–	2	7	**13**	18	24	30	36	**43**	**49**	55	61
19	–	**3**	**8**	**14**	**20**	**26**	32	**39**	45	**52**	**59**	65
20	–	**3**	8	14	**21**	**28**	34	41	48	55	62	69
21	–	**3**	**9**	**15**	22	29	36	**44**	**51**	58	**66**	73
22	–	3	9	16	23	**31**	38	**46**	**54**	**62**	69	77
23	–	3	**10**	17	**23**	32	40	48	56	**65**	73	81
24	–	**4**	10	**18**	24	**34**	42	**50**	**59**	**68**	**77**	85
25	–	**4**	**11**	**19**	27	**36**	44	53	62	71	80	89

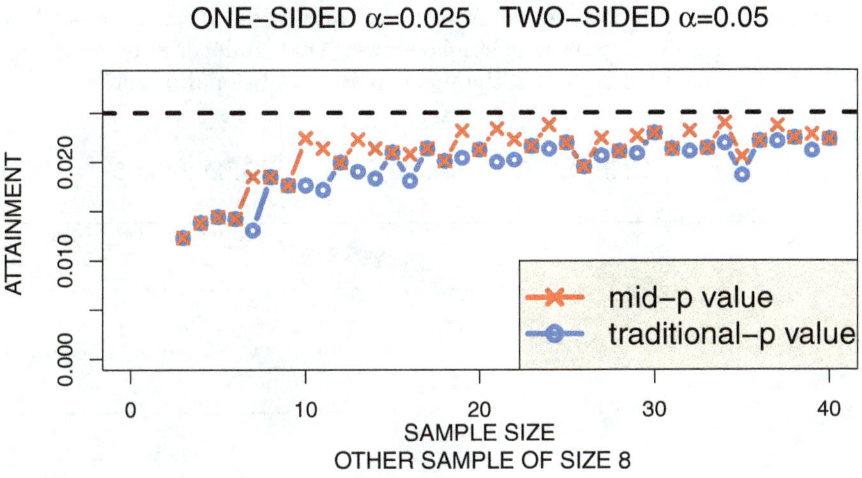

Fig. 3. Attainment: Wilcoxon-Mann-Whitney test, one sample of size eight.

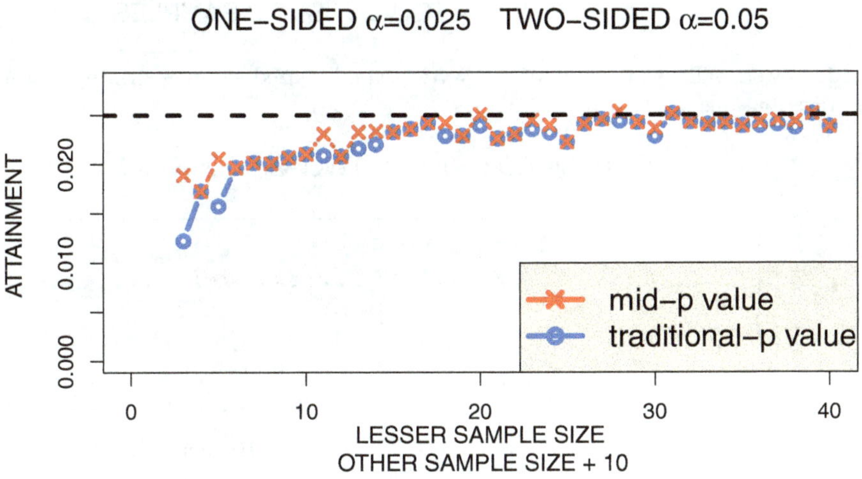

Fig. 4. Attainment: Wilcoxon-Mann-Whitney test

4 Power

Figure 5 compares the powers obtained when under both traditional- and mid-quantile methods when Wilcoxon-Mann-Whitney tests, are performed on two equally sized samples drawn from uniform distributions on (1, 4) and (2, 5) respectively. Figure 6 compares the powers obtained under both traditional- and mid-quantile methods when Wilcoxon-Mann-Whitney tests, are performed on two equally sized samples drawn from $\chi^2(3)$ and $\chi^2(5)$ distributions. Again, both methods result in extremely similar power, that under mid-quantile either equalling or being slightly better than that under traditional quantile.

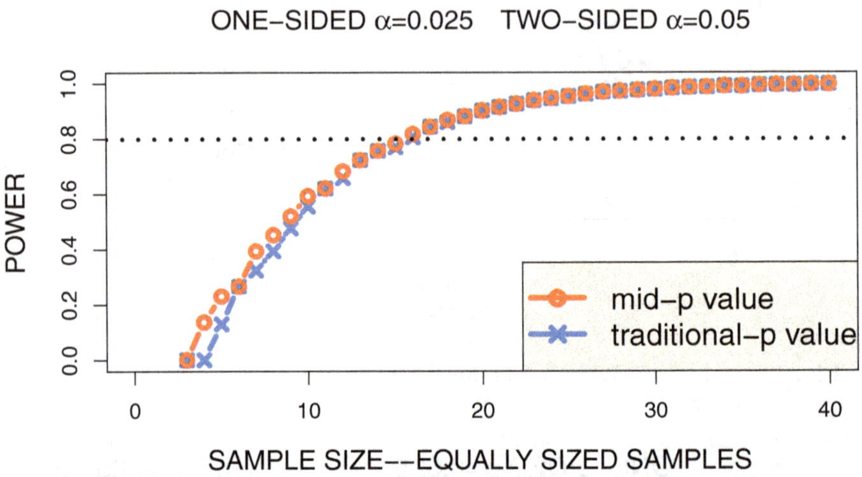

Fig. 5. Power: Wilcoxon-Mann-Whitney test, equally sized samples drawn from uniform distributions of $(1, 4)$ and $(2, 5)$.

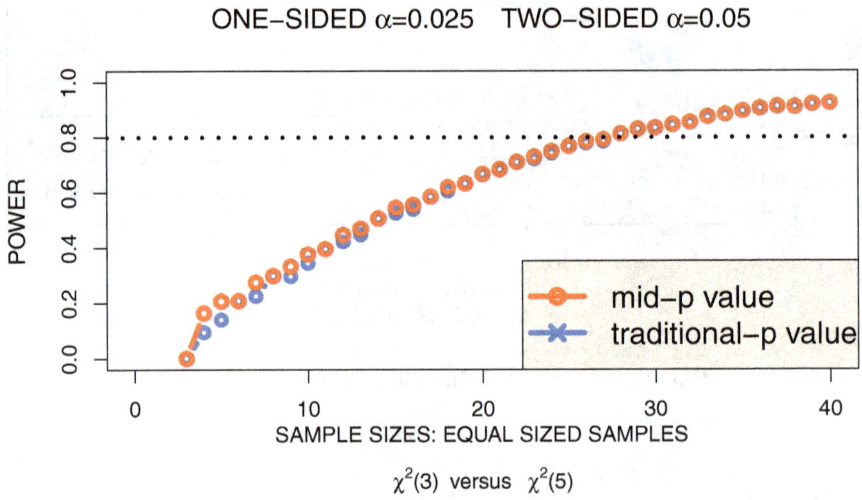

Fig. 6. Power: Wilcoxon-Mann-Whitney test, equally sized samples drawn from $\chi^2(3)$ and $\chi^2(5)$ distributions.

5 Conclusion

For tests with discrete test statistics, the use of mid-quantiles and mid p-values, as opposed to their traditional counterparts is advantageous. The Mann-Whitney-Wilcoxon test is one such test, and is one of the "classic" tests of statistics. Both the power and attainment of the Wilcoxon-Mann-Whitney test are improved by the employment of critical values based upon mid-quantile techniques; it is recommended that going forward such techniques are utilised. As a by product of this research we notice that unexpectedly it is not necessarily the case that attainment of the nominal level of significance improves with increased sample size, (see for example Fig. 3). As mentioned in Sect. 1, throughout this paper we have used the exact distribution of the test statistic. The comparison of the performance of mid-quantile based test statistics to that of the normal approximation is a topic for future research.

References

Franck, W.: P-values for discrete test statistics. Biometr. J. **28**, 403–406 (1986)

Ma, Y., Genton, M., Parzen, E.: Asymptotic properties of sample quantiles of discrete distributions. Ann. Inst. Stat. Math. **63**, 227–243 (2011)

Mann, H., Whitney, D.: On a test of whether one of two random variables is stochastically larger than the other. Ann. Math. Stat. **18**(1), 50–60 (1947)

Wilcoxon, F.: Individual comparisons by ranking methods. Biometr. Bull. **1**(6), 80–83 (1945)

Wilson, P., Einbeck, J.: Sample quantiles corresponding to mid p–values for zero-modification tests. In: Grzegorczyk, M., Ceoldo, G. (eds.) Proceedings of the 32nd IWSM, Groningen, The Netherlands, vol. 1, pp. 275–279 (2017)

Wilson, P., Einbeck, J.: A new and intuitive test for zero-modification. Stat. Model. **19**(4), 341–361 (2018). https://doi.org/10.1177/1471082x18762277

Wilson, P., Einbeck, J.: A consistent way to define p-values. In: Bergherr, G., Meyr (eds). Proceedings of the 37th IWSM, Dortmund, Germany, pp. 658–663 (2023)

Estimating a Lower Bound of the Population Size in Capture-Recapture Experiments with Right Censored Data

Anabel Blasco-Moreno[1] and Pere Puig[2(✉)]

[1] Departament de Matemàtiques and Servei d'Estadística de la UAB, Cerdanyola del Vallés, Spain
[2] Departament de Matemàtiques de la UAB, and CRM, Cerdanyola del Vallés, Spain
pere.puig@uab.cat

Abstract. In this work, we present a new non-parametric approach for estimating a lower bound of the population size in capture-recapture experiments with right-censored observations, along with several applications in ecology and social sciences. ...

Keywords: Censored data · Chao's estimator · Mixed-binomial distributions

1 Introduction

The estimation of the population size N or, equivalently, the frequency of unseen individuals is the goal of a capture-recapture model. Let f_0 represent the frequency of those who were never found during the study period and are not being observed, and let f_1, f_2, f_3,... f_m represent the frequencies of distinct individuals (or animals) identified exactly 1, 2, 3,..., m times during the study period, following T trapping occasions. Consequently, the population size N can be written as follows: $N = f_0 + f_1 + f_2 + \cdots + f_m = f_0 + n$, where $n = \sum_{i=1}^{m} f_i$ represents the total number of distinct individuals seen.

Table 1. Photographic sightings of dolphins in Sepetiba bay.

Sights	0	1	2	3	4^+
No. of dolphins (f_i)	–	228	110	19	25

The primary objective of this research is to present a new method for estimating the total number of animals or species when all that is known is the number that has been observed once (f_1), twice (f_2),..., and the number that has been

J. Einbeck et al. (Eds.): IWSM 2024, CONTRIB.STAT., pp. 166–171, 2024.
https://doi.org/10.1007/978-3-031-65723-8_26

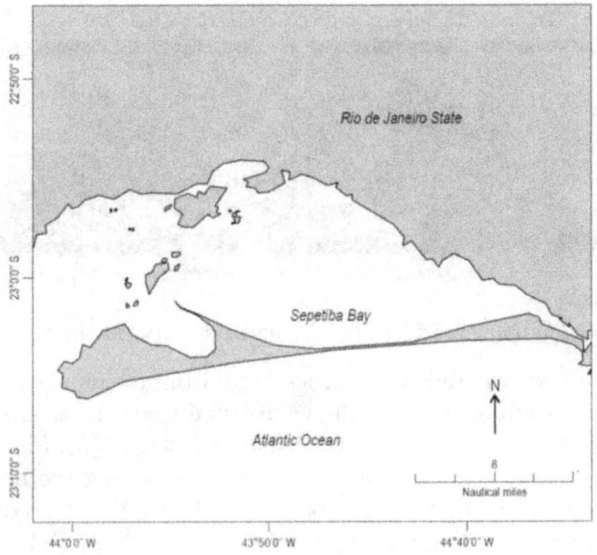

Fig. 1. Sepetiba bay (Brazil)

observed r and more than r times (f_{r+}). The frequency distribution of the observations is said to be right censored at r if this happens. Table 1 shows an example based on the research by [6] on the number of Guiana dolphins (*Sotalia guianensis*) in Sepetiba Bay, southeast Brazil (Fig. 1)). Using photo-identification and their inherent markings, dolphins can be identified. The shapes of the dolphins' dorsal fins were photographed and compared to those of previously known individuals, using tools like Darwin software (see Fig. 2). In this case the number of different dolphins observed was $n = f_1 + f_2 + ... + f_{4+} = 382$, obtained throughout $T = 14$ exploratory trips. Note that the frequency distribution of the observations is right censored at $r = 4$. This example is analysed in [4] without censorship using a non-parametric methodology based on the empirical probability generating function (epgf). Kokonendji and Puig (2018) [7] presented more non-parametric approaches based on the epgf.

The major question will now be: how can we estimate the total dolphin population using censored data?

2 The Model

Let Y_i be the random variable that represents the frequency with which the animal (or individual) i has been observed in T samples or trapping occasions. The probability of being observed k times is provided by the binomial distribution, assuming that the different samples are independent of one another, $P(Y_i = k) = \binom{T}{k}\lambda_i^k(1-\lambda_i)^{T-k}$, $i = 1, 2, ..., N$, where λ_i denotes the probability that the ith animal or individual will be captured or observed. We assume that there is only individual variation and no sample dependence. The probability

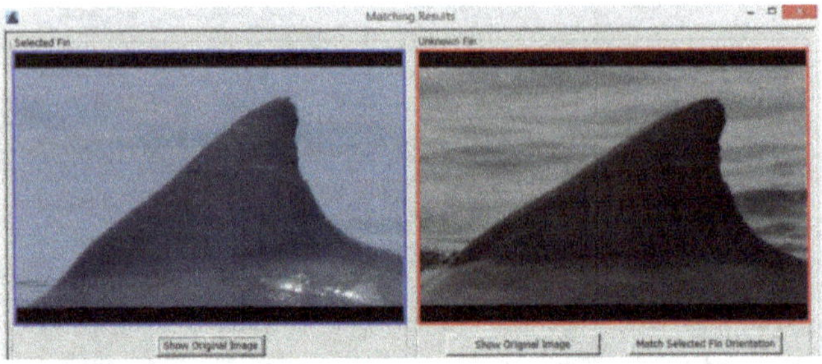

Fig. 2. Dolphins are identified by natural marks in the dorsal fin.

of catchability or identifiability λ_i varies across target population members in most application studies. As a result, we assume that the λ_i are taken from a probability distribution with unknown density function $f(\lambda)$, for λ belonging to the interval $(0,1)$. Let Y be the random variable counting the number of cases in which any animal or individual is observed. Thus, Y is mixed-binomial distributed with probability function, $p_k = P(Y=k) = \int_0^1 \binom{T}{k} \lambda^k (1-\lambda)^{T-k} f(\lambda) d\lambda$. We have to estimate f_0, or alternatively, p_0, in order to estimate the population size N. However, p_0 cannot be estimated because it is not identifiable. Nevertheless, certain lower bounds on p_0 can be found independent of the knowledge of $f(\lambda)$. One well-known example of this type of approach is the Chao inequality, which is expressed as $p_0 \geq (T-1)p_1^2/(2Tp_2)$. In reality, Chao inequality is a watershed moment, resulting in multiple developments and results during the last 30 years, as reported by [3]. It is important to note that, since the zero is not observable, what we actually have when we observe the frequencies f_1, f_2,..., f_{r+} is a sample of size n of the random variable Y truncated at zero. It can be represented by the random variable $Y_{zt} = Y|Y>0$, for which the probabilities are $P(Y_{zt}=k) = p_k/(1-p_0)$ for $k = 1, 2, ..., T$.

We have proven the following inequality for $F_{zt}(k) = P(Y_{zt} \leq k)$ that does not depend of the mixing density $f(\lambda)$:

$$F_{zt}(k) \leq G_k(p_0), \ k = 1, 2, ..., T \tag{1}$$

where,

$$G_k(p_0) = \frac{\sum_{i=1}^{k} \binom{T}{i} (1-p_0^{1/T})^i p_0^{1-i/T}}{1-p_0}.$$

Here is the lower bound estimator of p_0 that can be obtained using inequality (1):

$$\hat{p}_0 = \max_{1 \leq k \leq r-1} \{G_k^{-1}(\hat{F}_{zt}(k))\}, \tag{2}$$

where $\hat{F}_{zt}(k)$ is the empirical distribution function, that is,

$$\hat{F}_{zt}(k) = \frac{\sum_{i=1}^{k} f_i}{n}.$$

Blasco-Moreno and Puig (2024) [1] provide proof of these results as well as additional information regarding this methodology. From here, the population size N can be estimated through the following argument: $1 - p_0 \approx n/N$, leading to the so-called Horvitz-Thompson estimator,

$$\hat{N} = \frac{n}{1 - \hat{p}_0}. \tag{3}$$

We created a program in R to numerically solve the equations in (2) and calculate bootstrap confidence intervals. The script is available from the authors upon request.

3 Examples of Application

1. **Dolphins in Sepetiba bay:** In this example $T = 14$, $r = 4$, $n = 382$ and data are shown in Table 1. According to (2), $\hat{p}_0 = 0.3608$ is a lower bound estimate of p_0. By applying (3), we can determine a lower bound of the dolphin population size, which is $\hat{N} = 598$. We can compute a 95% confidence interval of this bound using a bootstrap sample of size 10,000, resulting, (554, 670). This result is consistent with that of [4], $\hat{N} = 632$, who used data that was not censored.
2. **Cubs-of-the-year in Yellowstone:** Keating et al. (2002) [5] examined the annual number of mothers with cubs-of-the-year in the Yellowstone grizzly bear population from 1986 to 2001. Table 2 shows the number of unique females with cubs-of-the-year that were sighted exactly one, two, three, and four or more times throughout 1998.
   In this case, T is regarded very huge, $r = 4$, $f_1 = 11$, $f_2 = 13$, $f_3 = 5$, $f_4^+ = 4$, and $n = 33$. According to (2), $\hat{p}_0 = 0.2009$ is a lower bound estimate of p_0. By applying (3), we may find a lower bound on the population size: $\hat{N} = 41$. We can construct a 95% confidence interval of this bound using a bootstrap sample of size 10,000, resulting in $(34, 58)$. The result is quite similar to that of [7], who used the complete dataset.

Table 2. Sights of unique females with cubs-of-the-year (1998).

Sights	0	1	2	3	4^+
No. of mothers (f_i)	–	11	13	5	4

The case $r = 2$ is especially interesting for its applications. In a generic way we can say that we only see one and more than one. When $r = 2$, only $F_{zt}(k)$ can be estimated for $k = 1$, obtaining $\hat{F}_{zt}(1) = f_1/n$. Therefore, from (2), the value of $\hat{p}_0$ is obtained solving numerically the equation,

$$\frac{T(1 - p_0^{1/T})p_0^{1-1/T}}{1 - p_0} = \frac{f_1}{n}. \tag{4}$$

When T is large, Eq. (4) remains,

$$\frac{-\log(p_0)p_0}{1-p_0} = \frac{f_1}{n}. \tag{5}$$

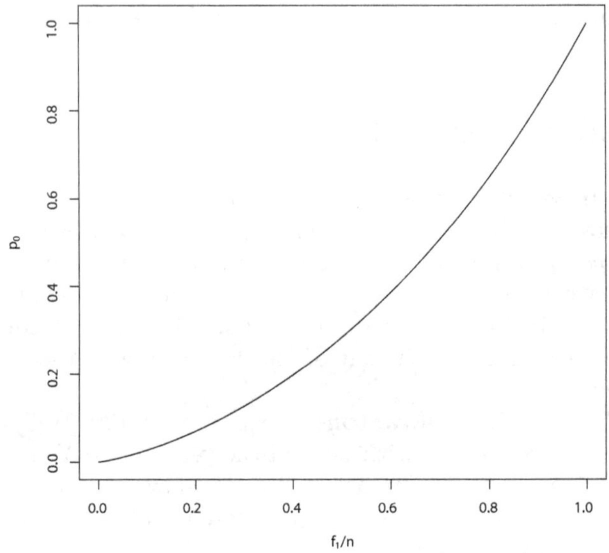

Fig. 3. Estimated lower-bounds of p_0 for different values of f_1/n

Figure 3 shows the solution of Eq. (5) for different values of f_1/n. Interestingly, the solutions to Eqs. (4) and (5) provide the maximum likelihood estimators of p_0 assuming data from binomial and Poisson distributions, respectively. We will now show two examples of applications with $r = 2$.

3. **Sexual assault offenders in North Wales:** The following information was reported in the Daily Post on August 13, 2018: "The 34 repeat offenders convicted since 2011 represent almost 10% of the total of 342 convictions for sexual assault". How many offenders were not caught (or not reported) and could have been found guilty? In this case, $n = 342$, $r = 2$, $f_{2+} = 34$ and $f_1 = 308$. Chao et al. (2017) [2] presented an alternative estimator of N for this particular censoring pattern with $r = 2$, based on the Good-Turing theory. Solving Eq. (5) we find that $\hat{p}_0 = 0.8139$, and $\hat{N} = 1838$, and the 95% bootstrap-CI is $(1381, 2629)$.
4. **Traffic Offenders in Tarragona:** The following information was published in the newspaper Diari de Tarragona on May 5, 2018. The news's subtitle reads, "Of the 546 drivers whose licences were revoked last year, 119 had already been left without one for the same reason at least once." In this situation, $n = 546$, $f_{2+} = 119$ and $f_1 = 427$. Once again, it would be interesting to

know how many potential offenders would have their licenses revoked. Solving Eq. (5) we find that $\hat{p}_0 = 0.6231$, and $\hat{N} = 1449$, and the 95% bootstrap-CI is $(1255, 1701)$.

References

1. Blasco-Moreno, A., Puig, P.: A non-parametric method of estimation of the population size in capture-recapture experiments with right censored data. In: Submitted to Methods in Ecology and Evolution (2024)
2. Chao, A., Colwell, R.K., Chiu, Ch., Townsend, D.: Seen once or more than once: applying good-turing theory to estimate species richness using only unique observations and a species list. Methods Ecol. Evol. **8**, 1221–1232 (2017)
3. Chao, A., Colwell, R.K.: Thirty years of progeny from chao's inequality: estimating and comparing richness with incidence data and incomplete sampling. SORT-Stat. Oper. Res. Transact. **41**, 3–54 (2017)
4. Jiménez-Gamero, M.D., Puig, P.: A nonparametric method of estimation of the population size in capture-recapture experiments. Biom. J. **62**, 970–988 (2020)
5. Keating, K.A., Schwartz, C.C., Haroldson, M.A., Moody, D.: Estimating numbers of females with cubs-of-the-year in the Yellowstone grizzlybear population. Ursus **13**, 161–174 (2002)
6. Nery, M.F., Simão, S.M.: Capture-recapture abundance estimate of Guiana dolphins in southeastern Brazil. Cienc. Mar. **38**, 529–541 (2012)
7. Puig, P., Kokonendji, C.C.: Non-parametric estimation of the number of zeros in truncated count distributions. Scand. J. Stat. **45**, 347–365 (2018)

Inference for Quasi-reaction Models with Covariate-Dependent Rates

Matteo Framba[1(✉)], Veronica Vinciotti[1], and Ernst C. Wit[2]

[1] Università degli Studi di Trento, Trento, Italy
{matteo.framba,veronica.vinciotti}@unitn.it
[2] Università della Svizzera Italiana, Lugano, Switzerland
ernst.jan.camiel.wit@usi.ch

Abstract. Statistical models of quasi-reaction systems are typically described by constant reaction rates. This assumption is too restrictive in many applications, as rates may vary dynamically, spatially or within groups of the population. In this paper, we capture this heterogeneity with the inclusion of covariates in the dynamic model. In particular, we propose an extension of a recently developed latent event history model, by allowing log-reaction rates to be linearly dependent on a vector of covariates. We describe an inferential approach for parameter estimation of the resulting model and evaluate its performance via a simulation study. Finally, we show an illustration on COVID-19 data, where the approach is able to measure the effect of environmental factors and governmental interventions on the disease spreading and severity.

Keywords: Quasi-reaction models · EM algorithm · Kalman filtering · latent event history models · epidemic modelling

1 Introduction

An increasing number of natural phenomena, such as infectious disease spreading (Britton et al. 2019), can be described by quasi-reaction systems of stochastic differential equations. A common modelling assumption is to associate a constant rate to each reaction. However, this assumption is too restrictive in many applications, leading to inferred dynamics that may be far from the true ones. Indeed, it is reasonable to assume that rates may vary dynamically or spatially, for example due to governmental imposed lockdowns, variations in the dynamics of contagion between geographical regions or between different groups of populations.

In the context of epidemic modelling, a certain level of heterogeneity can be achieved by adding new compartments and new reactions to the system. However, on the one hand, this is only a discrete approximation when the exogenous covariates are of a continuous nature, and, on the other hand, it may lead to overly complex models. As an alternative to this approach, in this paper, we propose to capture heterogeneity in the system dynamics by letting the rates

J. Einbeck et al. (Eds.): IWSM 2024, CONTRIB.STAT., pp. 172–178, 2024.
https://doi.org/10.1007/978-3-031-65723-8_27

of the quasi-reaction model depend directly on external covariates. In particular, we propose an extension of a recently developed latent event history model (Framba et al. 2023), by allowing log-reaction rates to be linearly dependent on a vector of covariates. In this way, the model is able to quantify the effect of covariates on the system dynamics. We adapt the Expectation-Maximization (EM) algorithm developed by Framba et al. (2023) to this new setting, and evaluate the effectiveness of this approach on simulated data and in the context of epidemic modelling.

The paper is organized as follows: Sect. 2 formalizes the proposed latent event history modelling approach. Section 3 evaluates the procedure on a simple SIR (Susceptible, Infected and Recovered) system, whose dynamics are affected by the start of a lockdown period. In Sect. 4, we show an illustration on COVID19 data from Italy, where the approach is able to assess the effect of environmental factors and public health interventions on the transmission and severity of the disease. Finally, in Sect. 5, we draw some conclusions.

2 Latent Event History Model

Consider a closed system in which p substrates, or compartments, interact via r reactions. Let k_{lj} be the stoichiometric coefficient, indicating the amount of substrate l needed for reaction j to occur, and let $\mathbf{Y}(t) = (Y_1(t), \ldots, Y_p(t))$ be the state of the system at time t. The hazard of reaction j occurring instantaneously at time t is given by

$$\lambda_j(t) = \theta_j \prod_{l=1}^{p} \binom{Y_l(t-1)}{k_{lj}} \mathbb{1}_{Y_l(t-1) > k_{lj}},$$

with θ_j the non-negative rate associated to reaction j, for $j = 1, \ldots, r$. These rates are typically assumed constant for each reaction (Framba et al. 2023). In contrast to this, in this paper, we propose to link the reaction rates to external covariates. In particular, given a vector of possibly time-dependent covariates $\mathbf{x} \in \mathbb{R}^q$, we assume

$$\theta_j = \exp(\mathbf{x}^t \boldsymbol{\beta}_j),$$

with $\boldsymbol{\beta}_j$ a q-dimensional vector of reaction-specific regression coefficients. In the following, we denote with $\boldsymbol{\beta}$ the vector of coefficients across all reactions. These are the parameters to be estimated.

The firing of reactions induces a change in the states of the system. In particular, if $\mathbf{Y}_i$, $i = 0, \ldots, N$, is the state of the process at $N+1$, not necessarily equispaced, time points, then $\mathbf{Y}_i - \mathbf{Y}_{i-1} = V\mathbf{N}_i$, with V the $p \times r$ net-effect matrix , indicating the variation of the lth substrate due to the occurrence of the jth reaction, and $\mathbf{N}_i$ the number of each reaction occurring in the interval $(t_{i-1}, t_i]$. Since the number of reactions is not observed, we follow Framba et al. (2023) and propose to infer the dynamics of the system via the following state-space model

$$\begin{cases} \mathbf{Z}_i = \boldsymbol{\mu}_i + \boldsymbol{\varepsilon}_i, & \boldsymbol{\varepsilon}_i \sim \mathcal{N}(0, \operatorname{diag}(\boldsymbol{\mu}_i)), \\ \mathbf{Y}_i = \mathbf{Y}_{i-1} + VG(\mathbf{Z}_i) + \boldsymbol{\psi}_i, & \boldsymbol{\psi}_i \sim \mathcal{N}(0, \sigma_i^2 \cdot \mathbb{I}_p), \quad i = 1, \ldots, N, \end{cases}$$

where ψ_i is a Gaussian measurement error, $\boldsymbol{\mu}_i = (t_i - t_{i-1})\boldsymbol{\lambda}(t_i; \boldsymbol{\beta})$ and $G(\mathbf{Z}_i)$, formally defined in Framba et al. (2023), is a continuous approximation to $\mathbf{N}_i$.

For the estimation of the parameters $\boldsymbol{\beta}$, we adapt the EM algorithm of Framba et al. (2023) to the presence of external covariates, making use of the extended Kalman filter for the prediction of the latent state variables at the E-step.

3 Simulation Study: SIR System Under Lockdown

We evaluate the performance of the method on a simple SIR epidemiological model, consisting of $p = 3$ substrates (Susceptible, Infected, Recovered), and $r = 2$ reactions, given by

$$S + I \xrightarrow{\theta_1} 2I$$
$$I \xrightarrow{\theta_2} R$$

The first reaction represents the contagion from an infected person to a susceptible individual, while the second reaction denotes the recovery of an infected individual.

We introduce a binary covariate x to represent the impact of a lockdown. The covariate is initially set to 0 to signify a non-serious pandemic situation and changes to 1 when the susceptible-to-infected ratio exceeds a critical threshold, indicating the necessity of implementing lockdown measures to reduce the spread. The lockdown will have an impact on the reaction rates. In particular, letting $\theta_j = \exp(\beta_{0j} + \beta_{1j}x)$, we expect the infection rate θ_1 to reduce after the lockdown, so we set $\beta_{11} = -2.303$, while we expect the recovery rate θ_2 to not be affected by lockdown measures, so we set $\beta_{12} = 0$. For the other two parameters, we set $\beta_{01} = -4.094$ and $\beta_{02} = -0.693$, respectively. Figure 1a represents a trajectory simulated from this system and indeed shows how the curve of infection counts shifts from increasing to decreasing at the start of lockdown, represented by a vertical line.

We utilize the Gillespie algorithm to simulate 50 stochastic processes over time from this system, starting with an initial particle count configuration of $\mathbf{y}_0 = (400, 20, 80)$. Data are collected at intervals of 10 time points, selected from the originally sampled trajectories, for a total of 41 observations. The EM algorithm starts from $\beta_0 = (0, 0, 0, 0)$. We set no measurement error, i.e., $\sigma_i^2 = 0$ for all i, the tolerance for convergence to 0.002, and the maximum number of iterations to 100. Figure 1b reports the accuracy of parameter estimates, by comparing the true values with their median across the 50 simulations. Overall, the results indicate a close proximity between the estimated and the true values for all parameters.

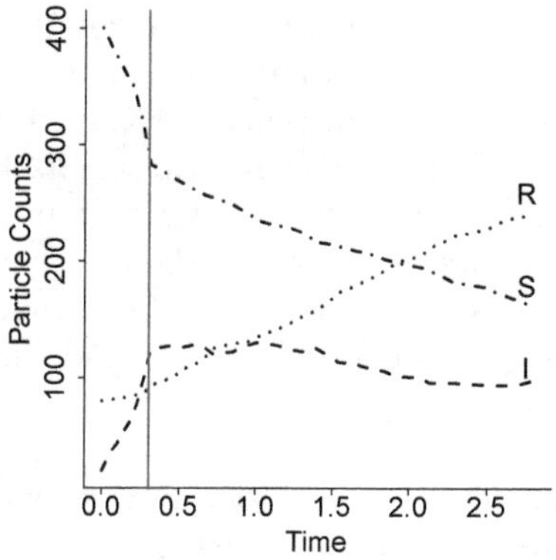

(a)

Parameters	True	Median	St. Dev.
β_{01}	-4.094	-4.424	0.096
β_{11}	-2.303	-2.029	0.138
β_{02}	-0.693	-0.611	0.256
β_{12}	0.000	-0.227	0.252

(b)

Fig. 1. (a) A trajectory of a stochastic SIR process. The vertical line denotes the beginning of lockdown, leading to a reduction in the infection rate; (b) Statistics of parameters across 50 simulations.

4 Epidemic Modelling of COVID-19

Italy was hit hard by the COVID-19 pandemic caused by the coronavirus SARS-CoV-2, and particularly so in the Lombardy region where the first cases were reported. The impact of the pandemic remains significant to these days: as of May 6th, 2024, the northern region has reported over 4.34 million confirmed cases and nearly 48,000 deaths (Guidotti and Ardia 2020). From day one of the pandemic, the Italian Institute of Health has started gathering a comprehensive dataset on the progression of the disease. In this section, we look closely at the data collected daily during the year 2021 (Guidotti and Ardia 2020).

Figure 2 shows the system that we consider for modelling the dynamics of COVID-19 progression. In particular, the total population is partitioned into the following five compartments, which define the states of the dynamic system: **I**, infected but not in serious condition (homebound); **H**, infected and hospitalised; **C**, critically ill (requiring respiratory support); **R**, recovered (no longer infected); **E**, extinct (dead). The arrows correspond to the 8 reactions that define the system. It seems natural to assume that the implementation of mass vaccination campaigns and rigorous public health measures that were put in place to contain the pandemic had indeed an effect on the virus progression and spread. From a modelling point of view, this results in reaction rates that vary over time due to external time-dependent covariates.

For the analysis, we consider in particular the following covariates:

1. **Vaccination Rate**: cumulative sum of the vaccines delivered at time t. SARS-CoV-2 vaccination is proven to protect against both infection and manifestation of severe and fatal symptoms of the disease (Corrao et al. 2022), so the dependence on this covariate has been included for all reactions.

2. **Temperature**: smoothed mean intensity of monthly temperatures retrieved from ARPA Lombardia (2022). Environmental factors have been found to have an impact on the transmissibility, severity, and mortality of COVID-19, so also this covariate has been considered for all reactions. (Kifer et al. 2021).
3. **% Time at Work**: smoothed variation of the percentage of time spent at work relative to its median value over the five weeks preceding the pandemic (Guidotti and Ardia 2020). Viral transmission is clearly influenced by the time people spend at work, so this covariate has been included only for modelling the rate of infection.
4. **Government Response Index (GRI)**: a measure of the severity of government policies to reduce interactions, accounting for school and workplace closures, bans on public gatherings, suspension of public transport, stay-at-home mandates, public information campaigns, and international travel controls (Hale et al. 2020). Similarly to the previous covariate, this index has been included only for the reaction representing new infections.

All covariates are rescaled to zero mean and unit standard deviation.

We use the proposed EM algorithm to estimate the regression coefficients associated to each reaction rate. As initial value, we run the method of Framba et al. (2023) and set these estimated values as the intercepts to all models, and zero for all the other regression parameters. We set the tolerance for convergence to 10^{-5} and the maximum number of iterations to 200. The variances σ_i^2 associated with the increments of the i-th state are estimated offline. The results are presented in Table 1 in terms of estimated regression coefficients and standard errors. Since the marginal log-likelihood is not a direct output of the EM algorithm, we use the Fisher information matrix associated with the Q-function for

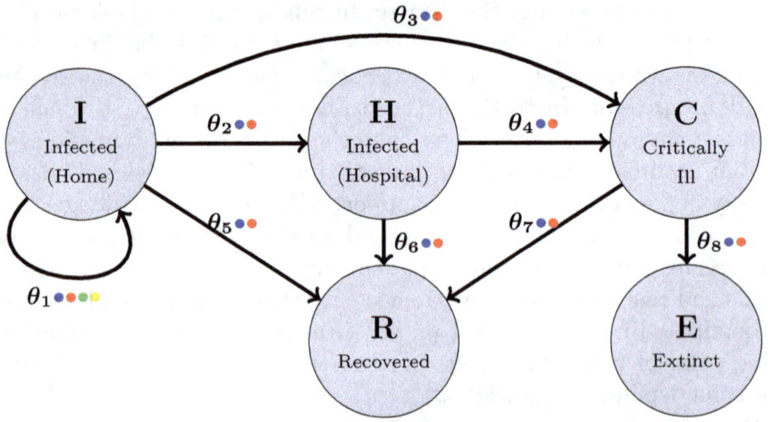

Fig. 2. Graphical illustration of the epidemic model for COVID-19 spreading: arrows correspond to the 8 reactions, associated to different stages of the infection; dependence of reaction rates on time covariates is represented with the following colours: • Vaccination Rate, • Temperature, • % Time at Work, • GRI. (Color figure online)

Table 1. Estimated regression coefficients and standard errors for the COVID-19 model in Fig. 2.

$\hat{\beta}$	$I \to 2I$	$I \to H$	$I \to C$	$H \to C$	$I \to R$	$H \to R$	$C \to R$	$C \to E$
Intercept	–1.82	–2.15	–4.04	0.006	–4.65	0.657	1.547	1.378
	(0.001)	(0.001)	(0.002)	(0.001)	(0.003)	(0.001)	(0.002)	(0.002)
Vaccination Rate	0.657	0.473	1.296	1.690	1.201	0.605	1.232	1.443
	(0.001)	(0.001)	(0.003)	(0.002)	(0.004)	(0.001)	(0.002)	(0.003)
Temperature	0.725	0.824	1.354	1.018	1.628	0.905	0.673	1.370
	(0.001)	(0.001)	(0.002)	(0.002)	(0.003)	(0.001)	(0.002)	(0.002)
% Time at Work	0.003	–	–	–	–	–	–	–
	(0.001)	–	–	–	–	–	–	–
GRI	0.573	–	–	–	–	–	–	–
	(0.001)	–	–	–	–	–	–	–

the calculation of the standard errors (Oakes 1999). The regression coefficients are all statistically significant and of a positive sign. As the variables are scaled, we deduce that temperature and vaccination have the strongest effects on the system dynamics while percentage of time at work has the smallest effect.

From the estimates of the reaction rates, it is possible to obtain the basic reproduction number, expressing the number of new infections that each infected individual produces on average. In particular, this is defined by

$$R_0(t) = \frac{\theta_1(t)}{\theta_2(t) + \theta_3(t) + \theta_5(t)}$$

and is shown in Fig. 3. The values estimated by our model (solid line) follow quite closely the ranges reported by the Italian government (Mattarella 2021b), which are depicted with different colours. In particular, we correctly detect the peak of infection in the spring of 2021 and the period of lowest infection in the summer of 2021. In the winter of 2021, the results show how the rates were

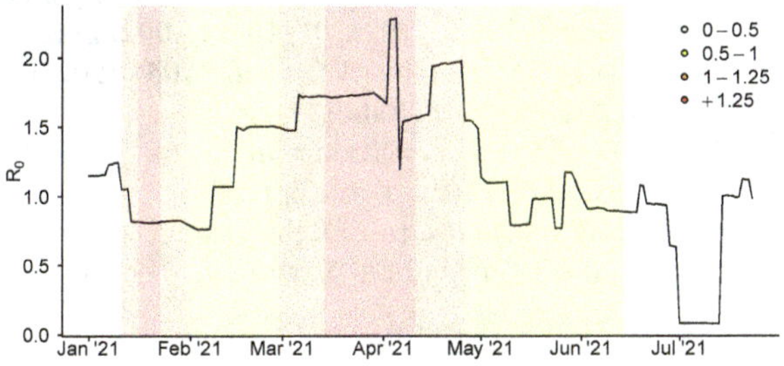

Fig. 3. Comparison of basic reproduction number estimated by the model (solid line) and reported by the government (background colours) (Mattarella 2021). (Color figure online)

decreasing already prior to the strict measures coming into force (red column). This phenomenon was also observed in the very early stages of the pandemic, as reported in Wood and Wit (2021).

5 Conclusion

In this paper, we have proposed an extension of existing quasi-reaction models to account for covariate-dependent reaction rates. We have evaluated the effectiveness of the proposed approach in modelling the dynamics of disease spreading and their changes due to environmental factors and governmental and public health interventions.

References

ARPA Lombardia. Temperatura minima media e massima mensili (2022). https://www.arpalombardia.it/indicatori/2021/meteo-e-clima/temperatura-minima-media-e-massima-mensili/

Britton, T., Pardoux, E., Ball, F., Laredo, C., Sirl, D., Tran, V.C.: Stochastic Epidemic Models with Inference, vol. 132. Springer, Heidelberg (2019). https://doi.org/10.1007/978-3-030-30900-8

Corrao, G., Franchi, M., Cereda, D., Bortolan, F., Zoli, A., et al.: Persistence of protection against SARS-CoV-2 clinical outcomes up to 9 months since vaccine completion: a retrospective observational analysis in Lombardy, Italy. Lancet Infect. Dis. **22**(5), 649–656 (2022)

Framba, M., Vinciotti, V., Wit, E.C.: Latent event history models for quasi-reaction systems. Comput. Stat. Data Anal., 107996 (2024). https://doi.org/10.1016/j.csda.2024.107996. Elsevier

Guidotti, E., Ardia, D.: COVID-19 data hub. J. Open Source Softw. **5**(51), 2376 (2020)

Hale, T., Webster, S., Petherick, A., Phillips, T., Kira, B.: Oxford COVID-19 government response tracker (OxCGRT). Last Updated **8**, 30 (2020)

Kifer, D., Bugada, D., Villar-Garcia, J., Gudelj, I., Menni, C., et al.: Effects of environmental factors on severity and mortality of COVID-19. Front. Med. **7**, 607786 (2021)

Mattarella, S.: Decreto del presidente del consiglio dei ministri 14 gennaio 2021 (2021a). https://www.gazzettaufficiale.it/eli/id/2021/01/15/21A00221/sg

Mattarella, S.: Decreto legge 23 luglio 2021, n. 105 (2021b). https://www.gazzettaufficiale.it/eli/id/2021/07/23/21G00117/sg

Oakes, D.: Direct calculation of the information matrix via the EM algorithm. J. R. Stat. Soc. Ser. B Stat Methodol. **61**(2), 479–482 (1999)

Wood, S.N., Wit, E.C.: Was R <1 before the English lockdowns? on modelling mechanistic detail, causality and inference about Covid-19. PLoS ONE **16**(9), e0257455 (2021)

Modelling of Overdispersed Count Rates

John Hinde[1(✉)], Alberto Alvarez-Iglesias[2], John Ferguson[1], Clarice G.B. Demétrio[3], John Crown[4,5], Bryan T. Hennessy[6], and Vicky Donachie[7]

[1] School of Mathematical and Statistical Sciences, University of Galway, Galway, Ireland
john.hinde@universityofgalway.ie
[2] HRB Clinical Research Facility Galway, University of Galway, Galway, Ireland
[3] ESALQ/USP, Piracicaba, Brazil
[4] Department of Medical Oncology, St Vincent's University Hospital, Dublin, Ireland
[5] Cancer Clinical Research Trust, National Institute for Cellular Biotechnology, Dublin City University, Dublin, Ireland
[6] Department of Medical Oncology/ICORG/Cancer Trials Ireland, Beaumont Hospital, Royal College of Surgeons in Ireland, Dublin, Ireland
[7] Cancer Trials Ireland/ICORG, Dublin, Ireland

Abstract. This paper revisits the common problem of analysing counts recorded over time through the modelling of the underlying rate, motivated by the analysis of a cancer treatment related study. The baseline Poisson model is simply implemented though the inclusion of an offset for the different exposure/recording times and the underlying Poisson process gives other nice well-known properties. We consider how this approach can be extended to models for overdispersed data. The use of a simple offset with a negative binomial model is common practice and we consider the appropriateness of this and the resulting implications. We discuss how these ideas extend to more general mixed Poisson models, including ZIP, to handle zero-inflation, and ZINB for zero-inflation and overdispersion. The simple offset approach does not extend to other extended count models such as the COM-Poisson and general weighted Poisson distributions.

Keywords: counts · rates · overdispersion models

1 Introduction

In many practical contexts counts for some particular event of interest are recorded over time (or some appropriate surrogate) for a sample of n individuals. It is very common for counts not to be recorded for each separate time unit (e.g, hour, day, etc.) but rather to just give a total count over the full observation period for each individual. Typically, the individual observation periods, T_i, differ and so the interest focusses on the underlying count rate and how this may depend on covariates of interest. The simplest model uses a Poisson distribution for the total counts, Y_i, over the observed time period T_i, assuming a

J. Einbeck et al. (Eds.): IWSM 2024, CONTRIB.STAT., pp. 179–184, 2024.
https://doi.org/10.1007/978-3-031-65723-8_28

time-homogeneous rate λ_i giving $Y_i \sim \text{Poisson}(T_i\lambda_i)$, where the individual rates λ_i depend on observed covariates $\mathbf{x}_i$ through a log-linear model $\log(\lambda_i) = \boldsymbol{\beta}^T\mathbf{x}_i$. While direct modelling of the observed rates Y_i/T_i is possible through an appropriately weighted pseudo-Poisson glm, the much simpler and common approach is to model the total counts Y_i with a Poisson glm where the means μ_i are given by

$$\log(\mu_i) = \log(T_i\lambda_i) = \log(T_i) + \log(\lambda_i) = \log(T_i) + \boldsymbol{\beta}^T\mathbf{x}_i$$

and $\log(T_i)$ is included as an *offset* in the linear predictor. The assumption of the Poisson distribution is the most basic count distribution based on a time-homogenous Poisson process and gives independent Poisson(λ_i) counts for each of the T_i unit subintervals. Additionally, conditional on the total observed count Y_i, the joint distribution for the counts in the T_i subintervals is multinomial with equal probabilities $1/T_i$. A consequence of this is that, conditional on the model being true, the total counts $\{Y_i\}$ are sufficient for $\boldsymbol{\beta}$ with no additional information from the individual subinterval counts, although they could provide a diagnostic check on the assumption of time homogeneity.

A feature of the Poisson distribution is that it is equi-dispersed, with the variance equal to the mean, while observed counts are frequently found to be more variable, that is *overdispersed*, see [4]. So an obvious question is which overdispersed count models easily extend to handle unequal observation times (exposures). The quasi-Poisson model with a scaled Poisson model and variance $\phi\mu_i$ is a simple fix for overdispersion and again handles the varying times through the $\log(T_i)$ offset, however as this is a quasi-likelihood approach there is no underlying probability distribution. A widely used overdispersed count probability model is the negative binomial, arising from the inclusion of a gamma mixing distribution to provide additional between-individual variation. Lawless [5] presents the negative binomial regression model as a natural extension of the Poisson rate model using the offset formulation; direct negative binomial modelling of the observed rate is not possible in any simple manner if the observation periods T_i differ. The consequences of this extension are not discussed by Lawless and this is also the case in other treatments of the negative binomial regression model, such as [2] and [3]. The aim of this paper is to look into this natural and simple extension of the Poisson rate model motivated by an example where quasi-Poisson and negative binomial results were surprisingly different. We then go on to consider how rates can be analysed on other extended Poisson models using the simple offset trick and also where this breaks down. The offset formulation is not restricted to counts over time but can be used with general exposure measures, such as geographic area, population, etc. More general models could include observation duration dependent rates, joint modelling of the counts and observation period, and mis-specification of the observed exposure (time). In the concluding discussion we return to why results and conclusions from different overdispersion rate models may differ.

2 Motivating Example

Data is from a randomised clinical trial in HER-2 positive breast cancer patients. During enrolment to the trial, evidence emerged of a high incidence of diarrhoea events in patients who were receiving lapatinib, an antineoplastic agent for the treatment of advanced breast cancer. These patients were treated with loperamide, a medicine to treat diarrhoea. A subsequent amendment to the protocol made mandatory the use of loperamide for all patients taking lapatinib. The aim of the analysis was to determine if the rate of diarrhoea-related adverse events that occurred during treatment was reduced after the introduction of the mandated prophylactic loperamide. For each patient, counts of diarrhoea events were recorded over time, although the observation periods (number of treatment cycles) were quite variable and differed over the two groups of interest, before and after loperamide use, and the observed rates displayed a marked difference between the two groups, see Fig. 1.

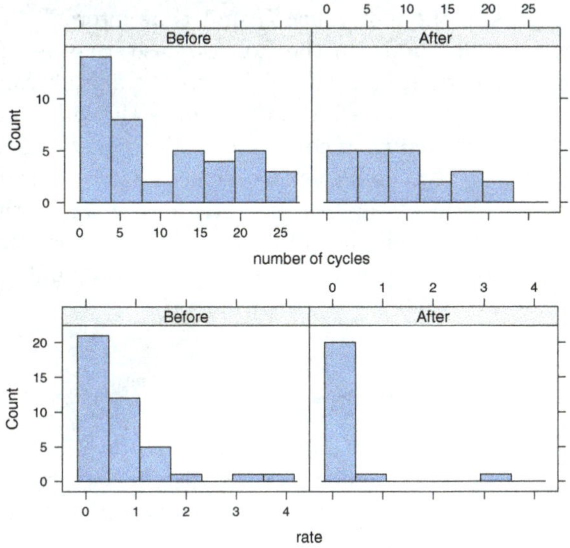

Fig. 1. Top: Comparison of observation periods for the two groups, before and after loperamide; Bottom: Comparison of rates for the two groups.

A simple Poisson rate model was fitted with an offset for the number of cycles and the treatment effect, but there was clear overdispersion; deviance = 235 on 61df and a half-normal diagnostic plot using **hnp** [6] showing a clear lack of fit. The quasi-Poisson model accounts for the overdispersion with an estimated scale parameter $\tilde{\phi} = 6.23$. Using a negative binomial rate model gave an adequate fit, and indeed a somewhat better half-normal diagnostic plot than for the quasi-Poisson, although both models accounted for the overdispersion. However, the treatment effect (on the log-scale) was now -1.02 (s.e. 0.38) compared to −0.41 (s.e. 0.19) for the Poisson model and −0.41 (s.e. 0.48) for the quasi-Poisson model, giving different conclusions from the two overdispersed models. The increased standard errors for the negative binomial and quasi-Poisson models are as expected and reflect the appreciable overdispersion. The large change in the parameter estimate for the negative binomial is more surprising and likely due to substantial variation in recording intervals within each group. Thinking about this led us to consider the role of the offset in the negative binomial and other overdispersed rate models.

3 Negative Binomial Rate Models

A simple formulation of the negative binomial rate model includes a gamma distributed random effect, U, for the individuals with conditionally a standard Poisson rate model, that is $Y_i|U_i \sim \text{Poisson}(T_i\lambda_iU_i)$, where the U_i are independent Gamma(θ, θ) distributed with mean 1 and variance $1/\theta$. Unconditionally, Y_i is negative binomial with mean $\mu_i = T_i\lambda_i$ and the usual quadratic variance $\mu_i + \mu_i^2/\theta$. The counts in the individual T_i unit time intervals are also negative binomial distributed, but, unlike in the Poisson case, they are no longer independent and have a common correlation due to the shared random effect U_i. However, conditional on the observed total counts the subinterval counts are still multinomially distributed with equal probabilities $1/T_i$, reflecting the time homogeneity of the assumed conditional Poisson rate model. In fact, this result is independent of the form of the assumed random effect as this is implicitly removed in the conditioning on the total count. So, for the negative binomial rate model the total counts are sufficient statistics with the $\log(T_i)$ being used as an offset in a log-linear model for the mean.

4 Extensions

From the specification of the multiplicative mixed rate model in the previous section, it is clear that the assumed gamma distribution can be replaced by any non-negative distribution. For an arbitrary distribution G with mean 1 and variance σ^2 we obtain the usual quadratic variance $\mu_i + \mu_i^2\sigma^2$ and the varying T_i can be handled with the offset. Taking G to be a two-point distribution on $\{0, 1\}$ leads to the zero-inflated Poisson (ZIP) model, while taking G to be a mixed distribution with a mass at 0 and a gamma distribution gives the zero-inflated negative binomial (ZINB) distribution. Such arguments show that the use of the offset is an appropriate way of handling different exposures in these extended mixed Poisson models.

Aside from the mixed Poisson there are many other extension of Poisson models that are used to account for overdispersion and excess zeros. Some of these models, such as the COM-Poisson (see for example [7]), can also account for underdispersion. One general class is the weighted Poisson distributions [1], but here it is not so simple to account for differing exposures and the modelling of rates.

Other potential extensions are more general Poisson exposure models, specifically when considering aggregate population rates over different regions. Between region-variation is easily handled with a region random effect, however, it is also possible to include individual level variation (overdispersion) within regions. Formulated as two nested random effects this gives a structured overdispersion model, that allows for correlation between individuals within the same region.

5 Discussion

In the above and in the analyses we have assumed that the counts are time-homogeneous, however, this is not necessary and one can think in terms of modelling the average rate over the observed time period. Furthermore, the dependence on time may not be directly proportional and models that include a simple power transformation of time are easily obtained by replacing the fixed offset term with a coefficient of 1 by a general regression term with a coefficient α that may even be allowed to depend on other covariates, although this destroys any simple interpretation. For the example, we obtain $\hat{\alpha} = 0.18$, very different from 1 for direct time proportionality implied by the offset model, and in fact there is some evidence that α also differs across the two groups.

More general mis-specification (or error) in the time variable could be incorporated by considering it as a random variable, which for the baseline Poisson model leads again to a mixed model or a negative binomial if the variation is taken to be gamma distributed. So evidence of overdispersion in such a mixed model could be due to variation in the individual rates or unknown variability in the recorded time periods; without more detailed data it would be impossible to separate out the cause of the overdispersion.

Returning to the example it is instructive to try to understand the reasons between the substantive different conclusions from the Poisson (or quasi-Poisson) and negative binomial models. Briefly, both Poisson regression and Negative binomial regression (assuming a fixed value for the dispersion parameter) can be fit using iterative re-weighted least squares, with the contribution of each individual observation to the overall fit being specified by differing weights for the two models. While the weights in the Poisson (or quasi-Poisson) model (for an individual) are proportional to that individual's exposure time, and are essentially unbounded if we consider arbitrarily long exposure periods, the weights in the negative binomial regression are bounded above.

A consequence of this is that a single individual, with an extremely long exposure period, can essentially determine the estimates from Poisson (or quasi-Poisson) regression. One may be easily fooled into believing that an appropriate correction for overdispersion can be made when using quasi-Poisson regression—but under the scenario of a single observation with long exposure period and the true distribution of counts being mixed Poisson, the quasi-Poisson estimator will be extremely unstable and the reported standard error will underestimate its sampling variability. We advise caution in using the quasi-Poisson method to account for overdispersion as a default option in count regression models where exposure times vary over observations. As in many other situations (in the context of excess zeros see for example Warton [8]) the negative binomial seems to be the sensible and simple choice for count data modelling.

Acknowledgments. This research was partially supported by FAPESP Project: 2024/01638-3, Brazil for John Hinde and by CNPq Project: 312645/2021-0, Brazil for Clarice G. B. Demétrio.

References

1. Del Castillo, J., Pérez-Casany, M.: Weighted Poisson distributions for overdispersion and underdispersion situations. Ann. Inst. Stat. Math. **50**(3), 567–585 (1998)
2. Cameron, A.C., Trivedi, P.K.: Regression Analysis of Count Data. Cambridge University Press, Cambridge (1998)
3. Hilbe, J.M.: Negative Binomial Regression. Cambridge University Press, Cambridge (2007)
4. Hinde, J., Demétrio, C.G.B.: Overdispersion: models and estimation. Comput. Stat. Data Anal. **27**, 151–170 (1998)
5. Lawless, J.F.: Negative binomial and mixed Poisson regression. Can. J. Stat. **15**, 209–225 (1987)
6. Moral, R.A., Hinde, J., Demétrio, C.G.B.: Half-normal plots and overdispersed models in R: the `hnp` package. J. Stat. Softw. **81**, 1–23 (2017)
7. Sellers, K.F., Borle, S., Shmueli, G.: The COM-Poisson model for count data: a survey of methods and applications. Appl. Stoch. Model. Bus. Ind. **28**(2), 104–116 (2012)
8. Warton, D.I.: Many zeros does not mean zero inflation: comparing the goodness-of-fit of parametric models to multivariate abundance data. Environmetrics **16**(3), 275–289 (2005)

Sparse Intrinsic Gaussian Processes for Prediction on Manifolds: Extending Applications to Environmental Contexts

Yuan Liu(✉), Mu Niu, and Claire Miller

School of Mathematics and Statistics, University of Glasgow, Glasgow, UK
y.liu.10@research.gla.ac.uk

Abstract. Traditional Gaussian Processes are limited in their application by complex boundaries and intricately structured manifolds, such as when predicting water quality in the Aral Sea. Intrinsic Gaussian Processes adequately accommodate these complex conditions. To address the computational complexity of Intrinsic Gaussian Processes, we employ the sparse approximation method known as Deterministic Inducing Conditionals (DIC). The Sparse Intrinsic Gaussian Processes approach we propose offers effective prediction over such manifolds.

Keywords: Sparse Intrinsic Gaussian Processes · Manifold · DIC

1 Introduction

In recent years, an increasing amount of research has been conducted in complex constrained domains, rather than being limited to the traditional Euclidean space. For example, researchers have been collecting chlorophyll concentration data in the Aral Sea, which has complex boundaries and intricate structures [1]. To model unknown functions and predict their values at unknown locations, Gaussian Processes (GPs) are widely used in such scenarios. Based on a series of random variables following joint Gaussian distributions, the GP can be specified by its mean function $m : \mathcal{X} \rightarrow \mathbb{R}$ and positive semi-definite covariance function $k : \mathcal{X} \times \mathcal{X} \rightarrow \mathbb{R}$. The GPs can be written as [2]:

$$f(\boldsymbol{x}) \sim \mathcal{GP}\left(m(\boldsymbol{x}), k\left(\boldsymbol{x}, \boldsymbol{x}'\right)\right), \tag{1}$$

where covariance function k is calculated as the kernel function, measuring the "distance" between any two points $\boldsymbol{x}$ and $\boldsymbol{x}'$. The most commonly used kernel function is the Radial Basis Function (RBF) kernel:

$$k\left(\boldsymbol{x}, \boldsymbol{x}'\right) = \alpha \exp\left(-\frac{\left|\boldsymbol{x} - \boldsymbol{x}'\right|_2^2}{2\ell^2}\right), \tag{2}$$

which has two parameters, length-scale parameter l and variance parameter α. Traditional kernels cannot accurately measure the intrinsic distance. Niu et al.

J. Einbeck et al. (Eds.): IWSM 2024, CONTRIB.STAT., pp. 185–190, 2024.
https://doi.org/10.1007/978-3-031-65723-8_29

(2019) proposed intrinsic GPs to adequately consider the intrinsic geometry of the spaces [3]. Intrinsic GPs are constructed using the heat kernel of the manifold which is estimated as the transition density of the Brownian Motion on manifolds. However, a significant limitation of intrinsic GPs is the expensive computational cost and memory requirements. As the number of training points n increases, the computational demand grows to $O(n^3)$ due to inversion of the covariance matrix [4]. To solve this issue, various computationally efficient approximation methods for GPs have been proposed, among which a representative one is DIC [5]. DIC reduces computational complexity by introducing inducing inputs. In this paper, we propose a Sparse Intrinsic GP that effectively predicts on manifolds while overcoming computational constraints, with applications to environmental contexts.

2 Construction of Sparse Intrinsic GP

2.1 Numerical Approximation of the Heat Kernel

In order to better evaluate the internal geometric features of the manifold, our Sparse Intrinsic GPs use the heat kernel as the covariance kernel. Let M be a d-dimensional complete and orientable Riemannian manifold. A heat kernel of M is a smooth function $K(x; y; t)$ on $M \times M \times R^+$ satisfying the heat equation, where the initial condition holds in a distributional sense:

$$\frac{\partial}{\partial t} K_{\text{heat}}\left(s_0, s, t\right) = \frac{1}{2} \Delta_s K_{\text{heat}}\left(s_0, s, t\right), \tag{3}$$

$$\lim_{t \to 0} K_{\text{heat}}\left(s_0, s, 0\right) = \delta\left(s_0, s\right), \quad s_0, s \in M, \tag{4}$$

which describes how heat is transferred from one point s_0 to another point s at a given time t. Letting $K_{\text{heat}}^t(x, y) = K^{\text{heat}}(x, y, t)$, $K_{\text{heat}}^t(x, y)$ represents the covariance kernel. However, for most cases, we cannot explicitly evaluate $K_{\text{heat}}^t(x, y)$. Here, we utilise the fact that heat kernels can be interpreted as transition densities of Brownian Motion (BM) on M. When BM path crosses the boundary, it will pause time and resample the next step until it remains within the boundary.

The probability of $S(t) \in A \subset M$, for any Borel set A, is given by

$$\mathbb{P}\left[S(t) \in A \mid S(0) = s_0\right] = \int_A K_{\text{heat}}^t\left(s_0, s\right) ds, \tag{5}$$

where the integral is specified in terms of the volume form of M. The transition density of $S(t)$ at s is approximated as:

$$K_{heat}^t\left(s_0, s\right) \approx \hat{K}^t = \mathbb{P}\left[S(t) \in A \mid S(0) = s_0\right] \approx \frac{1}{V(A)} \cdot \frac{k}{N}, \tag{6}$$

where $V(A)$ is the Riemannian volume of A, parameterised by the radius of A. Equation 6 provides an approximation for constructing the intrinsic GPs [3].

2.2 Sparse Method DIC Used for Intrinsic GP

Let $\mathbf{f}_*$ be a vector of values of $f(\cdot)$ at some test points that are not represented in the training sample. The joint distribution of $\mathbf{f}$ and $\mathbf{f}_*$ is

$$p(\mathbf{f}, \mathbf{f}_*) = \mathcal{N}\left\{0, \begin{pmatrix} \Sigma_{\mathbf{ff}} & \Sigma_{\mathbf{ff}_*} \\ \Sigma_{\mathbf{f}_*\mathbf{f}} & \Sigma_{\mathbf{f}_*\mathbf{f}_*} \end{pmatrix}\right\}, \tag{7}$$

where $\Sigma_{\mathbf{ff}_*}$ is the covariance matrix for training and test points. Without employing the sparse method, the predictive distribution is derived by marginalising out f:

$$\begin{aligned} p(\mathbf{f}_* \mid \boldsymbol{y}) &= \int p(\mathbf{f}_*\mathbf{f} \mid \boldsymbol{y})\, d\mathbf{f} \\ &= \mathcal{N}\left(\Sigma_{\mathbf{f}_*\mathbf{f}}\left(\Sigma_{\mathbf{ff}} + \sigma^2_{\text{noise}}\, I\right)^{-1} \boldsymbol{y}, \Sigma_{\mathbf{f}_*\mathbf{f}_*} - \Sigma_{\mathbf{f}_*\mathbf{f}}\left(\Sigma_{\mathbf{ff}} + \sigma^2_{\text{noise}}\, I\right)^{-1} \Sigma_{\mathbf{ff}_*}\right). \end{aligned} \tag{8}$$

When computing the variance, $\Sigma_{\mathbf{f}_*\mathbf{f}_*}$ needs to consider the BM originating from each grid point, which creates a significant computational burden. We introduce the sparse method DIC to address this issue [5].

The GPs prior can be extended by incorporating an additional set of m inducing points on the manifold M, $z = [z_1, z_2, ..., z_m], z_i \in M$, corresponding to m random variables $u = [f(z_1), \dots, f(z_m)]$. The prior distribution can be expressed in terms of $p(u)$ and the conditional distribution $p(\mathbf{f}|u)$.

$$p(\mathbf{f}) = \int p(\mathbf{f}|u)p(u)du, \quad p(u) = \mathcal{N}(0, \Sigma_{zz}), \tag{9}$$

where Σ_{zz} is the covariance matrix for inducing points. The effective prior implied by the DIC can be expressed as:

$$q_{\text{DIC}}(\mathbf{f}, \mathbf{f}_*) = \mathcal{N}\left(\mathbf{0}, \begin{bmatrix} Q_{\mathbf{f},\mathbf{f}} & Q_{\mathbf{f},*} \\ Q_{*,\mathbf{f}} & Q_{*,*} \end{bmatrix}\right), \tag{10}$$

where Q is defined as $Q_{\mathbf{f},*} = \Sigma_{\mathbf{f}_*\mathbf{u}} \Sigma_{\mathbf{uu}}^{-1} \Sigma_{\mathbf{uf}}$ and the predictive distribution can be derived as:

$$\begin{aligned} q_{\text{DIC}}(\mathbf{f}_* \mid \mathbf{y}) = \mathcal{N}\Big(& Q_{*,\mathbf{f}}\left(Q_{\mathbf{f},\mathbf{f}} + \sigma^2_{\text{noise}}\, \mathbf{I}\right)^{-1} \mathbf{y}, \\ & Q_{*,*} - Q_{*,\mathbf{f}}\left(Q_{\mathbf{f},\mathbf{f}} + \sigma^2_{\text{noise}}\, \mathbf{I}\right)^{-1} Q_{\mathbf{f},*}\Big). \end{aligned} \tag{11}$$

3 Implementation of Sparse Intrinsic GP

3.1 The Sparse Intrinsic GP on the U-Shape Domain

We implement the Sparse Intrinsic GP on the U-shape domain as shown in Fig. 1(a), where the value of the function varies smoothly from the lower right corner to the upper right corner of the domain ranging from –6.19 to 6.19. In our simulation study, we have 285 grid data points and 5 inducing points equally spaced within the boundary. The green crosses shown in Fig. 1(c) represents the inducing points' location and the black crosses in Fig. 1(b) and 1(c) show the randomly selected training points.

We randomly select 20 sets of training points from the grid points. Each set contains 15 training points. For each set, the results from the Sparse Intrinsic GP are compared with those from the traditional GP model. We selected one set of results for comparison as shown in Fig. 1(b) and 1(c). The calculated RMSEs are plotted in the boxplots in Fig. 1(d). The results of the traditional GP are substantively influenced by boundaries, whereas the sparse method is not. The RMSE results clearly demonstrate the improvement in precision of the sparse method, even with only 5 inducing points.

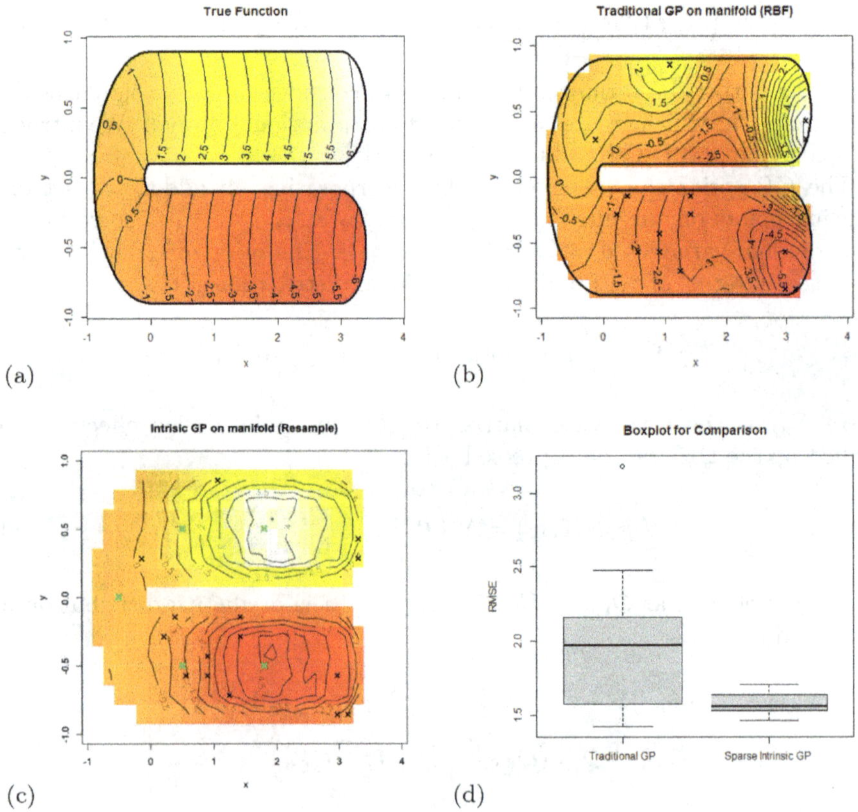

Fig. 1. (a) The true function in the U-shape domain; (b) Traditional GP predictions on U-shape domain with 15 training points (black crosses) and 5 inducing points (green crosses); (c) Sparse Intrinsic GP predictions on U-shape domain with 15 training points (black crosses) and 5 inducing points (green crosses); (d) RMSE results displayed in the boxplot form.

3.2 Impacted Predictive Distribution

Due to the degeneracy of the prior, the predictive distributions present inaccurate results. Specifically, as test points move further from the inducing points, $Q_{*,*}$ approaches zero. Thus the predicted variance goes to zero as test points become far from the inducing inputs. This is unreasonable because the predictive variance represents uncertainty; it should increase, indicating greater uncertainty, when moving away from the inducing points, rather than approaching zero. The issue lies within the sparse method DIC itself and is the subject of our future research

When we implemented the Sparse Intrinsic GP on the U-shape domain in the previous section, we have 5 inducing points equally spaced within the boundary. Figure 2 provides an example illustrating the issue we discussed above. Figure 2 shows the results for an increased number of training points, with 8 training points selected along the lower half of a U-shape. Figure 2(a) shows the corresponding predictive mean, while Fig. 2(b) shows the predictive variance. It is clear that the variance decreases to zero as the upper right part of the U-shape moves away from the inducing points.

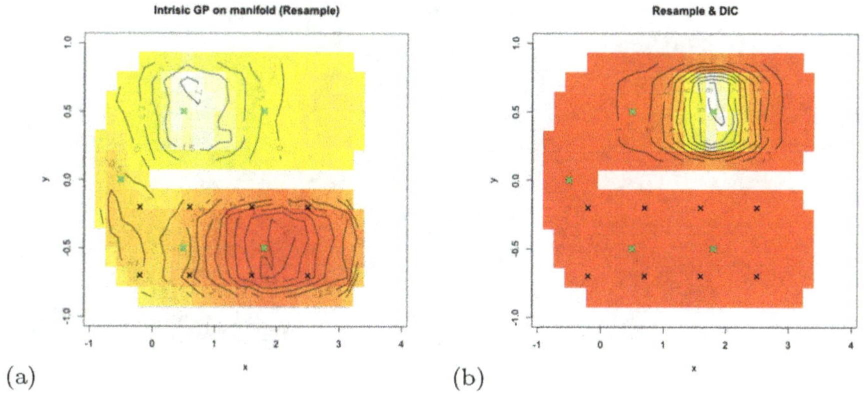

Fig. 2. (a) Sparse Intrinsic GP predictive mean on U-shape domain with 8 training points (black crosses) and 5 inducing points (green crosses); (b) the predictive variance of Sparse Intrinsic GP predictions with 8 training points (black crosses) and 5 inducing points (green crosses).

4 Discussion

Our main contribution lies in effectively employing the sparse method DIC to enhance the computational efficiency of intrinsic GPs on manifolds. Compared with traditional GPs on U-shaped data, we demonstrate the superiority of Sparse Intrinsic GPs. In the future work, the next steps include solving the inaccuracy issue of predictive variance when using DIC method.

References

1. Wood, S.N.: Generalized Additive Models: an Introduction with R. Chapman and hall/CRC, Boca Raton (2017)
2. Williams, C.K., Rasmussen, C.E.: Gaussian Processes for Machine Learning, vol. 2, no. 3. MIT press, Cambridge, MA (2006)
3. Niu, M., Cheung, P., Lin, L., Dai, Z., Lawrence, N., Dunson, D.: Intrinsic gaussian processes on complex constrained domains. J. Roy. Stat. Soc. Ser. B **81**(3), 603–627 (2019)
4. Park, C., Huang, J. Z., Ding, Y.: Domain decomposition approach for fast Gaussian process regression of large spatial data sets. In: 1foldr Import, 2019-10-08 Batch 12 (2011)
5. Quinonero-Candela, J., Rasmussen, C.E., Williams, C.K.: Approximation methods for Gaussian process regression. In: Large-Scale Kernel Machines, pp. 203–223. MIT Press, Cambridge (2007)

Functional Copula Graphical Regression Model for Analysing Brain-Body Rhythm

Rita Fici[1(✉)], Luigi Augugliaro[1], and Ernst C. Wit[2]

[1] University of Palermo, Palermo, Italy
[2] Università della Svizzera Italiana, Lugano, Switzerland

Abstract. In physiology, organ functions can be modelled as networks with individual regulatory mechanisms, forming a broader system through continuous interactions. The system not only interacts with itself, but can also respond to outside impulses. The paper proposes a functional graphical regression model to describe interconnected brain activities partly in response to other organs. The analysis focuses on the conditional independence structure of brain waves given the RR interval of the electrocardiographic waveform, the respiration amplitude and the blood volume pulse.

Keywords: EEG waves · network physiology · Functional Data Analysis · functional Graphical Regression Models · Gaussian copula

1 Introduction

This study contributes to exploring new statistical tools and advancing the comprehension of physiological interactions. The data originate from an investigation on network physiology by Pernice et al. (2021). Within their conceptual framework, the human organism is viewed as a network where coordinated interactions among organs are essential for generating distinct physiological states and maintaining health. Each organ is considered as a network with its own regulatory mechanisms, continuously interacting with other body organs to contribute to the broader system.

This analysis aims to recover the conditional independence structure of brain waves while simultaneously taking into account the effects of some external covariates. The response and the explanatory sets of variables constitute two functional stochastic processes, which take place in a closed interval of time. The conditional independence structure can be represented by an undirected graph. The vertices of the graph are the response variables, and the edges represent the conditional independence structure among them, given the values of external variables. For a parsimonious representation, we use the assumption of partial separability of the covariance operator defined in Zapata et al. (2022) . The estimation of the relationship between and within the response functions and the explanatory functions is performed by analyzing the relation between

J. Einbeck et al. (Eds.): IWSM 2024, CONTRIB.STAT., pp. 191–196, 2024.
https://doi.org/10.1007/978-3-031-65723-8_30

and within the elements of the vectorized Karhunen-Loéve expansions of the sets of functions. Following the methodology of Solea and Li (2022), the scores of the expansions are assumed to follow a Gaussian Copula distribution.

In Sect. 2, we provide a brief review of the methodological framework. The details of the analysis and the results are presented in Sect. 3. Finally, in Sect. 4, the main aspects of the analysis are summarized.

2 Metodology

Let us denote by $\mathbf{Y}(t)$ and $\mathbf{X}(t)$ the response and the explanatory sets of random functions of dimensions p and q, respectively. The time point, denoted by t, belongs to the closed time interval $\mathcal{T} \subset \mathbb{R}$. The graph $\mathcal{G} = \{\mathcal{V}, \mathcal{E}\}$ represents the conditional independence structure of $\mathbf{Y}(t)$, and it is conditioned on the effects of $\mathbf{X}(t)$.

To recover the effects of $\mathbf{X}(t)$ on the expectation of the responses, we analyze the relations among the coefficients resulting from the vectorized Karhunen-Loéve expansions:

$$\mathbf{Y}(t) = \sum_{l=1}^{\infty} \gamma_l \varphi_l(t) \text{ and } \mathbf{X}(t) = \sum_{l=1}^{\infty} \chi_l \varphi_l(t)$$

where the orthonormal basis system $\{\varphi_l\}_{l=1}^{\infty}$ is common to all the variables. The scores are

$$\gamma_l = \int_{\mathcal{T}} \mathbf{Y}(t)\varphi_l(t)dt \text{ and } \chi_l = \int_{\mathcal{T}} \mathbf{X}(t)\varphi_l(t)dt.$$

The conditional expectation of the response functions is reflected in the relation between γ_l and χ_l. As demonstrated by Fici et al. (2024), the conditional expectation of the responses can be written as

$$\mathbb{E}[\mathbf{Y}(t) \mid \mathbf{X}(\cdot)] = \sum_{l=1}^{\infty} \mathbf{b}_l \chi_l \varphi_l(t)$$

where $\mathbf{b}_l = \mathbb{E}[\gamma_l \chi_l^\top]\mathbb{E}[\chi_l \chi_l^\top]^{-1}$ and $(\cdot)$ indicates the entire domain of the variables.

To study the conditional independence structure of $\mathbf{Y}(\cdot) \mid \mathbf{X}(\cdot)$, we assume that the residuals, $\kappa_{jl} = \gamma_{jl} - \mathbf{b}_l \chi_{jl}$, are linked to some latent variables by a copula structure. We consider

$$z_{jl} = \Phi^{-1}(\mathtt{F}_{jl}(\kappa_{jl})) \text{ with } z_{jl} \sim \mathtt{N}(0, 1),$$

where Φ is the cumulative distribution function of a univariate standard normal distribution and $\mathtt{F}_{jl}$ is the true absolutely continuous cumulative distribution of κ_{jl}. $\mathbf{z}_l$ and the residuals have correlation matrix R_l. The edge set is encoded by

$$\mathcal{E} = \{(j, j') : \theta_{jj',l} \neq 0 \text{ for at least one } l\}$$

where $\theta_{jj',l}$ is the jj'th-entry of the precision matrix $\Theta_l = R_l^{-1}$ of $\mathbf{z}_l$.

3 Analysis

Our analysis focuses on the interaction within and between two subnetworks. $\mathbf{Y}(t)$ is the network consisting of β-waves of the brain activity, and $\mathbf{X}(t)$ describes the activity of three organs, namely: (i) the heart, measured as the time interval between two successive R-waves on the electrocardiographic waveform (ECG), (ii) the lungs, quantified as the respiration amplitude, (iii) the peripheral vasculature, measured by blood volume pulse (BVP).

3.1 Measurement Protocol

Brain activity is recorded using the EPOC PLUS wireless headset, consisting of 14 electrodes that record signals from different brain regions (see Fig. 1). The ECG (sampled at 250 Hz) and respiration signals (sampled at 25 Hz) are acquired through a sensorized t-shirt, while the E4 wristband captures the BVP signal (sampled at 64 Hz) with a photoplethysmographic (PPG) sensor. Each electrode records different amplitudes of EEG waves. The data were collected by monitoring eighteen young, healthy volunteers during a measurement protocol consisting of three experimental conditions corresponding to different levels of mental stress. The present study is conducted on the data regarding the waves of amplitude β, predominant when a person is awake and actively thinking. The analyzed data concern the condition of rest, where the subjects watch a video showing landscapes with relaxing background music. The data are gathered at 300 instants in time, which belong to a time window of 12 min.

3.2 Graph Estimation

The orthonormal basis system is determined by the eigen-decomposition on the observed matrices of data (Hsing and Eubank, 2015). For each term of the expansion, there is a $(p \times N)$-dimensional matrix and a $(q \times N)$-dimensional matrix; where $p = 14$ is the number of response variables, $q = 3$ is the number of explanatory variables and $N = 18$ is the sample size. The expansions are truncated to the 28th element, which corresponds to the 99% of the total variability of the functions. As done by Fici et al. (2024), the regression matrices are estimated by

$$\hat{\boldsymbol{b}}_l = \arg\min_{\mathbf{b}_l} \frac{1}{N} \sum_{i=1}^{N} \|\gamma_{il} - \mathbf{b}_l \chi_{il}\|^2,$$

for $l = 1, \ldots, 28$. Following Liu et al. (2009), the empirical cumulative distribution functions are estimated as

$$\widehat{\mathrm{F}}_{jl}(\hat{\kappa}_{ijl}) = \begin{cases} \delta_N & \text{if } F_{il}(\hat{\kappa}_{ijl}) < \delta_N \\ F_{il}(\hat{\kappa}_{ijl}) & \text{if } \delta_N \leq F_{jl}(\hat{\kappa}_{ijl}) \leq 1 - \delta_N \\ 1 - \delta_N & \text{if } F_{jl}(\hat{\kappa}_{ijl}) > 1 - \delta_N \end{cases}$$

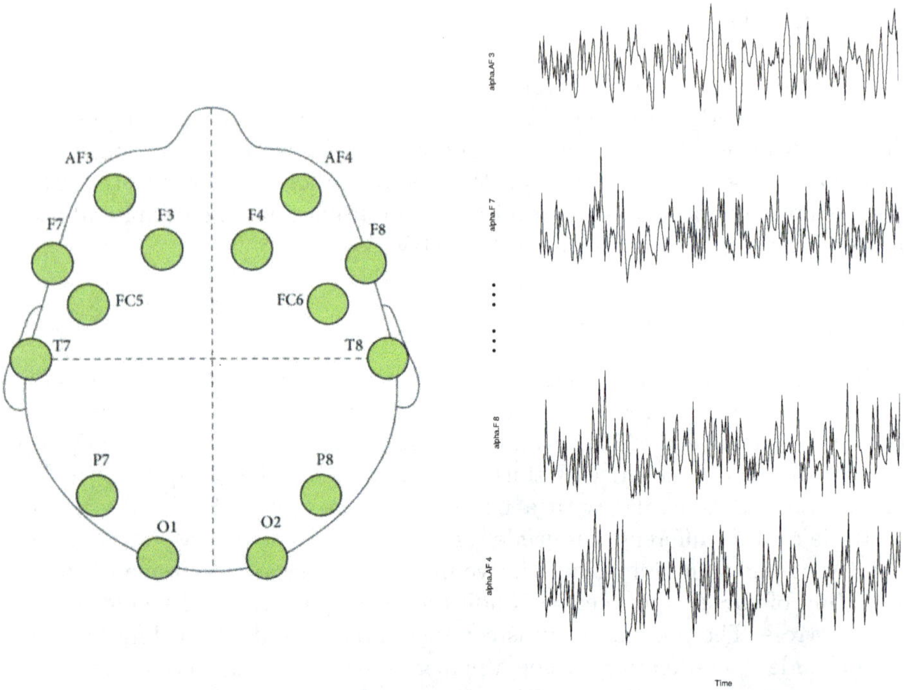

Fig. 1. Left: Graphical representation of the positioning of the 14 EEG electrodes over the scalp. Right: some of the vectors of data measured over the 12-min time window.

where

$$\delta_N = \frac{1}{4N^{1/4}\sqrt{\pi \log(N)}} \quad \text{and} \quad F_{il}(\hat{\kappa}_{ijl}) = \frac{1}{N}\sum_{i=1}^{N} 1_{\{\hat{\kappa}_{ijl} \leq \hat{\kappa}_{jl}\}}.$$

The estimation of $\mathcal{G}$ is performed using the group lasso estimator with penalty function on the set of precision matrices of $\{\widehat{\mathbf{z}}_l\}_{l=1}^{28}$,

$$\{\hat{\Theta}\} = \arg\max_{\Theta} \sum_{l=1}^{28} \Big\{\log \mid \Theta_l \mid - \text{tr}(\mathbf{S}(\hat{\boldsymbol{b}}_l)\Theta_l)\Big\} - \rho P(\{\Theta\}), \tag{1}$$

where $| \cdot |$ is the determinant and $\mathbf{S}(\hat{\boldsymbol{b}}_l) = \frac{1}{N}\sum_{i=1}^{N} \hat{\mathbf{z}}_{il}\hat{\mathbf{z}}_{il}^{\top}$ and ρ is the parameter that tunes the sparsity in the precision matrix. The penalty function is

$$P(\{\Theta\}) = \sum_{j \neq j'}^{p} (\sum_{l=1}^{28} \theta_{jj',l}^2)^{1/2}.$$

3.3 Model Selection and Results

The solution of (1) is found across 101 equally spaced values of ρ, from its maximum value to zero. For model selection, we use the Kullback-Leibler cross-

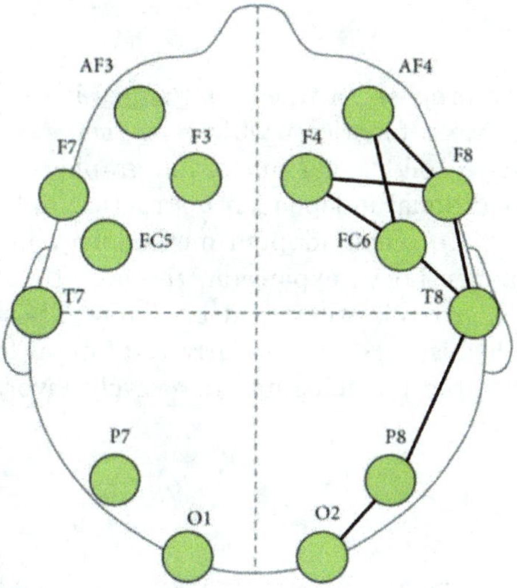

Fig. 2. jKLCV: conditional independence response network.

validation (KLCV) proposed by Vujačić et al. (2015). Figure 2 shows the selected graph.

The estimated graph is consistent with the fact that the participants are actively interpreting landscapes while listening to music; indeed, the right hemisphere results to be the most active. This hemisphere is involved in spatial awareness, perception of spatial relationships and understanding of visual information. It plays a significant role in processing visual stimuli and interpreting nonverbal cues such as facial expressions and body language. Additionally, the right hemisphere is involved in appreciating and interpreting music and recognizing melodies, rhythms, and emotional nuances in musical compositions. In particular, the most active region of the right hemisphere turns out to be the frontal lobe, where there is the right frontal eye field, which is responsible for voluntary eye movements and visual attention. Other regions of the right hemisphere have functions related to the elaboration of visual and auditory inputs: the parietal lobe integrates sensory information to form a coherent perception of the environment; the temporal lobe processes auditory information, including sound perception and music appreciation; and the occipital lobe analyze and interpret visual information, including object recognition, spatial relationships, and scene perception.

On the side of the estimation of the regression parameters, the impact of ECG and BVP on the right hemisphere is stronger than on the left hemisphere, with a notable emphasis on the BVP effects. This pattern does not hold for the effects of respiration amplitude, and the coefficients associated with it tend to be smaller than those associated with the other two organs.

4 Conclusion

In this paper, we have proposed a functional regression framework in order to study relationships between functional objects, which is common in the field of physiology. Employing a conditional functional graphical model, the objective was to recover the conditional independence structure of brain waves given the effect of external covariates. The adopted methodology includes the truncated joint vectorized Karhunen-Loève expansion, the use of Gaussian copula structure and the penalized group lasso estimator. The results suggest a more dense network in the right hemisphere, particularly the frontal lobe, which is consistent with the fact that the participants are actively involved in both a visual and auditory experience.

References

Fici, R., Augugliaro, L., Wit, E.C.: Functional gaussian graphical regression models (2024). https://doi.org/10.48550/arXiv.2401.10196

Hsing, T., Eubank, R.: Theoretical Foundations of Functional Data Analysis, with an Introduction to Linear Operators. John Wiley & Sons, Ltd., Hoboken (2015)

Liu, H., Lafferty, J., Wasserman, L.: The nonparanormal: semiparametric estimation of high dimensional undirected graphs. J. Mach. Learn. Res. **10**(80), 2295–2328 (2009)

Pernice, R., et al.: Multivariate correlation measures reveal structure and strength of brain-body physiological networks at rest and during mental stress. Front. Neurosci. **14** (2021)

Solea, E., Li, B.: Copula Gaussian graphical models for functional data. J. Am. Stat. Assoc. **117**(538), 781–793 (2022)

Vujačić, I., Abbruzzo, A., Wit, E.C.: A computationally fast alternative to cross-validation in penalized gaussian graphical models. J. Stat. Comput. Simul. **85**(18), 3628–3640 (2015)

Zapata, J., Oh, S.-Y., Petersen, A.: Partial separability and functional graphical models for multivariate gaussian processes. Biometrika **109**(3), 665–681 (2022)

State-Space Models for Clustering of Compositional Trajectories

Andrea Panarotto[1(✉)], Manuela Cattelan[1], and Ruggero Bellio[2]

[1] Department of Statistical Sciences, University of Padova, 35121 Padova, Italy
andrea.panarotto@phd.unipd.it
[2] Department of Economics and Statistics, University of Udine, 33100 Udine, Italy

Abstract. Compositional data are drawing increasing interest for their ability to depict interdependent and constrained observations. While time series analysis has sometimes been employed for the study of individual compositional trajectories, little attention has been given to finding and modeling groups of trajectories. Driven by a sustainable mobility motivation, we propose a model-based approach, relying on a state space model representation and an Expectation-Maximization algorithm, for clustering compositional trajectories according to their evolution in the simplex. Trajectory covariates, not captured by the compositional representation, can be included in the component weights in a mixture of experts fashion. The method is applied to urban movement data, where people's movements are represented in the simplex by the proportions of road types in their surroundings.

Keywords: compositional data · Expectation-Maximization algorithm · mixture of experts model · model-based clustering · state-space models

1 Introduction

Compositional data [1] consist of measurements of the proportions of elements in a total. Compositional trajectories represent dynamics of quantities that relate not only with each other but also with the previous and following elements in the sequences. In presence of a large amount of these trajectories, it is interesting to cluster them in meaningful groups where they share similar characteristics.

In this work, we propose two state space representations for compositional trajectories, one classic and one tailored to interpretability, and a related algorithm for the model-based clustering of such trajectories.

2 State Space Representations for Compositions

Let $\mathbb{S}^{d-1} = \left\{ \boldsymbol{y} \in \mathbb{R}^d_{>0} \mid \sum_{i=1}^d y_i = 1 \right\}$ be the d-dimensional simplex. The usual way to deal with compositional data is to exploit logratio transformations which

J. Einbeck et al. (Eds.): IWSM 2024, CONTRIB.STAT., pp. 197–203, 2024.
https://doi.org/10.1007/978-3-031-65723-8_31

map the data from the constrained simplex space $\mathbb{S}^{d-1}$ to the unconstrained Euclidean space $\mathbb{R}^{d-1}$. Assuming a Normal distribution on the transformed data allows to induce flexible variance structures on the data, which is not possible when modeling data via common simplex supported distributions, e.g. the Dirichlet. We adopt the isometric logratio (ilr) transformation [4], for its metric-preserving properties. Let $\mathbf{y}$ be a d-dimensional compositional vector. The ilr-transformed vector $\text{ilr}(\mathbf{y}) = \mathbf{z} = (z_1, \ldots, z_{d-1})$ is defined through

$$z_i = \left(\sqrt{\frac{i}{i+1}} \log \frac{\sqrt[i]{\prod_{j=1}^{i} y_j}}{y_{i+1}} \right), \qquad i = 1, \ldots, d-1 \, .$$

A compositional trajectory is an ordered sequence of compositional vectors, represented as $\mathbf{Y} = \{\mathbf{y}_t\}_{t=1,2,\ldots}$, with $\mathbf{y}_t \in \mathbb{S}^{d-1}$ for $t = 1, 2, \ldots$. In our first model-based clustering approach we will employ a modification of the linear Gaussian state space model from [3], referred to as the "ilr-Gaussian" model. Suppose we have n compositional trajectories, $\{\mathbf{Y}^{(1)}, \ldots, \mathbf{Y}^{(n)}\}$. We will work with the ilr-transformed trajectories, that is,

$$\mathbf{Z}^{(i)} = \{\mathbf{z}_t^{(i)}\}_{t=1,2,\ldots}, \qquad \mathbf{z}_t^{(i)} = \text{ilr}(\mathbf{y}_t^{(i)}), \qquad t = 1, 2, \ldots \, ,$$

for $i = 1, \ldots, n$. Let K be the total number of components in the mixture, and $k = 1, \ldots, K$. Given an initial state $\boldsymbol{\alpha}_0^{(i)}$, the Gaussian state space model reads

$$\begin{aligned} \boldsymbol{\alpha}_t^{(i)} &= \mathbf{T}^{(k)} \boldsymbol{\alpha}_{t-1}^{(i)} + \boldsymbol{\xi}_t^{(i)} \, , \quad \boldsymbol{\xi}_t^{(i)} \sim \mathcal{N}\left(0, \, \boldsymbol{Q}^{(k)}\right), \\ \mathbf{z}_t^{(i)} &= \boldsymbol{\alpha}_t^{(i)} + \boldsymbol{\zeta}_t^{(i)} \, , \qquad \boldsymbol{\zeta}_t^{(i)} \sim \mathcal{N}\left(0, \, \mathbf{H}^{(k)}\right). \end{aligned}$$

We assume that, for all k, the variance matrices $\mathbf{Q}^{(k)}$ and $\mathbf{H}^{(k)}$ are diagonal. We also assume that the system matrices $\mathbf{T}^{(k)}$, $\mathbf{Q}^{(k)}$, and $\mathbf{H}^{(k)}$ do not depend on time; instead, they are component-specific and are the elements on which the model-based clustering is performed. So, the groups will contain trajectories that "evolve" in a similar way, even if distant in the simplex.

An important phase of unsupervised model-based clustering is the interpretation of the clusters obtained in the end. In this interpretability framework, we move away from the literature and the convoluted ilr-transformation, and we attempt to model the trajectories directly on the simplex. In this "non-Gaussian" case, we adopt the state space extension from [2], where the state equation remains Gaussian, but the observations belong to whatever exponential family distribution, as

$$\begin{aligned} &\boldsymbol{\eta}_t = \mathbf{T}^{(k)} \boldsymbol{\eta}_{t-1} + \boldsymbol{\xi}_t \, , \ \boldsymbol{\xi}_t \sim \mathcal{N}(0, \, \mathbf{Q}^{(k)}) \, ; \\ &\mathbf{y}_t \sim p(\mathbf{y}_t \mid \boldsymbol{\eta}_t) \, , \qquad p\left(\mathbf{y} \mid \boldsymbol{\eta}\right) = \exp\left\{\boldsymbol{\eta}^\top \mathbf{y} - b\left(\boldsymbol{\eta}\right) + c_t\left(\mathbf{y}\right)\right\}. \end{aligned}$$

Again, a possible choice for the observation distribution would be the Dirichlet, but we prefer to adopt the continuous categorical distribution [5], with natural representation

$$p(\mathbf{y} \mid \boldsymbol{\eta}) \propto \exp\left\{\boldsymbol{\eta}^\top \mathbf{y}\right\}, \quad \boldsymbol{\eta} = (\eta_1, \ldots, \eta_{d-1}, 0) \, .$$

Such distribution extends the domain to the closure of the simplex, $\overline{\mathbb{S}^{d-1}} = \left\{ \mathbf{y} \in \mathbb{R}^d_{\geq 0} \mid \sum_{i=1}^d y_i = 1 \right\}$, allowing the presence of 0 measurements.

3 ECM Algorithm for Model-Based Clustering

Our clustering procedure consists of an Expectation Conditional Maximization algorithm. We assume a simple mixture of experts model [6], which allows us to model the probability of a time series to belong to each group as a function of both its component likelihood and its covariates. Let $i = 1, \ldots, n$ indicate the series and $k = 1, \ldots, K$ indicate the groups or mixture components. With a slight abuse of notation, let $\mathbf{Y}^{(i)}$ indicate both the original series and their ilr transformation, since most of the following holds both for the ilr-Gaussian and the non-Gaussian representations. At each iteration, as in [6], in the outer expectation step, we estimate the latent cluster membership of the series i as the probability

$$\hat{p}_{ik} \propto \pi_k \left(\mathbf{x}_i \mid \mathbf{\Gamma} \right) \phi \left(\mathbf{Y}^{(i)} \mid \mathbf{\Theta}^{(k)} \right), \quad k = 1, \ldots, K.$$

Here, the π_k, as k varies, indicate the component weights of the simple ME model, depending on the series covariates $\mathbf{x}_i$ and the current associated parameters in $\mathbf{\Gamma} = (\gamma_1, \ldots, \gamma_K)$, as

$$\pi_k \left(\mathbf{x}_i \mid \mathbf{\Gamma} \right) = \frac{\exp \left(\gamma_{k0} + \mathbf{x}_i^\top \gamma_{k1} \right)}{\sum_{k'=1}^K \exp \left(\gamma_{k'0} + \mathbf{x}_i^\top \gamma_{k'1} \right)}.$$

Meanwhile, $\phi \left(\mathbf{Y}^{(i)} \mid \mathbf{\Theta}^{(k)} \right)$ is the likelihood of the series $\mathbf{Y}^{(i)}$, computed via Kalman filter, given the current k-th set of system matrices $\mathbf{\Theta}^{(k)} = \{\mathbf{T}^{(k)}, \mathbf{Q}^{(k)}, \mathbf{H}^{(k)}\}$, in the ilr-Gaussian case, or $\mathbf{\Theta}^{(k)} = \{\mathbf{T}^{(k)}, \mathbf{Q}^{(k)}\}$, in the non-Gaussian case.

In the outer maximization step, the expectation of the complete data loglikelihood is computed as the Q-function

$$Q = \sum_{i=1}^n \sum_{k=1}^K \hat{p}_{ik} \left[\gamma_{k0} + \mathbf{x}_i^\top \gamma_{k1} - \log \left\{ \sum_{k'=1}^K \exp \left(\gamma_{k'0} + \mathbf{x}_i^\top \gamma_{k'1} \right) \right\} + \right. \left. + \log \phi \left(\mathbf{Y}^{(i)} \mid \mathbf{\Theta}^{(k)} \right) \right],$$

which is then maximized with respect to the set $\mathbf{\Gamma}$ and the sets $\mathbf{\Theta}^{(k)}$, $k = 1, \ldots, K$. While the estimation of $\mathbf{\Gamma}$ requires numerical optimization, the update of the system matrices can be performed, in the ilr-Gaussian case, through an inner EM algorithm, proposed in [8]. In the inner expectation phase, they use the Kalman Filter and Smoother (see e.g. [3]) to obtain the smoothed states

$$\hat{\boldsymbol{\alpha}}_t^{(i)} = E \left[\boldsymbol{\alpha}_t^{(i)} \middle| \left\{ \mathbf{y}_t^{(i)} \right\}_{t=1,2,\ldots}, \mathbf{\Theta}^{(k)} \right], \quad t = 0, 1, 2, \ldots$$

and their associated variances, which are then used to update the system matrices in the inner maximization step and provide starting points for the following iterations. The original EM algorithm aimed at estimating the system matrices of a single time series, but the extension to the case of multiple time series sharing the system matrices is straightforward.

In the non-Gaussian case, the EM algorithm from [8] requires to adopt an approximate Kalman Filter and Smoother, based on the linearization proposed in [2]. This iterative process is more expensive than the exact one, but it is guaranteed to converge when dealing with distributions from the exponential family. The linearization requires the computation of the Hessian of the normalizing constant with respect to the parameters. A simple and stable recursive way to calculate it is provided for the continuous categorical distribution.

Once the components weights parameters in $\mathbf{\Gamma}$ and the sets of system matrices have been updated, we can check if we reached convergence and, if it is not the case, proceed with the recursive iterations, going to the outer expectation step and recomputing the cluster membership probabilities.

4 Application

Our motivating application involves the analysis of urban mobility trajectories and their classification into mobility subgroups. We use mobile phone cell connections as a proxy for users' positions. The simplex is the space of road proportion in the surroundings of a user's position: we count the meters of walkable pathways, cycle lanes, and different road types in a circle of a certain radius around the estimated position, and normalize the obtained quantities to get a point in the simplex. As a user moves, he draws a trajectory in the simplex.

Our state space representation and clustering are motivated by the need to deal with high-variability observations, due to the noisy nature of telephonic data, while modeling in a simple way the evolution of the underlying state. Clustering on the system matrices is used to group together trajectories which are not "geographically close", but which show similar moving behaviors. The presence of measurements where some road types are absent is another justification for the future use of the continuous categorical distribution.

We show the application of the ilr-Gaussian version of our algorithm to $n = 927$ trajectories in the municipality of Padova, Italy, while the non-Gaussian version will be employed in future applications. We keep trajectories with at least 15 observations and consider $d = 4$ as we measure the following road types: fast-paced roads, such as motorways, trunks, or primary roads; smaller types of roads; cycle lanes; and walkable pathways. Since the true number of clusters is unknown, we run the algorithm multiple times varying $K = 3, \ldots, 7$ and computing the BIC to determine which number of clusters best fits the data. For each K, starting points for the elements of the system matrices of each group are obtained with the following procedure. We get an initial grouping of the trajectories, purely based on their location in the simplex, by performing a time series clustering based on Dynamic Time Warping distance [7]. The extension of the EM algorithm in [8] to the multiple series case can then be used group-wise to obtain both initial estimates for the matrices in $\mathbf{\Theta}^{(k)}$, $k = 1, \ldots, K$, and to get starting values for the state $\boldsymbol{\alpha}_0^{(i)}$ and its associated variance, for all the series $i = 1, \ldots, n$. In this approach, we do not employ external covariates in the mixture of experts, that is, we only base the clustering on the evolution of the trajectories in the simplex. This also means that the component weights π_k only depend on the intercepts $\gamma_{10}, \ldots, \gamma_{k0}$ and can be updated at the maximization step as

$$\hat{\pi}_k = \frac{1}{n} \sum_{i=1}^{n} \hat{p}_{ik}, \quad k = 1, \ldots, K,$$

without requiring numerical optimization.

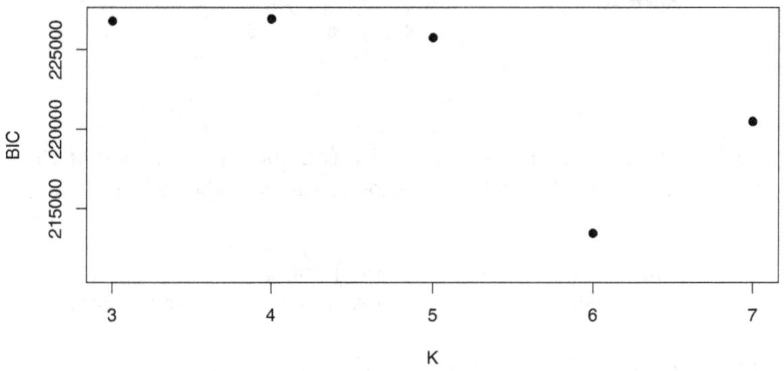

Fig. 1. BIC for different values of K

The optimal number of groups is obtained for $K = 6$, as shown in Fig. 1. From the final values of $\hat{p}_{ik}$, we get the clusters by assigning the series $i = 1, \ldots, 927$ to the mixture component that maximizes its inclusion probability, that is, the one corresponding to $k = \text{argmax}_{j=1,\ldots,6}\, \hat{p}_{ij}$. Figure 2 shows the inclusion probability of the trajectories to each of the mixture components. The algorithm unambiguously assigns most of the series to a single group.

In Table 1, we collect some descriptive statistics of the so-generated groups of trajectories. We can see that, even though the covariate information is not included in the clustering procedure, the algorithm can generate groups with large differences in the trajectories travel distance, radius of gyration, or average speed. For instance, we observe that Cluster 3 contains shorter trajectories lying in the city center, while the large Cluster 6 contains fast travelers trajectories, most likely corresponding to car drivers.

5 Ongoing Research

Further developments will focus on the refinement of the mixture of experts models, including some useful covariates, such as the traveled distance and the

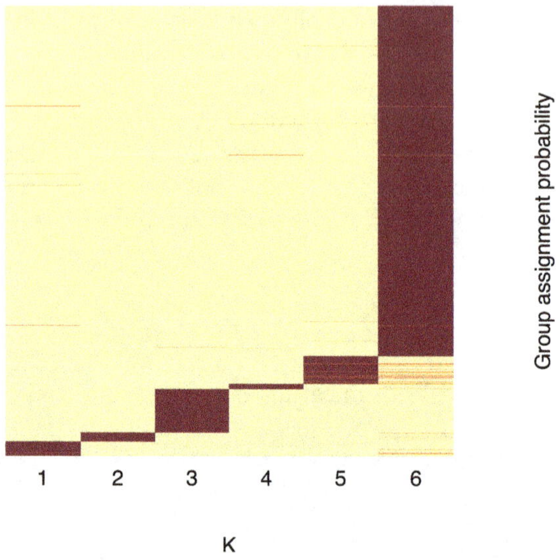

Fig. 2. Inclusion probability of the trajectories (one per row) in each of the 6 components of the mixture. A darker color corresponds to a higher assignment probability

Table 1. Sample means (standard deviations) for the travel distances, radius's of gyration, and average speeds of the trajectories in each obtained cluster

Cluster	Count	Travel distance	Radius of gyration	Average speed
1	30	10.6 (3.6)	2.6 (0.7)	19.3 (5.1)
2	19	8.4 (3.3)	1.9 (0.7)	20.4 (5.9)
3	89	5.1 (2.9)	1.3 (0.7)	13.3 (7.2)
4	11	14.5 (4.4)	3.4 (0.9)	22.3 (7.6)
5	57	7.7 (3.0)	2.0 (0.8)	17.9 (6.5)
6	721	15.0 (5.9)	3.4 (1.2)	39.3 (17.6)

average speed, in the mixture of experts component weights. Such variables represent some information that is not captured by the compositional representation, therefore their inclusion may improve the model performances. Another planned development concerns the implementation of model-based clustering on the continuous categorical state space representation of the trajectories, and the comparison of the results with those based on the ilr-Gaussian version.

Acknowledgments. Andrea Panarotto's scholarship is funded by PON "Research and Innovation" 2014–2020 Action IV.5 "PhDs on Green issues." — Ministerial Decree 1061/2021.

References

1. Aitchison, J.: The statistical analysis of compositional data. J. Roy. Stat. Soc.: Ser. B (Methodol.) **44**(2), 139–160 (1982)
2. Durbin, J., Koopman, S.J.: Time series analysis of non-gaussian observations based on state space models from both classical and Bayesian perspectives. J. R. Stat. Soc. Ser. B Stat Methodol. **62**(1), 3–56 (2000)
3. Durbin, J., Koopman, S.J.: Time Series Analysis by State Space Methods, vol. 38. Oxford: OUP (2012)
4. Egozcue, J.J., Pawlowsky-Glahn, V., Mateu-Figueras, G., Barcelo-Vidal, C.: Isometric logratio transformations for compositional data analysis. Math. Geol. **5**(3), 279–300 (2003)
5. Gordon-Rodriguez, E., Loaiza-Ganem, G., Cunningham, J.: The continuous categorical: a novel simplex-valued exponential family. In: International Conference on Machine Learning, pp. 3637–3647. PMLR (2020)
6. Gormley, I.C., Frühwirth-Schnatter, S.: Mixture of experts models. In: Handbook of Mixture Analysis, pp. 271–307. Chapman and Hall/CRC (2019)
7. Sardá-Espinosa, A.: Time-series clustering in R using the dtwclust package. R J. **11**(1), 22–43 (2019)
8. Shumway, R.H., Stoffer, D.S.: An approach to time series smoothing and forecasting using the EM algorithm. J. Time Ser. Anal. **3**(4), 253–264 (1982)

Approximated Gaussian Random Field Under Different Parameterizations for MCMC

Joaquin Cavieres[1](✉), Cole C. Monnahan[2], David Bolin[3], and Elisabeth Bergherr[1]

[1] Chair of Spatial Data Science and Statistical Learning, University of Göttingen, Göttingen, Germany
joaquin.cavieres@uni-goettingen.de
[2] National Marine Fisheries Service (NOAA), Alaska Fisheries Science Center, Seattle, Washington, USA
[3] King Abdullah University of Science and Technology (KAUST), Thuwal, Saudi Arabia

Abstract. Fitting spatial models with a Gaussian random field as spatial random effect poses computational challenges for Markov Chain Monte Carlo (MCMC) methods, primarily due to two factors: computational speed and convergence of chains for the hyperparameters. To deal with this, a Gaussian random field can be approximated by a Gaussian Markov random field using stochastic partial differential equations. This methodology is commonly used in "latent Gaussian models", where the inference is done by the Integrated Nested Laplace Approximations, but rarely used in an MCMC method. In this contribution, we evaluated different parameterizations of the approximated Gaussian random field, specifically using the Hamiltonian Monte Carlo algorithm of the Stan software. A simulation study demonstrated that models using the hyperparameters ρ and σ_u were better able to estimate the values used to simulate the spatial random field. Their speed computation were faster compared to models parameterized with κ and τ. In real data application, the index of relative abundance estimated for Pollock indicates similar trends for the six models proposed. However, models incorporating ρ and σ_u demonstrated faster computation compared to those utilizing κ and τ, corroborating the results found in the simulation. Even more important, none of these models encountered convergence issues, as indicated by the Rhat statistic.

Keywords: Approximated Gaussian random field · index of relative abundance · Bayesian spatial modelling

1 Introduction

In recent years, the interest in spatial statistics has grown within the scientific community. These methods enable us to establish spatial dependencies between

J. Einbeck et al. (Eds.): IWSM 2024, CONTRIB.STAT., pp. 204–210, 2024.
https://doi.org/10.1007/978-3-031-65723-8_32

environmental phenomena. To do so, several spatial methods have been used to estimate relative indices of abundance in fisheries science [1]. The indices of relative abundance rely on fishery catch-per-unit-of-effort (CPUE) data and serve as key inputs for stock assessment models, aiming to depict the proportion of the population captured in fishery. One of the most common methodologies to incorporate the uncertainty associated with a particular phenomenon is to approximate the Gaussian random field (≈GRF) by a Gaussian markov random field using stochastic partial differential equations (SPDE method, [2]). This approximation demonstrates good performance, particularly in "latent Gaussian models" (R-INLA; [3]). Although R-INLA serves as a computationally efficient approximation method with favorable properties, the most widely utilized approach for Bayesian inference remains Markov Chain Monte Carlo (MCMC). However, a spatial random field characterized by the hyperparameters κ and τ (scale and variance, respectively), faces convergence challenges for this type of methodology. In this work, we will compare and evaluate different parameterizations of the approximated GRF (≈GRF) using the Hamiltonian Monte Carlo (HMC) algorithm of the Stan software [4]. Specifically, to parameterize the ≈GRF we will use; (κ, τ), (ρ, σ_u) and Penalised complexity priors (PC prior's, [5]). For this comparison, we conduct both a simulation study and an application to real data, aiming to estimate an index of relative abundance for a fishery resource.

2 Spatial Modelling

A continuous spatial random process in d dimensions is defined by $\{Y(\boldsymbol{s}) : \boldsymbol{s} \in D \subset \mathcal{R}^d\}$, where $\boldsymbol{s}$ is the location of process $Y(\boldsymbol{s})$ in the domain D. We say that the spatial process is a GRF if $\{Y(\boldsymbol{s}_1), \ldots, Y(\boldsymbol{s}_n)\} \sim \mathcal{N}_n(0, \Sigma)$ and the process is completely specified by its mean function $\mu = \mathbb{E}(Y(\boldsymbol{s}))$ and the covariance function $C(\boldsymbol{s}_1, \boldsymbol{s}_2) = Cov(Y(\boldsymbol{s}_1), Y(\boldsymbol{s}_2))$. The GRF also is assumed stationary and isotropic.

2.1 The SPDE Method

Consider a spatial stochastic field $u(\mathrm{s}) \in \mathcal{R}^2$ with covariance function determined by

$$\mathrm{COV}(\boldsymbol{s}_i, \boldsymbol{s}_j) = \frac{\sigma_u^2}{2^{\nu-1}\Gamma(\nu)}(\kappa||\boldsymbol{s}_i - \boldsymbol{s}_j||)^{\nu} K_\nu(\kappa||\boldsymbol{s}_i - \boldsymbol{s}_j||). \tag{1}$$

In Eq. (1); Γ is the Gamma function, κ is a scale parameter, σ_u is the marginal standard deviation of the spatial process, ν is a smoothness parameter and K_ν is the modified Bessel function of second kind. A GRF with covariance (1) can be viewed as a solution to the SPDE

$$(\kappa^2 - \Delta)^{\alpha/2}(\tau u(\boldsymbol{s})) = \mathcal{W}(\boldsymbol{s}), \quad \boldsymbol{s} \in \mathbb{R}^d,$$

where $\tau > 0$ scales the variance, $\alpha > d/2$, Δ is the Laplacian and $\mathcal{W}$ is a Gaussian white noise. Finally, if $\alpha = 2$, the spatial random field $u(\mathbf{s})$ can be approximated as

$$u(\boldsymbol{s}) = \sum_{k=1}^{n} \psi_k(\boldsymbol{s}) u_k,$$

where $\{\psi_k\}$ are piecewise linear basis functions defined by some triangulation of D and the vector of weights $\boldsymbol{u} = (u_1, \ldots, u_n)^T$ is normally distributed, $\mathcal{N}(\boldsymbol{u}, \boldsymbol{Q}^{-1})$, where $\boldsymbol{Q}$ is sparse and represented by other sparse matrices $\boldsymbol{C}$, $\boldsymbol{G}_1$ and $\boldsymbol{G}_2$ such as

$$\boldsymbol{Q} = \tau^2(\kappa^4 \boldsymbol{C} + 2\kappa^2 \boldsymbol{G}_1 + \boldsymbol{G}_2).$$

2.2 Spatial Random Field Parameterization

Table 1 shows five different parameterizations of the spatial random field. For GRF_1, GRF_2, GRF_3 and GRF_4, the input parameters are in log scale, that means; $(\log(\tau), \log(\kappa))$ and $(\log(\rho), \log(\sigma_u))$. Internally, they are transformed to (τ, κ) and (ρ, σ_u) respectively. In GRF_3, the input parameters are $(\log(\tau), \log(\kappa))$ but the spatial random field is parameterized using ρ and σ_u. A similar transformation was done in GRF_4, the input parameters are $(\log(\rho), \log(\sigma_u))$ but τ and κ were used for modelling. Finally, GRF_5 is parameterized using PC prior's.

Table 1. Input hyperparameters of the spatial random field.

Cases	Hyperparameters	Prior distribution
GRF_1	τ and κ	$\mathcal{N}(0, 1.0)$ for τ and κ
GRF_2	ρ and σ_u	$\mathcal{N}(0, 1.0)$ for ρ and σ_u
GRF_3	τ and $\kappa \Longrightarrow \rho$ and σ_u	$\mathcal{N}(0, 1.0)$ for ρ and σ_u
GRF_4	ρ and $\sigma_u \Longrightarrow \tau$ and κ	$\mathcal{N}(0, 1.0)$ for τ and κ
GRF_5	ρ and σ_u	$\text{Wei}(1, \rho_0^{-1})$ for ρ and $\text{Exp}(\sigma_{u0})$ for σ_u

3 Simulation

Spatial data were simulated considering the following model:

$$\mathbf{y} \mid \mathbf{u}, \sigma_e^2 \sim \mathcal{N}(\mathbf{A}\mathbf{u}, \sigma_e^2) \tag{2}$$

$$\mathbf{u} \sim \text{GRF}(\mathbf{0}, \mathbf{Q}(\boldsymbol{\theta})^{-1}), \tag{3}$$

where $\mathbf{y} = (y_1, \ldots, y_n)^T$ denotes the response variable for $i, \ldots, n$, and n is the number of observations. Here, $\mathbf{A}$ is the projector matrix, $\mathbf{u}$ is the $\approx$GRF, $\boldsymbol{\theta}$ is the vector of hyperparameters (τ, κ) or (ρ, σ_u), and $\mathbf{Q}(\boldsymbol{\theta})$ is the precision matrix. The prior distribution for the standard deviation $\sigma_e \sim \text{Cauchy}(0, 5)$. This comparative analysis was conducted across four different numbers of random spatial locations (50, 100, 150, 200), and for each of these, we built a mesh to represent the discretized spatial domain. To simulate the GRF's, the initial values were the following: $\kappa_0 = 11.31$, $\tau_0 = 0.01$, $\rho_0 = 0.25$, $\sigma_{u0} = 2.0$.

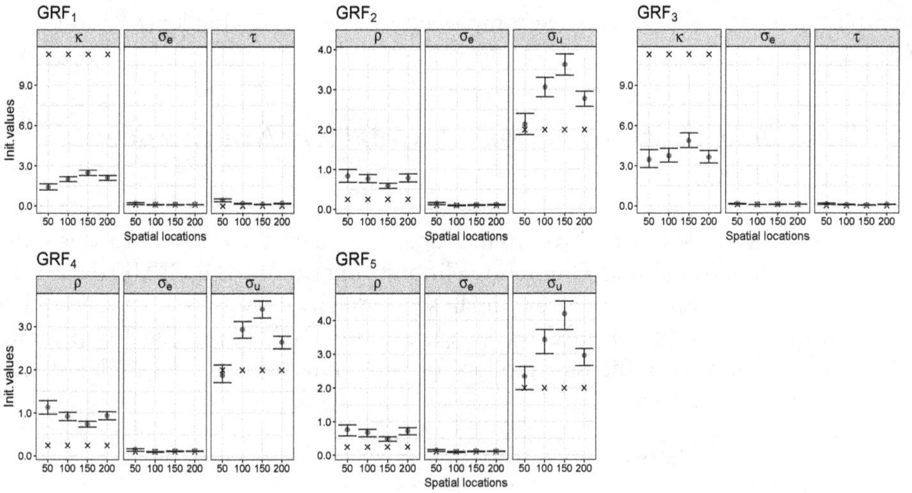

Fig. 1. Posterior means, 25% and 75% credible intervals in the cases evaluated for the different number of simulated spatial points (locations).

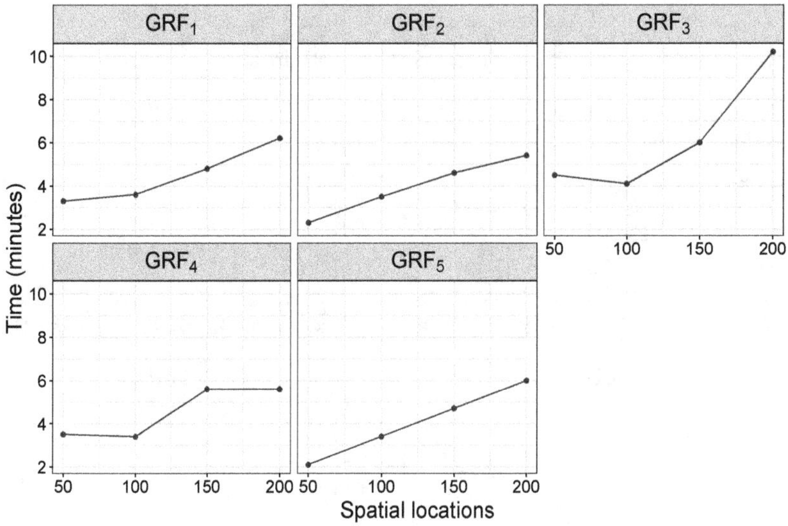

Fig. 2. Speed computation for the proposed models in the different number of simulated spatial locations.

3.1 Simulation Results

Figure 1 shows the posterior means of the hyperparameters estimated for each case. As we can see, the posterior distribution of the hyperparameters in GRF_5 are closer to the initial values used in simulated spatial random field. Moreover, it is important to highlight that all models utilizing ρ and σ_u as hyperparameters exhibit better speed performance compared to those employing $\log(\kappa)$ and $\log(\tau)$ (Fig. 2).

4 Real Application: Index of Relative Abundance for Pollock

We estimate an index of relative abundance (per year) for Pollock. In this case, we will fit a lognormal and Gamma likelihood function to the CPUE data with the purpose to obtain the indexes. In those models, we parameterize the ≈GRF as following: GRF_1 (τ, κ), GRF_2 (ρ, σ_u), and GRF_3 (ρ, σ_u using PC prior's). Thus, we will have two different models for each parameterization of the ≈GRF for comparative analysis.

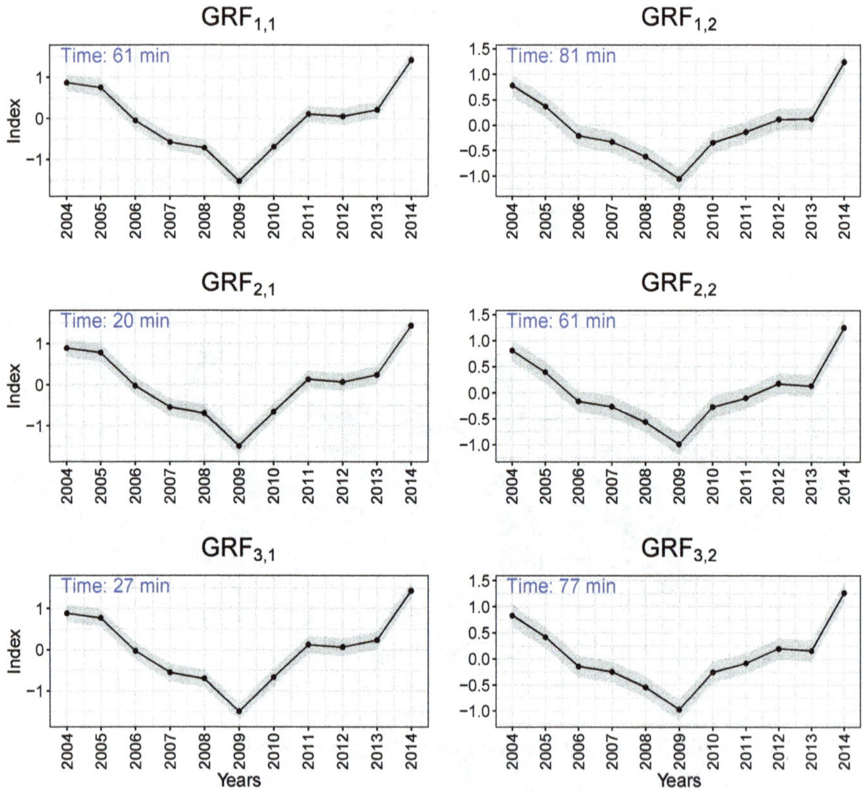

Fig. 3. Indexes of relative abundance estimated with lognormal (left side) and Gamma (right side) likelihood for the different parameterizations of the ≈GRF. The points are the values for the coefficients and the grey bands are uncertainty intervals computed from posterior draws with all chains merged in the MCMC method (25% and 75% credible intervals).

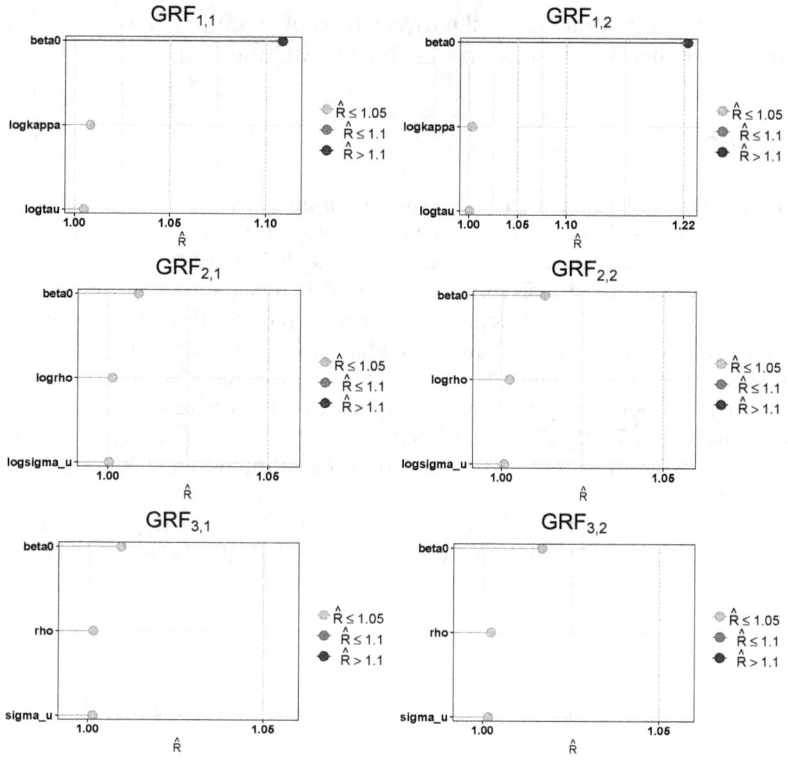

Fig. 4. Rhat ($\hat{R}$) values associated to the intercept and hyperparameters in the models.

4.1 Real Application Results

Although the trends of the estimated indexes are similar between models (Fig. 3), the Rhat ($\hat{R}$) statistic (which measures the degree of mixing of the chains and its convergence, based in a threshold $\hat{R} < 1.05$), allows us to identify that models utilizing κ and τ present convergence problems in the iterative process of estimation, specifically for the intercept (Fig. 4).

5 Conclusion

We evaluated the statistical performance and speed computation of different parameterizations in an approximated Gaussian random field. Computing the posterior distribution of these hyperparameters is often challenging for MCMC methods. Therefore, we suggest employing the parameterization utilizing ρ and σ_u due to its speed computation and the quick convergence of chains. While further analysis is necessary, such as incorporating more predictors or utilizing others real data, employing penalized complexity priors appears to be the optimal parameterization, since the direct uses of ρ and σ_u have some issues in calculating the effective sample size in the MCMC method.

References

1. Maunder, M.N., et al.: The need for spatio-temporal modeling to determine catch-per-unit effort based indices of abundance and associated composition data for inclusion in stock assessment models. Fish. Res. **229**, 105594 (2020)
2. Lindgren, F., Rue, H., Lindström, J.: An explicit link between Gaussian fields and Gaussian Markov random fields: the stochastic partial differential equation approach. J. R. Stat. Soc. Ser. B Stat Methodol. **73**(4), 423–498 (2011)
3. Rue, H., Martino, S., Chopin, N.: Approximate Bayesian inference for latent Gaussian models by using integrated nested laplace approximations. J. R. Stat. Soc. Ser. B Stat Methodol. **71**(2), 319–392 (2009)
4. Carpenter, B., et al.: Stan: a probabilistic programming language. J. Stat. Softw. **76**, 319–392 (2017)
5. Fuglstad, G.A., Simpson, D., Lindgren, F., Rue, H.: Constructing priors that penalize the complexity of Gaussian random fields. J. Am. Stat. Assoc. **114**(525), 445–452 (2019)

Shape Analysis of AF Segments for Rapid Assessment of Mohs Layers for BCC Presence by AF-Raman Microscopy

Alexey A. Koloydenko[1(✉)], Ioan Notingher[2], Radu Boitor[2], and Jüri Lember[3]

[1] Department of Mathematics, Royal Holloway, University of London, Egham TW20 0EX, UK
alexey.koloydenko@rhul.ac.uk

[2] School of Physics and Astronomy, University of Nottingham, Nottingham NG7 2RD, UK

[3] Institute of Mathematics and Statistics, University of Tartu, Narva mnt 18, 51009 Tartu, Estonia

https://pure.royalholloway.ac.uk/en/persons/alexey-koloydenko

Abstract. An automated method to detect Basal Cell Carcinoma (BCC) relies on Autofluorescence (AF) imaging guiding Raman microscopy to obtain biochemical information for tissue classification. The guidance is provided via an image segmentation technique aiming to reduce the risk of missing cancer. We present evidence that shape of an AF segment may be useful for 'trimming' 6–8% of non-BCC segments in an essentially coordinate free manner, without compromising BCC detection. By allowing the AF-Raman method to direct the more time consuming Raman analysis toward more relevant regions, the proposed trimming of unnecessary segments should ultimately improve the overall accuracy. The presented shape analysis uses the recently introduced Weighted Euler Curve Transform (WECT). WECT embeds segments in a space of real matrices of fixed dimensions, where a shape is an equivalence class of segments with WECTs matching under a cyclic permutation of columns. The induced rotation invariant distance is non-Hilbertian, which requires special care in using it with kernel methods (e.g. Kernel PCA, Kernel LDA, SVMs). Our currently best results are achieved by L_1 SVMs based on the Laplace 'kernel'.

Keywords: Autofluorescence imaging · Raman spectroscopy · skin cancer · Weighted Euler Curve Transform · shape analysis

1 Motivation and Objectives

Basal cell carcinoma (BCC) is the most common type of cancer in humans, with about 5.9 million cases diagnosed worldwide. Although BCC is usually not deadly, diagnosis and treatment costs are very high, involving several stages of mostly manual processing. In [2,3], and references therein, we described autofluorescence (AF)-Raman spectroscopy as a novel technology to detect BCC

J. Einbeck et al. (Eds.): IWSM 2024, CONTRIB.STAT., pp. 211–217, 2024.
https://doi.org/10.1007/978-3-031-65723-8_33

in surgically excised skin specimens. Currently, the most effective surgical treatment of BCC is Mohs micrographic surgery, where sequential thin layers of skin are removed and checked by frozen section histology to detect residual tumour in 30 – 60 min.

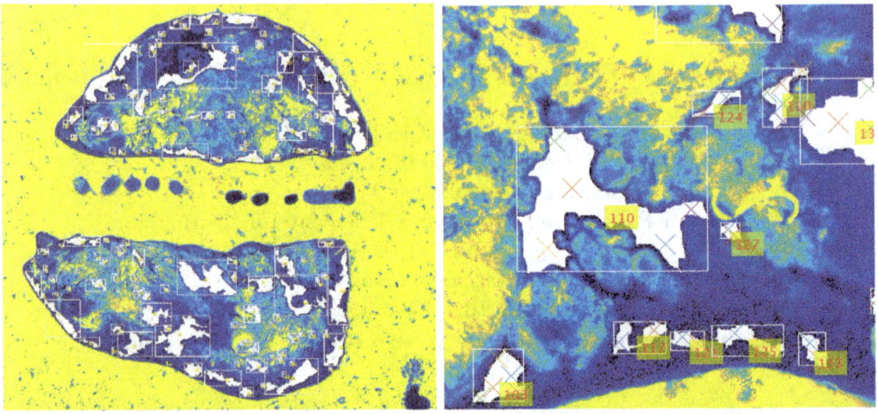

Fig. 1. Segmented AF image of patient X (left), zoomed in on segment 110 (right). Colour crosses mark sites selected for Raman microscopy.

However, the availability of Mohs surgery is not universal because of limited capacity to process and assess histologically stained tissue sections and scarcity of specialist surgeons trained to interpret histopathology slides. Mohs surgery could be more widely adopted in practices if the surgical margins could be analysed faster and without requiring tissue processing. Although Raman spectra of BCC and healthy tissue molecules tend to look different, quantifying such differences has been a challenge. In particular, Raman spectroscopic analysis of an entire surgical margin is too slow for clinical use in real time. Combining Raman spectroscopy with AF microscopy, which is fast and inexpensive, speeds up the analysis by probing only a relatively small number of 'promising' locations, yet allowing investigation of entire surgical margins of excised Mohs specimens intra-operatively. Figure 1 illustrates AF image segmentation resulting in tissue sites for examination with Raman spectroscopy. The segments are the complements of the regions deemed BCC free. There is a large variation in size and shape of the segments. With no evidence that size of a segment is relevant for tissue classification, we investigate if shape contains any cue about the tissue type. Here we analyze shape as a sole predictor of BCC for effective exclusion of non-BCCs from the Raman analysis, and a combined use of shape and Raman spectroscopic features for BCC prediction is subject of our ongoing investigation.

2 Data

Tissue specimens used in this work were obtained from 50 patients undergoing Mohs surgery at the Nottingham NUH NHS Treatment Centre. Ethical approval

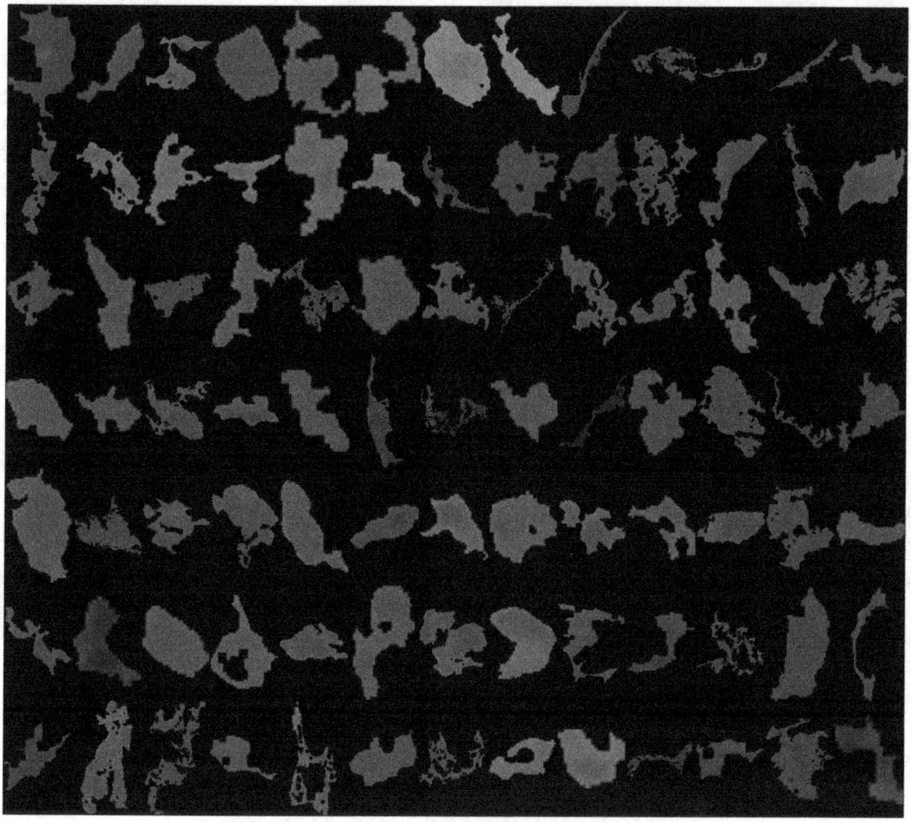

Fig. 2. The complete set of 91 BCC segments scaled to match the size of the largest BCC segment.

was granted by the Health Research Authority (HRA) and Health and Care Research Wales (HCRW) (18/WM/0105). All participating patients have given written informed consent for participation in the study and the use of their deidentified, anonymised, aggregated data and their case details for publication. Patients were recruited randomly, regardless of sex, age or anatomical characteristics. Batch 2, our training set, consists of 11,516 AF segments, $n_1 = 68$ of which are BCC. We have excluded 179 of the largest segments, all non-BCC, retaining $n_0 = 11,269$ non-BCC instances. Batch 3g, our test set, consists of 5,487 segments, 23 of which are BCC. Figure 2 shows all 91 BCC segments (in their original poses) scaled to match the size of the largest BCC segment.

3 Methods, Related Work

We transform AF segments to $p \times m$ matrices using the *unnormalized* Smoothed Weighted Euler Characteristic Curve Transform (SWECT) of Jiang et al. [9], which extends the Smoothed Euler Characteristic Transform (SECT) of Crawford et al. [5] by including image intensity in its topological summary. We use $m = 25$ directions and $p = 50$ points along each curve. Our shape space is the quotient of the set of segments under the discrete rotation equivalence of SWECTs: $A, B \in \mathbb{R}^{pm}$, $A \sim B$ iff $A = BR$ for some $R \in \mathcal{P}_m$, where $\mathcal{P}_m$ is the matrix representation of the cyclic group generated by the permutation $\langle 1, 2, \ldots, m \rangle$. The suitability of the method is not least due to the ease of computing the rotation invariant (up to discretization) equivalence class/orbit of a segment in the SWECT space and, subsequently, the distance between shapes. Thus, to compare shapes, the 'natural' segment similarity measure $K(A, B) = \langle A, B \rangle_F = \mathrm{tr}(A^T B)$ and the associated to it Euclidean distance $d_E(A, B) = \sqrt{K(A, A) - 2K(A, B) + K(B, B)}$ are replaced by their rotation invariant counterparts $K_{inv}(A, B) = \max_{R \in \mathcal{P}_m} \langle A, BR \rangle_F$ and $d_{inv}(A, B) = \sqrt{\min_{R \in \mathcal{P}_m} \|A - BR\|_F^2}$ respectively. We use d_{inv} directly and also via Laplace and Gaussian RBFs $K_L(A, B; d, \sigma) = \exp\{-d(A, B)/\sigma\}$, $K_G(A, B; d, \sigma^2) = \exp\{-d^2(A, B)/2\sigma^2\}$, respectively. To compute the SWECT of mean shape and enable k-means for unsupervised clustering of shapes, we adapt the Generalized Procrustes Analysis algorithm (see [7, Section 7.4]).

Crawford et al. [5] applied SECT to MRI data of Glioblastoma Multiforme (GBM) patients using Gaussian Process regression, finding the SECT to be 'a better predictor of clinical outcomes than both existing tumor shape quantifications and common molecular assays'. Jiang et al. [9] illustrated suitability of the (S)WECT for (also supervised) image classification by using WEC transformed gray scale images of hand-written digits (MNIST data) as inputs to a linear kernel classifier, and also to `t-SNE`, to visualize the (W)ECT data for overall assessment of class separation. They also illustrated WECT on the task of unsupervised clustering of MRI data of GBM subjects, this time using the rotation invariant L_2 distance on SWECTs, and reporting improvements over SECT. As their former example, our current problem is also supervised classification (at this stage, BCC versus all other tissue types), albeit harder (due to highly unbalanced and poorly separable classes and noisier data). As their latter, i.e. GBM, example, our problem also calls for rotation invariant solutions, which we also seek using the distance data directly.

Wang et al. [10] are also concerned with statistical classification of shapes without relying on pre-specified landmarks, and without constructing diffeomorphisms between shapes. Their SINATRA pipeline also uses the Euler Characteristic transform but their input is '3D shapes (represented as triangular meshes)' and their classifier is based on '(weight-space) Gaussian process probit regression', which is particularly suitable for variable selection. In principle, we could convert our 2D segments (with variable intensities) to triangulated 3D surfaces. However, such pseudo-3D shapes will remain essentially surfaces (either with planar bases or artificially closed by symmetric reflections), and this feature alone (not to mention frequently encountered holes) will likely dominate any other mode of variation. Furthermore, given that our present work is only a small part of our larger project where the Raman spectroscopy features already provide substantial power for tissue classification, we first need proof of concept that the segment data have the potential to improve our existing method. Currently, our AF segments were obtained in a rather crude way, and our ECT resolution of 25 directions/Euler curves (14.4° apart) with 50 sampling point granularity (the same as in [9]) is significantly lower than 72 curves (5° apart) by 100 sampling points, the resolution used in [5]. Nonetheless, we observe that for several kernel methods considered, a reliable trimming of a fraction of non-BCC segments is possible.

Calissano et al. [4] use a non-Euclidean metric, which is similar to ours, on graph space representing networks, where they do statistics with generalized geodesic principal components and "align-all-and-compute algorithms" instead of using kernels.

As a sanity check, we use a simple heuristic to assess the effect of the kernel-based non-linear embeddings, which, due to the kernel function being Gaussian or Laplace, make the implicit feature space infinite dimensional. We also wanted to assess consistency of our samples by a 'model-free' approach. We sought this extra assurance after an episode where a batch of data appeared significantly different from others while the observed variations were impossible to interpret in terms of medical or physical conditions. The cause of the discrepancy was established in a visual inspection of a 3D `t-SNE` representation of Raman spectral features used for classification. Namely, the diagnostic device had been accidentally dropped while in use by a hospital. The initial repairs (re-calibration of the damaged laser to the highest engineering standards) proved insufficient for our needs and the `t-SNE` revealed segregation of the affected batch into the subsets collected before the accident and after the initial repairs. Subsequently, the manufacturer re-calibrated the laser to a substantially higher standard, eliminating the cause of the problem. Our present test data is exactly the 'good' subset of the affected batch, Batch 3. The proposed naïve heuristic, which we call 'Balls', is similar to *one-class nearest neighbour classification*, and is as follows: For BCC instance i, $i = 1, 2, \ldots, n_1$, of the training set (Batch 2, $n_1 = 68$), consider a succession of nested balls centred at this instance and having as their radii the distances to the other BCC instances, which, in ascending order, we write as $r_i^{(1)} \leq r_i^{(2)} \leq \ldots \leq r_i^{(n_1-1)}$. Next, for each rank $j = 1, 2, \ldots, n_1 - 1$, consider the BCC detector that classifies all data that belong to the union of the balls of radii $r_i^{(j)}$ as BCC (and everything else as non BCC). Using a 'leave one BCC out' cross-validation, choose the lowest such rank that attains 100% sensitivity on all n_1 rounds, which gives $j = 43$.

4 Results and Discussion

We establish that for 'large' values of $\sigma > 0$, $K_L(\cdot, \cdot; d_{inv}, \sigma)$ and $K_G(\cdot, \cdot; d_{inv}, \sigma)$ lose conditional positive semi-definiteness, which is essential for SVMs and other kernel methods. Thus, our shape metric space, just as the graph metric space in [4], is fundamentally non-Euclidean i.e. it cannot be isometrically embedded into a Hilbert space, see [8]. Restrictions on σ hinder model optimization in cross-validation and pose risk to semisupervised application of the kernel methods. However, in our SVM experiments, quadratic programming tolerates a certain degree of indefiniteness, which allows `LapMRL1SVM`, the L_1-norm K_L-based SVM and its semisupervised counterpart that is additionally regularized with respect to the K_L-weighted and symmetrically normalized Graph Laplacian eigenmaps [1] to achieve our currently highest trimming rates. To enforce the 100% sensitivity regime, threshold of 0 is replaced by the minimum score of the BCC instances on the training set. With our severely unbalanced data, we scale up the side length of the SVM box constraint for the BCC class by n_0/n_1. As forthcoming data reveal previously unseen tissue types, new experiments will be needed to re-validate this approach on the expanded data. To this end, we have also experimented with *bagged ensembles*, training each SVM learner on the training BCCs and equally many randomly sampled non-BCCs. As a benchmark, we have used the Kernel Minimum Volume Enclosing Ellipsoid (`KMVEE`) of Dolia et al. [6], which is essentially a *one-class* classifier. Table 1 summarizes results of our currently best performing and select other non-BCC 'trimmers'. Figure 3 displays our data, with the best results, using KPCA.

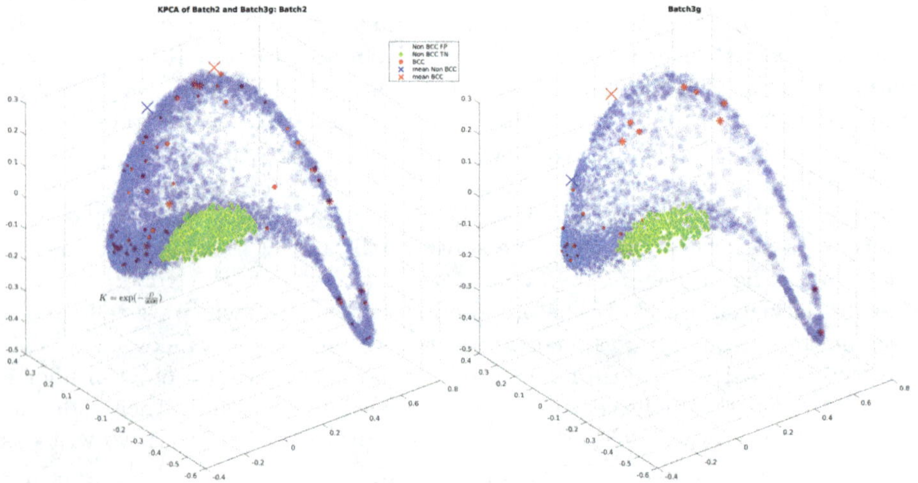

Fig. 3. The currently best trimming results displayed using the Laplace Kernel PCA. Marker size is proportionate to root area of the segment. Sample means computed using the adaptation of the Generalized Procrustes Algorithm.

Table 1. 'Trimming' rates (sensitivity 100%); Gaussian (G) and Laplace (L).

Method	train, %	test, %	Method	train, %	test, %
Balls	0.36	0.22	BaggedL1SVM/G	6.42	6.39
KLDA/L	5.82	6.02	L1SVM/L	7.96	6.61
KMVEE/G	3.29	4.06	LapMRL1SVM/L	8.08	6.68

This work was supported by the Engineering and Physical Sciences Research Council grant number EP/W031779/1.

References

1. Belkin, M., Niyogi, P., Sindhwani, V.: Manifold regularization: a geometric framework for learning from labeled and unlabeled examples. J. Mach. Learn. Res. **7**(85), 2399–2434 (2006). http://jmlr.org/papers/v7/belkin06a.html
2. Boitor, R., et al.: Diagnostic accuracy of auto-fluorescence-Raman spectroscopy for surgical margin assessment during Mohs micrographic surgery of basal cell carcinoma. Br. J. Dermatol. **5**, ljae196 (2024). https://doi.org/10.1093/bjd/ljae196
3. Boitor, R., et al.: Ex vivo assessment of basal cell carcinoma surgical margins in Mohs surgery by autofluorescence-Raman spectroscopy: a pilot study. JEADV Clin. Pract. **3**(2), 498–507 (2023). https://doi.org/10.1002/jvc2.336
4. Calissano, A., Feragen, A., Vantini, S.: Populations of unlabelled networks: graph space geometry and generalized geodesic principal components. Biometrika **111**(1), 147–170 (2023). https://doi.org/10.1093/biomet/asad024
5. Crawford, L., Anthea Monod, A., Andrew, X., Chen, A.X., Mukherjee, S., Rabadán, R.: Predicting clinical outcomes in glioblastoma: an application of topological and functional data analysis. J. Am. Stat. Assoc. **115**(531), 1139–1150 (2020). https://doi.org/10.1080/01621459.2019.1671198
6. Dolia, A.N., Harris, C.J., Shawe-Taylor, J.S., Titterington, D.M.: Kernel ellipsoidal trimming. Comp. Stat. Data. Anal. **52**(1), 309–324 (2007). https://doi.org/10.1016/j.csda.2007.03.020
7. Dryden, I.L., Mardia, K.V.: Statistical Shape Analysis, with Applications in R, 2nd edn. John Wiley and Sons, Chichester (2016). https://doi.org/10.1002/9781119072492
8. Hein, M., Bousquet, O., Schölkopf, B.: Maximal margin classification for metric spaces. J. Comput. Syst. Sci. **71**(3), 333–359 (2005). https://doi.org/10.1016/j.jcss.2004.10.013
9. Jiang, Q., Kurtek, S., Needham, T.: The weighted Euler curve transform for shape and image analysis. In: 2020 IEEE/CVF Conference on Computer Vision and Pattern Recognition Workshops (CVPRW), pp. 3685–3694. Seattle, Washington (2020). https://doi.org/10.1109/CVPRW50498.2020.00430
10. Wang, B., et al.: A statistical pipeline for identifying physical features that differentiate classes of 3D shapes. Ann. Appl. Stat. **15**(2), 638–661 (2021). https://doi.org/10.1214/20-AOAS1430

Additive Mixed Models for Location, Scale and Shape via Gradient Boosting Techniques

Colin Griesbach(✉) and Elisabeth Bergherr

Georg-August-Universität Göttingen, Göttingen, Germany
colin.griesbach@uni-goettingen.de

Abstract. In this work we adapt recent findings from statistical boosting in order to construct an estimation approach for distributional regression including random effects. The algorithm is applied to registry data provided by the German Cystic Fibrosis Registry where the subject-specific evolution of each patients lung function and its corresponding distributional parameters are modelled.

Keywords: Statistical Boosting · Distributional Regression · Random Effects

1 Overview

Cystic fibrosis (CF) is a severe genetic disorder, leading to several health related problems, one of which is the malfunctioning of the lung. A widely-used indicator for disease progression is forced expiratory volume in one second (%FEV1) which the German Cystic Fibrosis Registry collects together with other patient related variables of CF patients in Germany [3]. The registry includes longitudinal data spanning over the course of several decades which we will use to predict lung function decline. As the mean of %FEV1 alone is not enough to describe the state of the patients, there is also an interest in other distributional parameters, e.g. its variability like shown in Fig. 1, which depicts varying variabilities of %FEV1 values for different patients in the registry data. Concepts from distributional regression are established tools for these questions and while the `gamboostLSS` framework [2] offers a fast performing fitting routine for larger data sets and in addition includes base-learners for random effects in longitudinal data, [1] discovered a crucial potential for bias in the random effects estimation and proposed a solution for ordinary linear mixed models. The focus of this contribution will be to adapt these findings to distributional regression.

J. Einbeck et al. (Eds.): IWSM 2024, CONTRIB.STAT., pp. 218–223, 2024.
https://doi.org/10.1007/978-3-031-65723-8_34

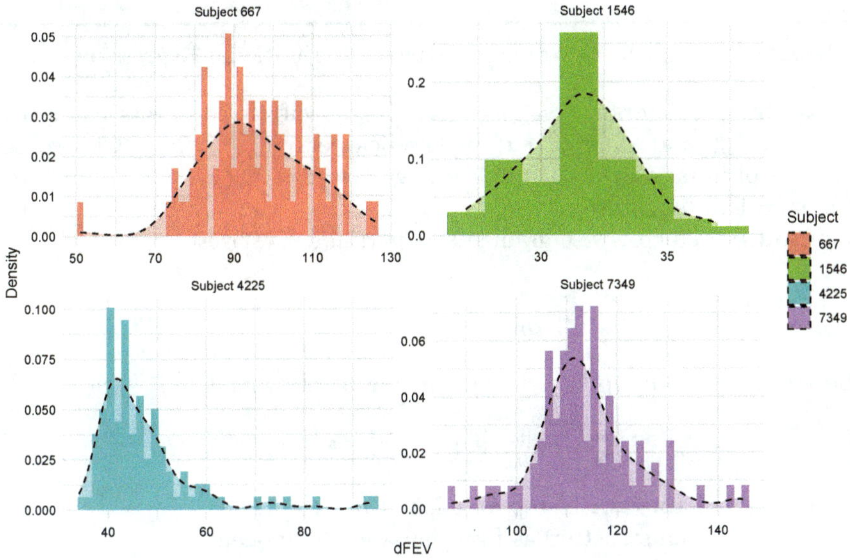

Fig. 1. Varying distributions of the %FEV1 lung function values for four subjects from the German Cystic Fibrosis Registry data.

2 Methods

2.1 Model Formulation

For groups $i = 1, \ldots, n$ each distributional parameter θ_k, $k = 1, \ldots, 4$, is modelled by

$$g_k(\theta_{ki}) = \beta_{k0} + \sum_{j=1}^{p_k} f_{kj}(x_{kj}) + \boldsymbol{Z}_{ki}\boldsymbol{\gamma}_{ki} = \eta_{\theta_k i}$$

with appropriate link functions g_k, where the f_{kj} denote a set of $p_k \in \mathbb{N}$ possibly non-linear population effects and $\boldsymbol{\gamma}_{ki}$ sets of $q_k \in \mathbb{N}$ group-specific random effects, which are assumed to be normally distributed with mean $\boldsymbol{0}$ and covariance $\boldsymbol{Q}$, i.e. $\boldsymbol{\gamma}_{ki} \sim \mathcal{N}^{\otimes q_k}(\boldsymbol{0}, \boldsymbol{Q})$. Based on the negative log-likelihood a loss function is given by

$$\rho(y, \eta_{\theta_1}, \ldots, \eta_{\theta_4}) = -\sum_{i=1}^{n} \log f_{\text{dens}}(y_i | \theta_{1i}, \ldots, \theta_{4i})$$

with corresponding density f_{dens}. We consider the full likelihood as penalization of the random effects takes place within the baselearner for the random structure which is defined below.

2.2 Boosting Algorithm

The following algorithm gives a rough overview of the concepts to optimize the loss ρ using model-based gradient boosting.

`gammboostLSS` Gradient Boosting for Mixed Distributional Regression

- **Initialize** predictors $\hat{\boldsymbol{\eta}}^{[0]} = (\hat{\eta}_{\theta_1}^{[0]}, \ldots, \hat{\eta}_{\theta_4}^{[0]})$, specify fixed effects baselearners $h_{11}, \ldots, h_{4p_4}$ and random effects base-learners $h_{1\gamma}, \ldots, h_{4\gamma}$. Choose total amount of iterations m_{stop} and learning rate ν.
- **for** $m = 1$ to m_{stop} **do**
- **Compute** predictor-wise gradients as partial derivatives

$$\boldsymbol{u}_k^{[m]} = -\frac{\partial}{\partial \eta_{\theta_k}} \rho(y, \hat{\boldsymbol{\eta}}^{[m-1]}), \quad k = 1, \ldots, 4.$$

Select and weakly update the best fitting baselearner $1 \leq j_k^* \leq p_k$

$$\tilde{\eta}_{\theta_k}^{[m]} = \hat{\eta}_{\theta_k}^{[m-1]} + \nu \hat{h}_{kj*}, \quad k = 1, \ldots, 4,$$

for each predictor k with step-length factor $\nu \in (0, 1)$.
Update random structure as fixed nuisance-component

$$\hat{\eta}_{\theta_k}^{[m]} = \tilde{\eta}_{\theta_k}^{[m]} + \nu \hat{h}_{k\gamma}, \quad k = 1, \ldots, 4.$$

- **end for**
- **Return** final fits $\hat{\eta}_{\theta_k}^{[m_{\text{stop}}]}$ or $\hat{\eta}_{\theta_k}^{[m_*]}$ for some tuned number of total iterations m_*.

Tuning for the optimal number m_* of total iterations is usually achieved via resampling strategies like cross-validation or bootstrapping, but other methods, e.g. probing [4] or various information criteria, are possible.

2.3 Computational Details

We will briefly highlight some computational details regarding the random effects estimation.

Random Effects Baselearner. Instead of being incorporated within the selection-cycle, the random structure is treated as nuisance parameter and updated in every iteration similar to Algorithm 2 in [6]. While not stated explicitly in the formulation above, the routine can be made more flexible by introducing separate stopping iterations $m_{\text{stop},k}$ per predictor. For each predictor, a random effect baselearner h_γ can be formulated as ridge penalized group effect via a corresponding projection matrix

$$\boldsymbol{H}_\gamma = \boldsymbol{Z}\boldsymbol{C}(\boldsymbol{Z}^T\boldsymbol{Z} + \lambda \boldsymbol{I})\boldsymbol{Z}^T,$$

where $\boldsymbol{Z}$ is a convenient random effects design matrix linking a set of covariates to each group and the penalization parameter λ, inversely linked to the random effect variance, is chosen to match a desired and usually rather low degree of flexibility. This penalization parameter λ is only tuned indirectly via the amount of optimal iterations m_*, i.e. reapplying the learner $\boldsymbol{H}_\gamma$ with sufficiently small λ for an increasing amount of iterations yields decreasing penalization overall. The correction matrix $\boldsymbol{C}$ corrects the random effects estimates for potential correlations with observed covariates and is motivated in the following.

Random Effects Correction Matrix. The ensemble scheme consisting of multiple weak baselearners states a problem when random effects are included, as each random effects fit is conducted without the presence of the remaining covariates and, thus, can lead to identification problems. To overcome this, a correction matrix $\boldsymbol{C}$ can be formulated in terms of

$$\boldsymbol{C} = \boldsymbol{I} - \bar{\boldsymbol{X}}(\bar{\boldsymbol{X}}^T\bar{\boldsymbol{X}})^{-1}\bar{\boldsymbol{X}},$$

where $\bar{\boldsymbol{X}}$ denotes a subset of covariates the random effects should be corrected for. In short, $\boldsymbol{C}$ denotes a residual maker matrix counting out any potential correlations to a vector by the product $\boldsymbol{C}\boldsymbol{\gamma}$. The so obtained corrected random effects are ensured to be independent of any observed covariates included into the fitting process.

3 Cystis Fibrosis Application

The `gammboostLSS` routine is showcased via a small subset of the German Cystic Fibrosis Registry to keep it comparable to the well-established `gamlss` library. Overall we consider $n = 49$ individuals with a total of $N = 1301$ observations and outcome Δ%FEV1 with corresponding observation time t in years. `gammboostLSS` as well as `gamlss` are specified with a Gaussian distribution and identical predictors for each parameter where time t is modelled via a P-spline as population effect and in addition as monomial basis expansion of degree 3 for the individual-specific random effects. Computation time was 6.2 seconds for `gammboostLSS` and 101.4 for `gamlss`. Figure 2 showcases both model fits based on four subjects highlighted from the data. It is already revealed that the boosting approach tends to fit the individual specific trajectories more closely while also preserving a competitive computational effort. This may be due to an increasingly unstable performance by `gamlss` regarding the quite flexible random structure which turns out to be underdeveloped while the robust design of the refined boosting routine produces more reliable fits.

4 Outlook

Overall, the `gammboostLSS` routine shows high potential regarding distributional regression for clustered and possibly large data. Apart from more thorough evaluations of the method via extensive simulations, some crucial steps to take will be

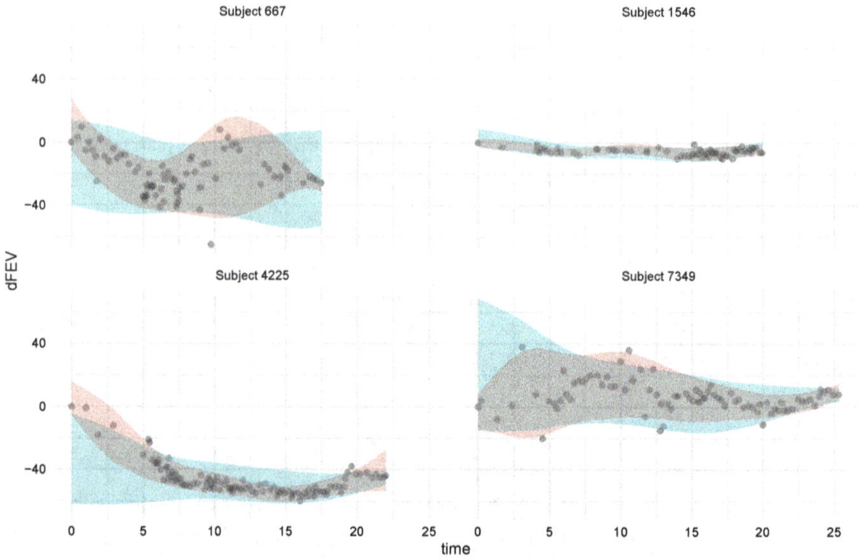

Fig. 2. Fitted distributions (indicated by 0.025 and 0.975 quantiles) of four subjects from the German Cystic Fibrosis Registry data. Blue depicts the fit by `gamlss` and red by `gammboostLSS`.

an incorporation of the method within the convenient `gamboostLSS` framework to bring the method on `CRAN` and benefit from the large collection of baselearners and regression families, as well as the implementation of non-cyclical updates [5] for faster and improved tuning properties.

Acknowledgments. The work on this contribution was supported by the DFG (Deutsche Forschungsgemeinschaft - Projektnummer 426493614).

References

1. Griesbach, C., Säfken, B., Waldmann, E.: Gradient boosting for linear mixed models. Int. J. Biostat. **17**(2), 317–329 (2021). https://doi.org/10.1515/ijb-2020-0136
2. Mayr, A., Fenske, N., Hofner, B., et al.: Generalized additive models for location, scale and shape for high dimensional data - a flexible approach based on boosting. J. R. Stat. Soc. Ser. C **61**(3), 403–427 (2012). https://doi.org/10.1111/j.1467-9876.2011.01033.x
3. Nährlich, L., Burkhart, M., Wosniok, J.: Deutsches Mukoviszidose-Register - Berichtsband 2022. Mukoviszidose e.V. & Mukoviszidose Institut gGmbH, Bonn (2022)
4. Thomas, J., Hepp, T., Mayr, A., Bischl, B.: Probing for sparse and fast variable selection with model-based boosting. Comput. Math. Methods Med. **2017**, 1421409 (2017). https://doi.org/10.1155/2017/1421409

5. Thomas, J., Mayr, A., Bischl, B., et al.: Gradient boosting for distributional regression: faster tuning and improved variable selection via noncyclical updates. Stat. Comput. **28**, 673–687 (2018). https://doi.org/10.1007/s11222-017-9754-6
6. Waldmann, E., Taylor-Robinson, D., Klein, N., et al.: Boosting joint models for longitudinal and time-to-event data. Biom. J. **59**(6), 1104–1121 (2017). https://doi.org/10.1002/bimj.201600158

Regression Analysis with Missing Data Using Interval Imputation

Tathagata Basu(✉)

University of Strathclyde, Glasgow G1 1XQ, UK
tathagata.basu@strath.ac.uk

Abstract. Regression analysis with missing data is a common problem in statistical modelling. Majority of the available methods use point imputation strategy to get rid of the missing entries. However, such methods rely on different observational assumptions. In this paper, we propose a novel approach based on interval imputation, that is, instead of a single value imputation, we replace the missing entries with the range of the variables obtained from the observational data. This way, we avoid any distributional assumption on the data and formulate our model based only on the information in hand. For estimation, we rely on the interval matrix algebra. We also introduce regularisation terms with Bayesian analysis which also allows us to incorporate our subjective belief and avoid singularity in the estimation process similar to ridge regression. We evaluate the maximum a posteriori estimates of these regression coefficients to obtain the approximate posterior bounds. Once we have these posterior bounds, we use cross validation to obtain mixing parameters between the lower and upper bounds of the posterior estimates for model fitting. Finally, we illustrate our method with real-life dataset and compare with other state of the art methods to showcase our methods applicability.

Keywords: Bayesian Analysis · Linear Regression · Missing Data · Interval Arithmetic

1 Introduction

Linear regression is one of the most common methods for modelling with input-output data. Let $x := (x_1, x_2, \cdots x_n)^T$ be a design matrix with dimensions $n \times p$ and let $y := (y_1, y_2, \cdots, y_n)^T$ be corresponding n real responses. Then assuming a Gaussian noise on the observations, we can define a linear model in the following way

$$y := \beta_0 + x\beta + \epsilon \tag{1}$$

where β_0 is the intercept term, $\beta := (\beta_1, \beta_2, \cdots, \beta_p)^T$ is the vector of regression coefficients and $\epsilon := (\epsilon_1, \epsilon_2, \cdots, \epsilon_n)^T$ is the vector of Gaussian error such that $\epsilon_i \sim \mathcal{N}(0, \sigma^2)$ for $i = 1, 2, \cdots, n$.

J. Einbeck et al. (Eds.): IWSM 2024, CONTRIB.STAT., pp. 224–230, 2024.
https://doi.org/10.1007/978-3-031-65723-8_35

Parameter estimation for linear models is a well investigated topic in the field of statistical modelling. Least squares method, LASSO, ridge regression, and Bayesian approaches are a few of the commonly used methods. However the problem becomes difficult to solve when some of the inputs are missing. In those cases we have to rely on imputation techniques to make the data complete. A comprehensive review of imputation methods can be found in [1,4]. The latter being focused on the linear regression problems. However, these techniques are restrictive as they come with certain assumptions. To avoid that, we are interested in interval imputation, i.e. we seek to replace the missing entries with intervals and treat the problem as linear regression with interval valued observations.

The rest of the paper is organised as follows: in Sect. 2 we present the notion of interval imputation relevant preliminaries. Followed by a simple hierarchical model for our Bayesian analysis in Sect. 3. Section 4 illustrates our method with both real and synthetic datasets to show the applicability of our method and finally we conclude this paper in Sect. 5.

2 Interval Imputation

Let x and y be n inputs and outputs with missing entries. We impute those entries with an interval, which is bounded by the observed minimum value and observed maximum value of that variable. That is, for the i-th missing entry of the j-th input, we can write $x_{ij} \in [\underline{x}_j, \overline{x}_j]$, where $\underline{x}_j = \min_{1\leq k\leq n}\{x_{kj}\}$ and $\overline{x}_j = \max_{1\leq k\leq n}\{x_{kj}\}$. Similarly, we have $y_i \in [\underline{y}, \overline{y}]$, where $\underline{y} = \min_{1\leq k\leq n}\{y_k\}$ and $\overline{y} = \max_{1\leq k\leq n}\{y_k\}$.

Definition 1 (Interval Arithmetic). *Given two intervals $i_1 = [\underline{i}_1, \overline{i}_1]$ and $i_2 = [\underline{i}_2, \overline{i}_2]$, the standard algebraic operations are defined by the following way [5]:*

- *addition:* $i_1 + i_2 = [\underline{i}_1 + \underline{i}_2, \overline{i}_1 + \overline{i}_2]$
- *subtraction:* $i_1 - i_2 = [\underline{i}_1 - \overline{i}_2, \overline{i}_1 - \underline{i}_2]$

Now, let $Ext(i_1 i_2) := \{\underline{i}_1\underline{i}_2, \underline{i}_1\overline{i}_2, \overline{i}_1\underline{i}_2, \overline{i}_1\overline{i}_2\}$ *then*

- *multiplication:* $i_1 \times i_2 = [\min Ext(i_1 i_2), \max Ext(i_1 i_2)]$
- *Division:* $i_1/i_2 = i_1 \times i_2^{-1} = [\min Ext(i_1 i_2^{-1}), \max Ext(i_1 i_2^{-1})]$ *when* $0 \notin [\underline{i}_2, \overline{i}_2]$.

Along with the above operations, for any scalar s and interval i_1

$$i_1 + s = [\underline{i}_1 + s, \overline{i}_1 + s] \quad \& \quad i_1 \times s = [\underline{i}_1 \times s, \overline{i}_1 \times s]$$

Definition 2 (Interval Valued Decomposition). *Let $M \in \mathbb{R}^{n\times p}$ be an interval valued matrix. An interval valued decomposition [3] is given by $M \approx U_M D_M V_M^T$ such that*

- $[\underline{U}_M, \overline{U}_M] = U_M \subset \mathbb{R}^{n \times n}$ *and* $[\underline{V}_M, \overline{V}_M] = V_M \subset \mathbb{R}^{p \times p}$ *are interval matrices such that columns of* U_I *and* V_I *are quasi orthonormal. That is, for* i, j

$$[U_M]_{\cdot i}[U_M]^T_{\cdot i} \approx 1; [V_M]_{\cdot i}[V_M]^T_{\cdot i} \approx 1 \quad \& \\ [U_M]_{\cdot i}[U_M]^T_{\cdot j} \approx 0; [V_M]_{\cdot i}[V_M]^T_{\cdot j} \approx 0 \quad \forall i \neq j.$$

- $D_M \subset \mathbb{R}^{n \times p}$ *is a diagonal matrix with interval-valued entries.*

3 Bayesian Analysis

We consider a simple hierarchical model given by:

$$\beta_0 \mid \sigma^2 \sim \mathcal{N}\left(0, c^2\sigma^2\right); \quad \beta \mid \sigma^2 \sim \mathcal{N}\left(0, c^2\sigma^2\mathbf{I}_p\right); \quad \sigma^2 \sim \mathrm{InvG}(a, b). \tag{2}$$

Such that, $a, b, c > 0$ and $y \in [\underline{y}, \overline{y}]$, $x \in [\underline{x}, \overline{x}]$ component-wise. With this formulation, we can easily obtain the analytical expression for the posteriors by exploiting the properties of conjugate priors [2].

Theorem 1. *Let* X, Y *be the interval imputed matrices corresponding to* x *and* y *and* $Z := [1\ X]$. *Let* $\mu \in [\underline{\mu}, \overline{\mu}]$, $\Sigma \in [\underline{\Sigma}, \overline{\Sigma}]$ *be the posterior expectation and variance of the regression coefficients. Then the following approximations hold.*

$$\mu \in [\underline{\mu}, \overline{\mu}] \approx V_Z \left(D_Z^T D_Z + \frac{1}{c^2}\mathbf{I}_{p+1}\right)^{-1} D_Z^T U_Z^T Y \tag{3}$$

$$r \in [\underline{r}, \overline{r}] = R \approx \frac{1}{2} Y^T U_Z \frac{1}{c^2}\mathbf{I}_n \left(D_Z D_Z^T + \frac{1}{c^2}\mathbf{I}_n\right)^{-1} U_Z^T Y + b \tag{4}$$

and

$$\Sigma \in [\underline{\Sigma}, \overline{\Sigma}] \approx \frac{2R}{\nu} V_Z \left(D_Z^2 + \frac{1}{c^2}\mathbf{I}_{p+1}\right)^{-1} V_Z^T \tag{5}$$

where $Z \approx U_Z D_Z V_Z^T$.

Note that this theorem ensures that we only need to invert interval matrix with diagonal entries.

Proof. For any fixed $y \in Y$ and $z \in Z$ we have

$$\mu = \left(z^T z + \frac{1}{c^2}\mathbf{I}_{p+1}\right)^{-1} z^T y.$$

Now, from interval valued decomposition we get

$$\left(Z^T Z + \frac{1}{c^2}\mathbf{I}_{p+1}\right)^{-1} Z^T Y \approx \left(V_Z D_Z^T U_Z^T U_Z D_Z V_Z^T + \frac{1}{c^2}\mathbf{I}_{p+1}\right)^{-1} V_Z D_Z^T U_Z^T Y$$

since U_Z and V_Z are quasi-orthonormal

$$\left(Z^TZ+\frac{1}{c^2}\mathbf{I}_{p+1}\right)^{-1}Z^TY\approx\left(V_Z\left(D_Z^TD_Z+\frac{1}{c^2}\mathbf{I}_{p+1}\right)V_Z^T\right)^{-1}V_ZD_Z^TU_Z^TY.$$

Therefore applying Lemma 1 we get

$$\left(Z^TZ+\frac{1}{c^2}\mathbf{I}_{p+1}\right)^{-1}Z^TY\approx V_Z\left(D_Z^TD_Z+\frac{1}{c^2}\mathbf{I}_{p+1}\right)^{-1}D_Z^TU_Z^TY\approx\left[\underline{\mu},\overline{\mu}\right].$$

Similarly, for any fixed $y\in Y$ and $z\in Z$ we have

$$2r=y^Ty-y^TzL^{-1}z^Ty+2b\quad\&\quad\Sigma=\frac{2r}{\nu}L^{-1}.$$

Therefore, proceeding as before we get,

$$2R\approx Y^TU_Z\frac{1}{c^2}\mathbf{I}_n\left(D_ZD_Z^T+\frac{1}{c^2}\mathbf{I}_n\right)^{-1}U_Z^TY+2b.$$

and

$$\Sigma\in\left[\underline{\Sigma},\overline{\Sigma}\right]\approx\frac{2R}{\nu}V_Z\left(D_Z^TD_Z+\frac{1}{c^2}\mathbf{I}_{p+1}\right)^{-1}V_Z^T.$$

Lemma 1. *Let $U_ZD_ZV_Z^T$ be the interval-valued decomposition of Z where U_Z and V_Z are quasi-orthonormal matrices. Then the following approximations hold:*

$$\left(V_Z\left(D_Z^TD_Z+\frac{1}{c^2}\mathbf{I}_{p+1}\right)V_Z^T\right)^{-1}\approx V_Z\left(D_Z^TD_Z+\frac{1}{c^2}\mathbf{I}_{p+1}\right)^{-1}V_Z^T \qquad (6)$$

and

$$\mathbf{I}_n-D_Z\left(D_Z^TD_Z+\frac{1}{c^2}\mathbf{I}_{p+1}\right)^{-1}D_Z^T=\frac{1}{c^2}\mathbf{I}_n\left(D_ZD_Z^T+\frac{1}{c^2}\mathbf{I}_n\right)^{-1}. \qquad (7)$$

Proof. Let

$$A{:=}V_Z\left(D_Z^TD_Z+\frac{1}{c^2}\mathbf{I}_{p+1}\right)V_Z^T$$

Now, using the right hand side of Eq. (6), we have

$$AV_Z\left(D_Z^TD_Z+\frac{1}{c^2}\mathbf{I}_{p+1}\right)^{-1}V_Z^T=V_Z\left(D_Z^TD_Z+\frac{1}{c^2}\mathbf{I}_{p+1}\right)V_Z^TV_Z\left(D_Z^TD_Z+\frac{1}{c^2}\mathbf{I}_{p+1}\right)^{-1}V_Z^T.$$

Since V_Z is quasi-orthonormal

$$\begin{aligned}AV_Z\left(D_Z^TD_Z+\frac{1}{c^2}\mathbf{I}_{p+1}\right)^{-1}V_Z^T&\approx V_Z\left(D_Z^TD_Z+\frac{1}{c^2}\mathbf{I}_{p+1}\right)\left(D_Z^TD_Z+\frac{1}{c^2}\mathbf{I}_{p+1}\right)^{-1}V_Z^T\\&\approx V_ZV_Z^T\approx\mathbf{I}_{p+1}.\end{aligned}$$

Similarly, we can show that,

$$V_Z\left(D_Z^T D_Z + \frac{1}{c^2}\mathbf{I}_{p+1}\right)^{-1} V_Z^T A \approx \mathbf{I}_{p+1}.$$

Therefore,

$$A^{-1} \approx V_Z\left(D_Z^T D_Z + \frac{1}{c^2}\mathbf{I}_{p+1}\right)^{-1} V_Z^T.$$

This proves the claim in Eq. (6).

To prove Eq. (7), we only need to consider the diagonal entries of $\underline{D}_Z$ and $\overline{D}_Z$. Let $q{:=}\min(n, p+1)$ and $d_{ii} \in \left[\underline{d}_{ii}, \overline{d}_{ii}\right]$, from the left hand side of Eq. (7), we have

$$\left[\mathbf{I}_n - D_Z\left(D_Z^T D_Z + \frac{1}{c^2}\mathbf{I}_{p+1}\right)^{-1} D_Z^T\right]_{ij} = \begin{cases} 1 - \frac{d_{ii}^2}{d_{ii}^2 + \frac{1}{c^2}} & \text{for } 1 \le i = j \le q \\ 0 \quad \text{for } n \ge i = j \ge q \\ 0 \quad \text{for } i \ne j, 1 \le i, j, \le n \end{cases}$$
$$= \frac{1}{c^2}\left[\mathbf{I}_n\left(D_Z D_Z^T + \frac{1}{c^2}\mathbf{I}_n\right)^{-1}\right]_{ij}.$$

3.1 Point Estimation from Intervals

We perform cross validation following algorithm to find the set of mixing parameters.

1. Estimate $\underline{\hat{\beta}}_j, \hat{\overline{\beta}}_j$ and choose α_j for $j = 0, 1, 2, \cdots, p$.
2. Compute: $\hat{y}_i = \alpha_0\underline{\hat{\beta}}_0 + (1-\alpha_0)\hat{\overline{\beta}}_0 + \sum_{j=1}^p \alpha_j \min\left\{\underline{X}_{ij}\underline{\hat{\beta}}_j, \overline{X}_{ij}\underline{\hat{\beta}}_j\right\} + \sum_{j=1}^p (1-\alpha_j)\max\left\{\underline{X}_{ij}\hat{\overline{\beta}}_j, \overline{X}_{ij}\hat{\overline{\beta}}_j\right\}$
3. Compute and minimise $L(Y, \hat{y}) = \sum(\underline{Y}_i - \hat{y}_i)^2 + \sum(\underline{Y}_i - \hat{y}_i)^2$ w.r.t. α_j's
4. Compute: $\beta_j^{\alpha_j} = \alpha_j\underline{\hat{\beta}}_j + (1-\alpha_j)\hat{\overline{\beta}}_j$

4 Illustration

We illustrate our result with synthetic dataset as well as Naval Propulsion Plants Data Set from UCI repository for real-life example. For comparison we use: k-Nearest Neighbour (kNN), iterative EM PCA (imPCA) and Iterative robust model-based imputation (irmi). We use the imputed datasets to perform Bayesian analyses with the standard hierarchical model mentioned in Eq. (2) with $a = 0.001, b = 0.001$ and $c = 1$.

4.1 Synthetic Dataset

We construct 2 synthetic datasets with 20 input variables and 100 observations. In the first synthetic dataset all the variables are related to the output. However, in the second dataset, only first 15 variables have an effect on the output and the rest have no effect. We consider three different training scenarios: A) only 1% entries are missing, B) 5% entries are missing and C) 10% entries are missing.

We show our prediction accuracy in Table 1 with root mean-squared error as the loss function. Here we provide our method in the first row and denote it by IntImp (interval imputation). The first three columns show the results for setting 1, whereas the next three column represent results for setting 2. We also show our method's performance in estimating the regression coefficients in Table 2 and compare with other methods.

Table 1. Summary of prediction accuracy

	1st			2nd		
Missing %	1	5	10	1	5	10
IntImp	**0.359**	0.577	**0.352**	**0.584**	1.016	**0.303**
imPCA	0.659	**0.488**	0.651	1.359	**0.934**	1.082
Irmi	0.646	0.505	0.653	1.373	1.173	1.270
kNN	0.595	0.565	0.650	1.332	1.287	1.271

Table 2. Summary of estimation accuracy w.r.t. true regression effect

	1st			2nd		
Missing %	1	5	10	1	5	10
IntImp	0.296	0.426	0.523	0.707	0.469	0.845
imPCA	0.067	0.183	0.157	0.223	0.376	0.445
Irmi	0.064	0.083	0.101	**0.222**	0.273	0.269
kNN	**0.061**	**0.063**	**0.074**	0.225	**0.240**	**0.232**

4.2 Naval Propulsion Plants Data Set

There are 16 input variables related to the naval vessel system and two output variables: compressor decay state coefficient and turbine decay state coefficient (CDS and TDS) in the dataset. Out of the 16 input variables, we remove 7th, 9th and 12th variables. We sample a total of 100 observations for training and

10 observations for testing. We follow similar training scenarios as of the our analyses with synthetic dataset.

For real data, we only show prediction accuracy of different methods in Table 3. The basic structure of the table is the same as Table 1, except the first three columns show the results for CDS whereas the next three column represent results for TDS in the table.

Table 3. Summary of prediction accuracy

	CDS			TDS		
Missing %	1	5	10	1	5	10
IntImp	1.286	**0.772**	**0.652**	0.993	**0.538**	0.853
imPCA	**0.933**	0.897	0.974	**0.856**	0.809	**0.769**
Irmi	0.940	0.922	0.938	0.870	0.859	0.851
kNN	0.943	0.924	0.939	0.862	0.847	0.876

5 Conclusion

We presented an approximate algorithm for linear regression with interval imputation. We notice that with 10-fold cross-validation, our method performs well and often outperforms other methods, with imPCA being the only method with similar performance in prediction. However, we also notice an unexpected behaviour of our method. We see that for synthetic datasets, the regression coefficient estimates are far from the true values, despite outperforming other methods in terms of prediction accuracy. This shows the need of performing further analysis to investigate overfitting effect through changing the level of additional noise in the model. But this also motivates us to look for further analytical properties of the method and understand if the regression coefficient estimates gets closer to the true values as we increase the sample size of the training dataset.

References

1. Emmanuel, T., Maupong, T.M., Mpoeleng, D., Semong, T., Banyatsang, M., Tabona, O.: A survey on missing data in machine learning. J. Big Data **8**, 1–37 (2021)
2. Gelman, A., Carlin, J.B., Stern, H.S., Rubin, D.B.: Bayesian Data Analysis, 2nd edn. Chapman and Hall/CRC (2004)
3. Li, M.L., Mauro, F.D., Candan, K.S., Sapino, M.L.: Matrix factorization with interval-valued data. IEEE Trans. Knowl. Data Eng. **33**(4), 1644–1658 (2019)
4. Little, R.J.A.: Regression with missing x's: a review. J. Am. Stat. Assoc. **87**(420), 1227–1237 (1992)
5. Sunaga, T.: Theory of an interval algebra and its application to numerical analysis [Reprint of Res. Assoc. Appl. Geom. Mem. 2 (1958), 29-46]. Japan J. Ind. Appl. Math. **26**(2–3), 125–143 (2009)

Models of Network Delay

Ronan Wallace(✉), Xabier Garcia Andrade, Pedro Kayser, Zhao Luo, Hrishav Mukherjee, Ruan Nunes, and Marc Warrior

Amazon Web Services, Seattle, USA
ronanw@amazon.com

Abstract. In this paper several mathematical models for end-to-end network delay are derived, where exponential wait times at intermediate network routers are assumed. The feasibility of using these models to extract parameters related to the routers is investigated by performing closure tests using synthetic data generated from the models themselves. Data from an experimental test bed is used to compare the different models. The fits are used to estimate the difference between network probe latencies. Specifically, a difference of 4.67 ± 0.27 μs is measured between a distinct pair of measurement probes across an experimental test bed.

Keywords: IP Networks · Packet Delay

1 Introduction

One important characteristic of a communications network is the delay that is experienced in delivering a message from sender to receiver [1]. There are several distinct contributions to this delay: propagation delay, switching delay, queuing delay, transmission delay and application delay.

Propagation delay is a function of distance and the speed of light in the transmission medium. Switching delay is the time it takes intermediate routers to make their forwarding decision. Queuing delay accounts for time that messages may be waiting due to intermediate routers being busy and unable to forward messages. Transmission delay refers to the time between the first and last bytes of the packet are emitted by the router. Application specific delays account for details related to the events at sender and receiver that trigger timestamping.

In this paper we consider the queuing delay at intermediate routers to be the main driver of end-to-end latency variability. We derive probability distributions for end-to-end latency variability by assuming that the queueing delays at intermediate routers are exponentially distributed. The rate at which routers process incoming data depends on the speed of the interfaces; routers with similar/different interface speeds will have similar/different exponential rate parameters. The feasibility of extracting the rate parameters is investigated using synthetic data generated by these models. Real data from an experimental test bed is also fitted using the models.

J. Einbeck et al. (Eds.): IWSM 2024, CONTRIB.STAT., pp. 231–238, 2024.
https://doi.org/10.1007/978-3-031-65723-8_36

The rest of this paper is organised as follows. Section 2 gives a short overview of queuing theory and related work; Sect. 3 outlines our notation; Sect. 4 derives a probability distribution for the sum of groups of n and m exponential random variables, where the rate parameters are the same within each group; Sect. 5 discusses fits to real data; and Sect. 6 concludes the paper.

2 Queuing Theory and Related Work

The work presented here builds on concepts from queuing theory. In this framework, queuing systems are characterised by: the probability distributions of the number of packets arriving at the server; the probability distribution of the packet service time; and the number of servers [1]. In Kendall's notation, the distributions are denoted by M, G or D depending on whether the distribution is exponential, general or deterministic. For example, the M/M/1 queue system is one where: the inter-arrival time of packets is exponential (or equivalently the number of packets arriving in a time interval is Poisson); the service time of packets is exponential; and there is one server. The M/G/n queue is one where the inter-arrival time of packets is exponential; the service time of packets follows a general distribution; and there are n servers in parallel. For these systems, Little's Theorem is used to express steady state quantities like the average number of packets in a queue, the average service time per packet etc [1]. In this work we are considering m G/M/1 systems in series: we are not concerned about the arrival rate, so we designate a general distribution; we are assuming that the service time is exponential; and we model each router as a single server. What we are interested in is overall delay distribution of the m G/M/1 systems in series.

The models described in this paper assume a dependence between the network delay and the number of network hops. The approach was considered before as a way to describe end-to-end internet latency data, but the assumption above was not consistent with this data and another kind of treatment was required [2,3]. In this work we look at data where this assumption does hold; the data has been collected on an experimental test bed, which is a more controlled environment than the internet.

The main assumption made in this paper is that the queueing delays are exponentially distributed. One consequence of this is that a delay of zero has the highest probability, yet for real systems this delay is non-zero. In other work the exponential wait time is only assumed to hold in the tail of the distribution [4].

Others have modeled end-to-end delay distributions with Normal, Lognormal and Pareto distributions directly [5]. While these often obtain good results, they are not built up from the delay distributions of the underlying routers and so don't provide an interpretation at the per hop level.

In this paper we look at models of end-to-end delay across several routers. We provide explicit derivations and comparisons to real data collected on an experimental test bed.

3 Notation and Convolution

Random variables are represented using capital letters like X, Y and Z. Lower cases x, y, z refer to particular values of the random variable. Probability density functions of random variables are represented by lower case letters such as f, g, and h. It should be obvious from the context when lower cases letters are used to represent functions or values of random variables.

Suppose we have two random variables X and Y. Suppose that their distributions are known. The distribution of their sum $Z = X + Y$ is given by the convolution. In the continuous case it is given by the integral

$$h(Z = z) = f * g(Z = z) \tag{1}$$

$$= \int_{-\infty}^{+\infty} f(X = z - t)g(Y = t)dt \tag{2}$$

The limits at infinity can be reduced to 0, t for functions supported on $[0, +\infty)$.

4 Combination of Gamma Random Variables

We now consider the end-to-end delay distributions that can occur when we assume the router delay distribution to be exponential. There are a number of different scenarios: all of the exponential rate parameters are the same, leading to a gamma distribution (this is a well-known result); all of the exponential rate parameters are different, leading to a hypoexponential distribution; all but one of the exponential rate parameters are the same; and two sets of exponential rate parameters, corresponding to the situation where there are two sets of several network routers, where the queue depths and processing rates are similar within a set but different between sets. To determine the result we convolve two gamma distribution of the form:

$$X \sim g(x) = \frac{\beta_1^{\alpha_1}}{\Gamma(\alpha_1)} x^{\alpha_1 - 1} e^{-\beta_1 x} \tag{3}$$

Implementing the convolution

$$h(z) = g * f(z) = \int_0^z g(t) f(z - t)dt \tag{4}$$

$$= \int_0^z \frac{\beta_1^{\alpha_1}}{\Gamma(\alpha_1)} t^{\alpha_1 - 1} e^{-\beta_1 t} \frac{\beta_2^{\alpha_2}}{\Gamma(\alpha_2)} (z - t)^{\alpha_2 - 1} e^{-\beta_2 (z - t)} dt \tag{5}$$

$$= \frac{\beta_1^{\alpha_1}}{\Gamma(\alpha_1)} \frac{\beta_2^{\alpha_2}}{\Gamma(\alpha_2)} e^{-\beta_2 z} \int_0^z t^{\alpha_1 - 1} e^{(\beta_2 - \beta_1)t} (z - t)^{\alpha_2 - 1} dt \tag{6}$$

Now make the subsititutions $u = t/z$ and $dt = zdu$.

$$h(z) = \frac{\beta_1^{\alpha_1}}{\Gamma(\alpha_1)} \frac{\beta_2^{\alpha_2}}{\Gamma(\alpha_2)} e^{-\beta_2 z} \int_0^1 (uz)^{\alpha_1 - 1} e^{(\beta_2 - \beta_1)zu} (z - zu)^{\alpha_2 - 1} z du \tag{7}$$

$$= \frac{\beta_1^{\alpha_1}}{\Gamma(\alpha_1)} \frac{\beta_2^{\alpha_2}}{\Gamma(\alpha_2)} e^{-\beta_2 z} z^{\alpha_1 - 1} z^{\alpha_2} \int_0^1 u^{\alpha_1 - 1} e^{[(\beta_2 - \beta_1)z]u} (1 - u)^{\alpha_2 - 1} du \tag{8}$$

$$= \frac{\beta_1^{\alpha_1}}{\Gamma(\alpha_1)} \frac{\beta_2^{\alpha_2}}{\Gamma(\alpha_2)} \frac{\Gamma(\alpha_1 + \alpha_2)}{\Gamma(\alpha_1 + \alpha_2)} e^{-\beta_2 z} z^{\alpha_1 - 1} z^{\alpha_2} \int_0^1 e^{[(\beta_2 - \beta_1)z]u} u^{\alpha_1 - 1} (1 - u)^{\alpha_1 + \alpha_2 - \alpha_1 - 1} du \tag{9}$$

$$= \frac{\beta_1^{\alpha_1} \beta_2^{\alpha_2}}{\Gamma(\alpha_1 + \alpha_2)} e^{-\beta_2 z} z^{\alpha_1 + \alpha_2 - 1} \frac{\Gamma(\alpha_1 + \alpha_2)}{\Gamma(\alpha_1)\Gamma(\alpha_2)} \int_0^1 e^{[(\beta_2 - \beta_1)z]u} u^{\alpha_1 - 1} (1 - u)^{\alpha_1 + \alpha_2 - \alpha_1 - 1} du \tag{10}$$

$$= \frac{\beta_1^{\alpha_1} \beta_2^{\alpha_2}}{\Gamma(\alpha_1 + \alpha_2)} e^{-\beta_2 z} z^{\alpha_1 + \alpha_2 - 1} {}_1F_1(\alpha_1; \alpha_1 + \alpha_2; (\beta_2 - \beta_1)z) \tag{11}$$

This shows that the convolution of two Gamma random variables can be written in terms of the confluent hypergeometric function of the 1st kind, ${}_1F_1$. Note that if $\beta_1 = \beta 2 = \beta$ then this reduces to $Z \sim Gamma(z; \alpha_1 + \alpha_2, \beta)$.

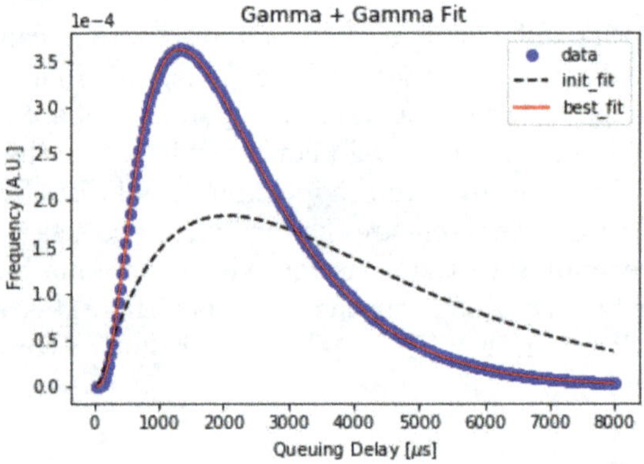

Fig. 1. The fit of the Gamma + Gamma distribution to one hundred million samples generated from the same distribution.

Synthetic data sampled according to a Gamma + Gamma distribition is shown in Fig. 1, where the parameters of the underlying exponential distributions are given in Table 1. The first Gamma is generated from 3 independent and identically distributed exponential functions, all with Rate parameter 0.01. The second Gamma is generated from 2 independent and identically distributed exponential functions, all with Rate parameter 0.001. We then fit the same function to the generated data and see that the Best Fit parameters are the same as the true Rate parameters.Thus, the fitting approach satisfies a closure test.

Table 1. Parameters of the Gamma + Gamma distribution. Note that the Mean Delay and Rate are reciprocal.

Parameter	Mean Delay [μs]	Rate $[\mu s]^{-1}$	Initial	Best Fit
α_1	-	-	3	3
β_1	100	0.01	0.04	0.01
α_2	-	-	2	2
β_2	1000	0.001	0.0005	0.001

5 Fits to Real Data

5.1 Data Set

Round trip time latency data between servers attached to an experimental test bed was collected on the 1st July 2022 between 2000 and 2100 UTC. Two specific network probes (we shall call them P1 and P2) were configured to collect this data. The two probes have a common source (sharing server and switch) but different destination racks; the network path differs in length by 8 network hops in the complete round trip. Both probes are generated by agents from servers of the same model type. The top-of-rack switches and network routers are also the same type.

There are thus three entity types for this probe - the server, the switch and the router. We can expect the hypoexponential, Gamma + Gamma or Gamma + Exp fits to perform best depending on how different the delays are for these different entity types.

Packets are sent at a rate of 1 packet per second so each of the data sets has 3600 samples from the hour of data taking. The latency measurement is obtained by combining four kernel timestamps, two from each of the sending and receiving servers.

The resulting data is summarised in Fig. 2. Both probe latency distributions have four peaks, 1 main peak and 3 smaller peaks. The main peak positions of the distributions are shifted relative to one another. The peak positions of the 3 smaller distributions are not shifted and are understood to be caused by batching/queuing of packets at the server network interface. Understanding the distribution of the main peak is the focus in this note.

5.2 Fits to Data

Before fitting, the minimum value is subtracted from all values. The effect of this is to subtract out the constant delays from each latency measurement, such as the propagation delay. Rather than fitting the latency we are then fitting the variable delay. This simplifies the form of the fitting function.

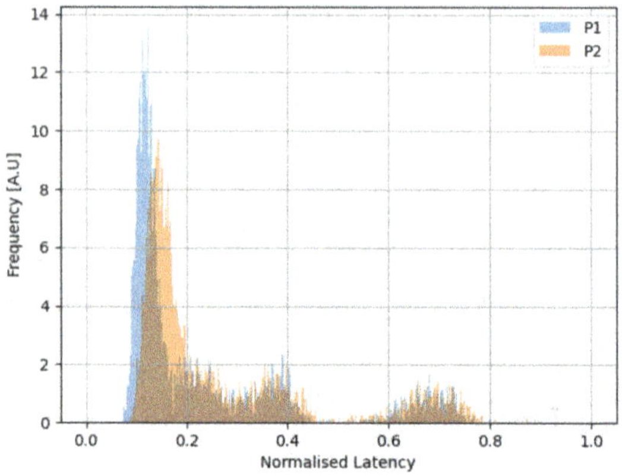

Fig. 2. The histograms of the two latency data sets used in the study. Note that the latency values have been mapped to the dimensionless interval [0,1].

We use the lmfit package with least square and Nelder-Mead methods.

First the data is fit with a combination of 4 Gaussian distributions, which serves as the baseline model. This model is not suitable for a network delay because it is not strictly positive. The Gaussian parameters extracted for the 3 smaller peaks are used for other fits whereas the Gaussian parameters for the main peak are swapped with the parameters from the models, like the ones described in Sect. 4.

Fits are compared using the reduced χ^2 test statistic. This is the usual χ^2 test statistic divided by the number of degrees of freedom, which in this case is the number of bins of the histogram minus the number of parameters in the model.

Table 2. Results of the fitting methods on the two different data sets.

Method	Data Set	χ^2	Parameters	$\chi^2/ndof$
4 Gaussian	P1	0.002	12	1.99e−06
Hypoexponential + 3 Gaussian	P1	0.011	11	1.14e−05
Gamma + Gamma + 3 Gaussian	P1	0.002	13	2.17e−06
Gamma + Exponential + 3 Gaussian	P1	0.006	13	6.38e−06
4 Gaussian	P2	0.002	12	1.85e−06
Hypoexponential + 3 Gaussian	P2	0.008	11	8.59e−06
Gamma + Gamma + 3 Gaussian	P2	0.002	13	1.98e−06
Gamma + Exponential + 3 Gaussian	P2	0.004	13	3.82e−06

The results of the fits are summarised in Table 2. The best performing model of those proposed in this note is the Gamma + Gamma + 3 Gaussian model.

5.3 Estimating the Latency Shift

Each Gaussian from the 4 Gaussian model has 3 parameters: a mean, a width and a normalisation. The 4 means correspond to the location of the peaks and can be used to quantify the offset between the P1 and P2 data sets (Table 3).

Table 3. 4 Gaussian peak positions and differences between P1 and P2 data.

Peak	P2 Mean	P1 Mean	Difference	Relative Uncertainty
Main	21.68 ± 0.22	17.01 ± 0.10	4.67 ± 0.24	5 %
Small 1	55.62 ± 1.98	54.03 ± 1.13	1.59 ± 2.28	143 %
Small 2	115.00 ± 1.28	118.25 ± 1.25	-3.25 ± 1.79	55 %
Small 3	240.00 ± 1.69	243.00 ± 1.75	-3.00 ± 2.43	81 %

Uncertaintaines are propagated to the difference by adding in quadrature, which amounts to assuming the uncertainties on the parameters are independent. This is reasonable since the data sets are independent. There is a 4.67 ± 0.24 microsecond difference between the P1 and P2 main peak positions. The differences between the small peak positions are not statistically significant given the uncertainites.

6 Conclusion

We have derived a number of models that can be used to explain the shapes of end-to-end delay distributions. Our derivations assumed exponential wait times at each router. Using these models we have tested the feasibility of extracting parameters related to the routers by performing closure tests using synthetic data generated from the models themselves.

The best fit to real data is with the baseline model of 4 Gaussians. Strictly speaking this model is not a correct description of network delay because the domain of the Gaussian function is the set of real numbers, including the negative ones. The models we have derived are correct in this sense as their domain is the set of positive real numbers. The second best fit is from the Gamma + Gamma + 3 Gaussian model.

We demonstrated a nice application of the fit results where the difference of latency between different probes can be estimated. In our case the measurement is 4.67 ± 0.27 μs. Since the only difference between these probes are the 8 networking hops, the difference is a pure measure of network performance. Contrast this with absolute latency measures that can include non-network components.

We have identified potential future work that includes: empirically measuring the router delay with timestamps for packets in and packets out; repeating the data collection while controlling for the queue lengths in the routers; repeating the data collection with more diverse sets of paths, different path lengths, and paths experiencing congestion.

References

1. Bertsekas, D.P., Gallager, R.G.: Data Networks. Prentice Hall, Hoboken (1992)
2. Hooghiemstra, G., Van Miegham, P.: Delay Distributions on Fixed Internet Paths (2001)
3. Van Mieghem, P.: A lower bound for the end-to-end delay in networks: application to voice over IP. In: Proceedings IEEE GLOBECOM (1998)
4. Abate, J., Whitt, W.: Exponential approximations for tail probabilities in queues, I: waiting times. Oper. Res. **43**, 885–901 (1995)
5. Zhang, W., He, J.: Statistical modeling and correlation analysis of end-to-end delay in wide area networks. In: Eighth ACIS International Conference on Software Engineering, Artificial Intelligence, Networking, and Parallel/Distributed Computing, vol. 3, pp. 968–973 (2007)

Estimating Dose and Time of Exposure from a Protein-Based Radiation Biomarker

Yilun Cai[1(✉)], Jochen Einbeck[1], Stephen Barnard[2], and Elizabeth Ainsbury[2]

[1] Durham University, Durham, UK
{yilun.cai,jochen.einbeck}@durham.ac.uk
[2] UKHSA Radiation, Chemicals and Environmental Hazards Division, Chilton, Didcot, UK
{stephen.barnard,liz.ainsbury}@ukhsa.gov.uk

Abstract. In order to analyze the potential damage to the human body caused by exposure to ionizing radiation, one needs to have an estimation of the dose of radiation received by the individual. In the context of a protein-based biomarker for radiation exposure, we present here a new method that, unlike the approaches that produce the estimation with data collected at a predetermined time after exposure, allows us to estimate the dose at any time within a reasonable time interval after exposure, as well as determine the time of exposure if needed. Namely, we take existing calibration curves and generalize them using the decay mechanism of γ-H2AX foci to build a model that describes the functional relationship between the count of γ-H2AX foci in exposed blood cells and the time and dose of exposure. This model is illustrated using both real and simulated data.

Keywords: Biological dosimetry · Poisson regression · Overdispersion

1 Introduction

In modern society, individuals are at risk of potentially harmful ionizing radiation exposure, such as occupational radiation workers (nuclear workers, medical staff, radiographers etc.) and also patients undergoing diagnostic or therapeutic radiation treatments to detect or treat cancers and other related health conditions (orthopaedics, cardiology etc.). Therefore, following a potential over-exposure to radiation, one needs a tool such as biodosimetry to estimate the dose of the exposure to inform on medical intervention and/or triage of patients for treatment following a mass-casualty radiological accident or incident.

Ionizing radiation exposure causes DNA double strand breaks (DSBs) which leads to the formation of chromosome aberrations during DNA replication [3]. The well established 'gold standard' method for accurate dose estimation is the dicentric chromosome assay (DCA). However, a drawback of the DCA, especially

J. Einbeck et al. (Eds.): IWSM 2024, CONTRIB.STAT., pp. 239–245, 2024.
https://doi.org/10.1007/978-3-031-65723-8_37

in the case of emergencies, is that it takes at least two days after the collection of samples to produce the dose estimation.

A more suitable biomarker for rapid dose estimation could be the γ-H2AX assay. γ-H2AX foci are phosphorylated proteins (histones) which form proportionally to DSBs to repair them and can be detected, visualized, and counted minutes after ionizing radiation exposure.

In order to utilize this biomarker, one produces a 'calibration curve' by exposing batches of blood to ionizing radiation at given 'design doses' (typically, at least 8 values weighted towards lower doses, such as $d = 0.1, 0.2, 0.5, ..., 1, 2,$ 4Gy), then counting the number of γ-H2AX foci in a set number of cells in each sample at a predetermined time after exposure such as $2h$ or $24h$, and fitting a count data model to these counts. There is solid evidence that these foci counts are overdispersed [1], so Negative Binomial models are preferable to Poisson models for this purpose.

These approaches are, however, limited by their time dependence. For instance, if blood samples from a potentially irradiated individual were to be examined 6 h after exposure, any dose estimate would inevitably carry a large bias if the lab decided to resort to a calibration curve from a different ('wrong') time of exposure. Similar problems would occur if this individual is unsure about the time of the possible exposure.

To address this issue, we present here a new method that allows us to estimate ionizing radiation dose at any time within a reasonable time interval after exposure, as well as determine the time of exposure if needed.

2 A Model Linking Calibration Curves with Foci Decay

We denote the average count of γ-H2AX foci in a sample of cells at a time after exposure as y, and refer to it as 'yield'. The basic idea is to take γ-H2AX foci count measurements twice, i.e. at different time points. This gives two pieces of information (two yields at unknown times with known time distance), which allow to estimate dose and time of exposure. We assume that two calibration curves

$$y_t = a_t + b_t d$$

at known times $t = t_c$, $c = 1, 2$, are available from the specific laboratory. We further assume that two measurements at times t_0, $t_0 + \Delta$ are taken from the potentially exposed individual, where t_0 is unknown (to be inferred) but Δ known. It is not necessary for t_0 or $t_0 + \Delta$ to correspond to any of the t_c. The behavior between the time points t_0 and $t_0 + \Delta$ can be assumed to be governed by a double-exponential decay mechanism [2]. In order to connect this decay mechanism with the two calibration curves, we build the model

$$y = a + bt + d(Ae^{ut} + Be^{vt}) \quad (1)$$

where a, b, A, B, u, v are constants, which we will show can be established in a certain way, and t_0 are d are to be inferred. We do have two realizations of model (1) available, namely at time points t_0 and $t_0 + \Delta$.

3 Parameter Elicitation

Here we describe how to find values for the parameters a, b, A, B, u, v. Firstly, we note that the parameters u and v can reasonably be assumed to be determined by the nature of the physical decay mechanism and hence we fix them at $u = -0.3495$ and $v = -0.01843$ according to [2]. The situation is, however, different with the parameters a, b, A, B which are related to the absolute magnitude of foci observed, and hence are likely to be lab-specific (e.g. depending on the filter settings of the foci detection software). Specifically, the 'linear intercept' $a + bt$ relates to the background yield of foci (i.e., when no exposure has taken place), and hence we can find a, b by solving the system of two linear equations $a_t = a + bt$ at $t = t_c$, $c = 1, 2$. Similarly, we equate

$$Ae^{-0.3495t} + Be^{-0.01843t} = b_t$$

for $t = t_c$, $c = 1, 2$, yielding values of A and B.

For instance, for the two calibration curves at $t_1 = 1h$ and $t_2 = 24h$ given in [1],

$$y_1 = 0.131 + 12.559d; \quad y_{24} = 0.179 + 1.937d, \tag{2}$$

this procedure yields $\hat{a} = 0.129$, $\hat{b} = 0.002$, $\hat{A} = 13.622$, $\hat{B} = 3.010$.

The final step is to set up a system of two equations of type (1) with our two yield measurements at times t_0 and $t_0 + \Delta$, and solve this system for d and t_0, for which we use the Mathematica solver "NSolve".

4 Simulation Test Results

A simulation study was carried out to verify the efficiency of the solving step for t_0 and d. We generate foci counts, for known (true) $d = 1$, at time points $t_0 = 1h$ and $t_1 = 24h$, from $n = 500$ cells via a Negative Binomial model with mean (yield) equal to the two calibration curves (2), and dispersion (variance/mean ratio) equal to 50. The resulting yields then give rise to two equations of type (1), as described above, for known $\Delta = 23h$, from which d and t_0 are estimated through Mathematica. We consider the settings $n = 200, 500, 1000$, and $n = 2000$. We repeat this procedure $N = 100$ times each and display two examples of the results(due to lack of room) in Fig. 1 (for the dose estimates) and Fig. 2 (for the estimates of t_0). We find that both dose and time are well estimated, and that the estimates approach the true values when n increases.

5 Real Data Bootstrap Test Results

The methods discussed above are applied to a real data set produced at the chromosome dosimetry unit at UKHSA. Four blood samples from a healthy volunteer were exposed *in vitro* to ionizing radiation with design doses $0, 0.5, 1, 2$. For each sample, the foci counts in $n = 200$ cells were scored at time points

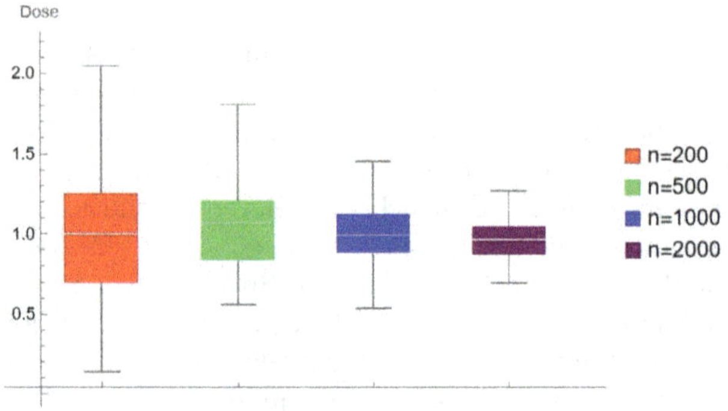

Fig. 1. Dose estimates $\hat{d}$ for simulated foci samples from a Negative Binomial distribution with true $d = 1$ and $t_0 = 1$

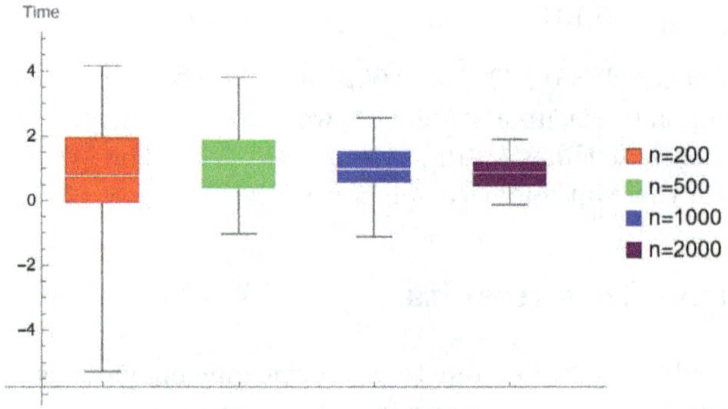

Fig. 2. Time estimates $\hat{t}_0$ for simulated foci samples from a Negative Binomial distribution with true $d = 1$ and $t_0 = 1$

Table 1. Laboratory data from UKHSA: Foci yields in batches of 200 cells

	design dose (Gy)			
time of scoring (h)	0	0.5	1	2
1	0.68	2.27	4.62	5.91
2	0.17	2.05	3.79	6.04
4	0.15	1.74	3.17	4.48
24	0.27	0.55	1.12	2.03
48	0.17	0.64	0.76	1.29

$1h, 2h, 4h, 24h, 48h$ after exposure. Table 1 displays the average foci count (yield) at each individual design dose and time point.

From a calibration point of view, this is a relatively small data set, where ideally one would like to have more than $n = 200$ scored cells per sample, and also more than one sample for each design dose (for instance, 32 samples were used in [1]). We also immediately notice two anomalies, namely the data with design dose $0.5Gy$ at time $48h$ and the data with design dose $2Gy$ at time $1h$.

We can still use this data set to apply the methodology. Firstly, we put the foci yields at times $2h$ and $24h$ aside, and use them as calibration data, giving rise to two calibration curves:

$$y_2 = 0.1954 + 3.2167d; \quad y_{24} = 0.2355 + 0.8609d.$$

Like illustrated in Sect. 3, these can be used to produce a time-and dose dependent model of type (1). Assuming now that yields y, y' at two unknown t_1 and $t_1 + \Delta$ are available, we obtain the system of two equations

$$y = 0.1918 + 0.001823t_1 + d(3.8760e^{-0.3495t_1} + 1.3385e^{-0.01843t_1})$$
$$y' = 0.1918 + 0.001823(t_1 + \Delta) + d(3.8760e^{-0.3495(t_1+\Delta)} + 1.3385e^{-0.01843(t_1+\Delta)})$$

We will first test the model on the average foci counts (except the two anomalies and the $2h$ and $24h$ data that were used to generate the calibration curves) so as to have a straightforward idea of the performance of the model. We take the yield of each sample to produce dose estimations of each design dose using each combination of data from t_1 and t_2 at each design dose. The results are displayed in Table 2.

We find that the model is quite good at detecting non-exposure and quite accurate at higher design doses, but generally overestimates the doses at lower design doses when using data from small t_1 and t_2. This is to be expected due to a well documented 'saturation effect' [4] in the foci counting process due to a more significant undercount of foci at its higher concentration.

Table 2. Dose estimations for different pairings of (unknown) exposure times (t_1, t_2) with known time distance Δ (in h).

t_1, t_2	Δ	design dose (Gy)			
		0	0.5	1	2
1, 4	3	0.00	1.12	1.90	
1, 48	37	0.00		0.86	
4, 48	34	0.00		0.84	1.81

Additionally, we employ the bootstrap [5] to assess the reliability of the model on real data. For each of the average foci count in consideration, we take 1000 bootstrap samples of its $n = 200$ cells' foci count where each sample consists of $n = 200$ counts that was drawn from the original data with replacement. We take the average of each sample which we use as yields to produce dose estimations of each design dose using each combination of data from t_1 and t_2 at each design dose, and repeat this process for each of the 1000 Bootstrap samples. We display two examples of resulting dose estimates in Fig. 3 and Fig. 4. We find that the estimated doses reasonably reliable considering the low amount of cells being counted.

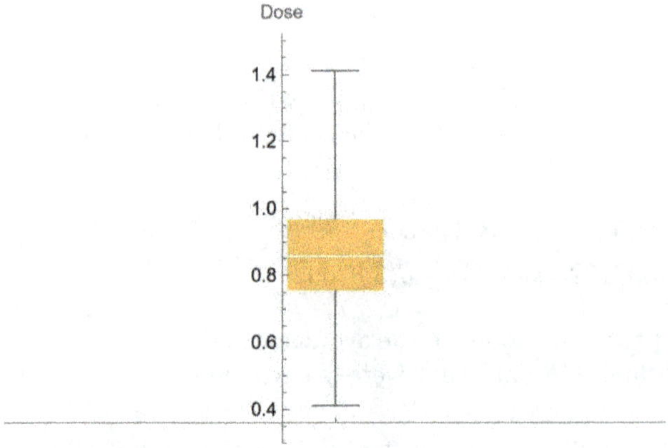

Fig. 3. Dose estimates $\hat{d}$ from bootstrap simulated data generated using real data with $d = 1$, $t_1 = 1$, $t_2 = 48$

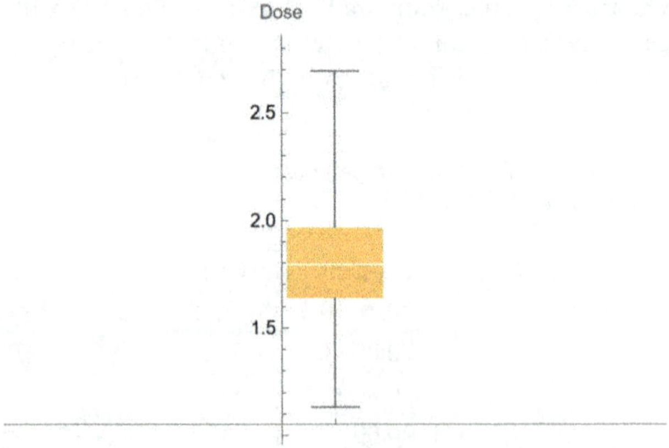

Fig. 4. Dose estimates $\hat{d}$ from bootstrap simulated data generated using real data with $d = 2$, $t_1 = 4$, $t_2 = 48$

6 Conclusion

We aimed to build a model that would allow us to determine ionizing radiation dose and exposure time using a sequence of biomarker measurements. We greatly reduced the time dependency of previous methods of ionizing radiation dose estimation that uses γ-H2AX foci as the biomarker, and we have also sped up the estimation process. We tested this model using both simulated and real data and can conclude from the results that the model performs well with reasonable discrepancies that can be expected, given the relatively low foci numbers involved.

References

1. Einbeck, J., Ainsbury, E. A., Sales, R., Barnard, S., Kaestle, F., Higueras, M.: A statistical framework for radiation dose estimation with uncertainty quantification from the *gamma*-H2AX assay. PloS One **13**(11), e0207464 (2018). https://doi.org/10.1371/journal.pone.0207464
2. Horn, S., Barnard, S., Rothkamm, K.: Gamma-H2AX-based dose estimation for whole and partial body radiation exposure. PloS One **6**(9), e25113 (2011). https://doi.org/10.1371/journal.pone.0025113
3. Pfeiffer, P., Goedecke, W., Obe, G.: Mechanisms of DNA double-strand break repair and their potential to induce chromosomal aberrations. Mutagenesis **15**(4), 289–302 (2000). https://doi.org/10.1093/mutage/15.4.289
4. Moquet, J., et al.: The second gamma-H2AX assay inter-comparison exercise carried out in the framework of the European biodosimetry network (RENEB). Int. J. Radiation Biol. **93**(1), 58–64 (2017). https://doi.org/10.1080/09553002.2016.1207822
5. Efron, B., Tibshirani, R.: An Introduction to the Bootstrap. Chapman and Hall, Boca Raton (1993)

Statistical Modelling for Big and Little Data

Robin Henderson(✉)

Newcastle University, Newcastle upon Tyne, UK
Robin.Henderson@ncl.ac.uk

Abstract. While the difference between "Data Science" and "Statistics" disciplines is, at best, blurred, many people associate machine learning methods and big data with the former, and modelling and inference for small samples (little data) with the latter. We present a big data application where no sophisticated method at all is needed, a small data application where a partial modelling approach seems useful, and a big-and-little data application where we can borrow strength from limited information in a large sample, to improve estimation based on more detailed data in a small sample.

Keywords: Data science · Extrapolation · Inference · Smoothing · Two cultures

1 Introduction

In his 1997 University of Michigan inaugural lecture, C.F. Jeff Wu stated that the term "Statistics" was too narrow in regard to the discipline (rather than a collection of numbers) and he suggested "Data Science" might be taken into common usage as a replacement [1]. Cleveland in 2001 set out a plan to enlarge the field of statistics and confidently defined "Data Science" as the name for his altered field [2]. Donoho [3] traced data science, as distinct from data engineering, to Tukey's work in the 1960s and 1970s, and in a wide-ranging essay recapped Breiman's two cultures: data modelling and algorithmic modelling [4]. Adherents of the former propose generative models and focus on inference whilst proponents of the latter are content with black box methods with success judged by predictive accuracy. Breiman estimated that 98% of academic statisticians were at that time in the data modelling group, while the algorithmic modelling group consisted of the remaining 2% of statisticians together with large numbers of others, many being computer scientists. It is fair to say that the two cultures still exist. ChatGPT for instance, when asked to distinguish statistical from machine learning methods, summarised as "statistical methods are rooted in theory and inference, whereas machine learning methods emphasise data-driven learning and prediction". Traditional statistical modellers argue the merits and necessity of having a firm mathematical base to any technique and asymptotic analysis remains an almost obligatory requirement for publication in the highest prestige

J. Einbeck et al. (Eds.): IWSM 2024, CONTRIB.STAT., pp. 246–254, 2024.
https://doi.org/10.1007/978-3-031-65723-8_38

statistical methodology journals. Meanwhile, unperturbed, computer scientists and engineers continue to develop methods that work.

Sometimes a claim is made that data science is about big data whereas statistics is not. Sometimes the claim seems to be reversed. Donoho draws attention to the definition in the professional code of conduct of the Data Science Association as "Statistics" being "the practice or science of collecting and analyzing numerical data in large quantities". Donoho rightly refutes the definition because "statisticians deal with data however it arrives – big or small". We agree but bear in mind that the choice of method should of course depend upon the information available. In the next two sections we discuss a big data example where standard statistical methods are inappropriate and a small data example where standard statistical methods are the only realistic option. In the final section we propose a method for combining limited information from big data with fuller information from little data.

2 Big Data

A key performance measure for UK Accident and Emergency departments is the *four hour standard*, which is a government pledge of a maximum four hour wait in A&E from arrival to admission, transfer or discharge [5]. A target of 98% compliance was set when the standard was introduced in 2004, lowered to 95% in 2010 [6]. Of interest is whether the change had an effect.

Comparing the full years immediately before and after the change was announced, a headline summary is that 114 of 144 A&E departments had a statistically significant decrease in the proportion of patients seen within four hours, when testing at the 5% level. At the 0.1% level there were 110 departments with a significant decline in performance. The effect of the intervention is apparently dramatic. Yet questions might be asked if, still concentrating on significance tests, we add that 24 departments had a significant improvement in performance (23 at the 0.1% level) and just 6 had no significant change. The reason for the high number of statistically significant results is of course that A&E departments see large numbers of patients, between 10,000 and 300,000 per year for the 144 under consideration. For all departments, a change in compliant proportion of just 0.4% would be declared statistically significant, with a much lower threshold for most. At large sample sizes, a "significant" change is the norm not the exception for observational data.

The point is that for really big data sets standard statistical inferential methods are rarely, and probably never, appropriate. What *is* appropriate, is to look at the data, which can reveal issues that would not arise through unthinking concentration on performance measures. Figure 1 shows the distribution of A&E waiting times for 2011: the distribution for other years is similar. The spike in the ten minutes before the four hour mark indicates that the performance measure strongly influences behaviour, and this should be of more concern than tiny changes in compliance rate.

A small addendum. A&E compliance with the four hour standard fell steadily year on year after 2012, as the number of patients using A&E increased. The four

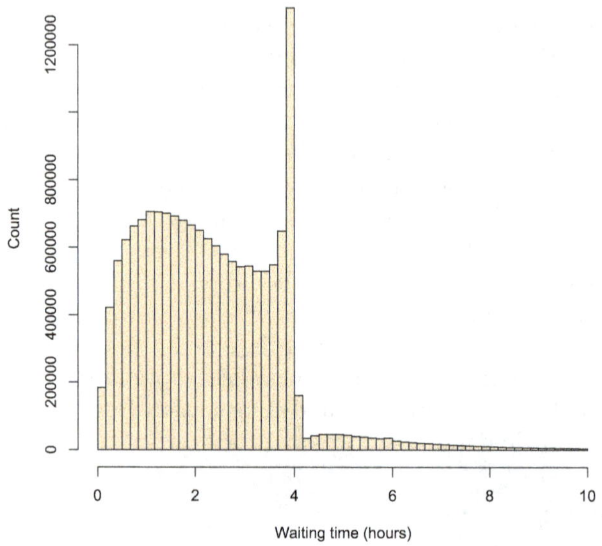

Fig. 1. 15.8 million A&E waiting times

hour pledge is still in place, albeit now included in a larger basket of measures, but the compliance target as of March 2024 is 76%. In 2003, the year before national standards were first introduced as part of a major NHS reform that promised "long waits in accident and emergency departments will be ended" [7], the estimated compliance rate was 84% [8].

3 Little Data

Figure 2 shows lifetime to date of 136 cooling coils, used in a bespoke facility for the long term storage of liquid hazardous waste. Since 2002 a review has taken place roughly every five years, with one purpose being to look ahead and predict the number of coil failures over the next five years. The latest review considered data to the end of 2023.

We work in discrete time. Let y denote calendar year and t refer to coil operating time. There are three types of coil and we can assume that coil lifetimes depend on t and coil type only, with independence between coils. The problem is unusual in that we wish to predict the total number of failures in year y over the population of coils, which will be at a range of different t.

We need some notation. Let $\mathcal{R}(t)$ be the number of coils known to have reached at least t years of operation. Let $\mathcal{N}_y(t, \tau)$ be the number of coils that were operational at the end of year y, that would be entering t years of experience in year $y+\tau$ if still operational. For example in 2024 there are three coils that are entering their 55th operational year, so $\mathcal{N}_{2023}(55, 1) = 3$. We have no experience of coils at this lifetime so $\mathcal{R}(55) = 0$. Table 1 gives all values for $y = 2023$.

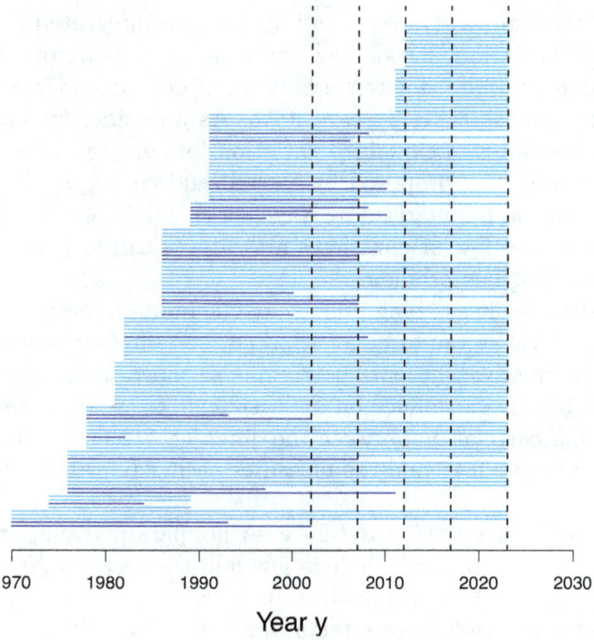

Fig. 2. Cooling coil timeline. Each horizontal line corresponds to a separate coil. Darker lines are for coils that have failed. Vertical lines mark review times

Table 1. Position in 2024

t	55	49	47	44	43	39	36	34	14	13
$\mathcal{N}_{2023}(t,1)$	3	9	9	12	11	17	3	18	12	12
$\mathcal{R}(t)$	0	3	12	21	33	44	62	65	108	120

No coils have reached lifetime $t = 55$ and hence some form of modelling and extrapolation is unavoidable. But at lower t, there is reasonable experience of coils and their failure rates and we might consider making use of this aspect of the data without parametric assumptions.

To explore we fitted six different fully parametric models together with a semiparametric Cox model and a fully nonparametric model. For the latter two we took a temporary working assumption of zero discrete hazard whenever $R(t) = 0$. We fitted at each of the five review years $y \in 2002, 2007, 2012, 2017, 2023$, with estimation of course based only on the information available to that time. For all reviews we can measure the fit of the model to the data available to that time, i.e. looking backwards. For the first four reviews we can also look forward and compare observed and predicted number of failures over the five years following y.

We used three measures to compare models looking backwards: i) the Akaike information criterion AIC, ii) integrated absolute differences IAD between observed and fitted survival curves, and iii) IBS, an integrated Brier score measure of explained variation [9]. Looking forwards, we measure predictive accuracy by the integrated absolute difference between observed and predicted cumulative failures for the following 5 years, PA5. As an aside, we note that by far the most-cited measures of explained variation for survival data are the c-index of concordance originally proposed by Harrell and colleagues [10] and a coefficient of determination popularised by Nagelkerke [11]. The c-index has problems when sample sizes are low or covariates are categorical, as here. The coefficient of determination just has problems.

No model stands out as being preferred. The nonparametric and Cox models provide the best IAD as would be anticipated, but they are worst on AIC given their lack of parsimony. The parametric models have mixed performance: five of the six have best performance on at least one of the measures at one of the reviews. The rank correlation between the different measures is low, particularly between the predictive PA5 and the measures of fit AIC (-0.18), IAD (0.20) and IBS (-0.06).

No coil failed between 2012 and 2023. A nonparametric approach reacts to this slowing of failure rate and predicts few failures between 2024 and 2028, for example an estimated 0.957 probability of fewer than 5 failures in that period (with 95% bootstrap confidence interval 0.952 to 0.971). The parametric models extrapolate earlier failure rates more severely and reduce the corresponding probability estimates, for example to 0.720 (0.696, 0.737) for the Burr distribution. Given the flattening-off of the coil lifetime survival distribution at high lifetimes one might be tempted to fit a cure model to these data. The temptation should be avoided. Instead, our recommendation is to take a hybrid approach, to obtain predictive probabilities using both a nonparametric and a parametric model, but then to weight them together. In brief, more weight can be given to the nonparametric estimates when based on hazards that can be reliably estimated, which means times t where $\mathcal{R}(t)$ is sufficiently large. As a simple example we tried using nonparametric estimates when $R(t) > 10$ and parametric otherwise. With Burr as the parametric choice, the estimated probability of fewer than 5 failures between 2024 and 2028 is 0.821 (0.801 to 0.835) which seems a reasonable solution.

4 Big and Little Data

We now turn to a more generic problem. Consider a response y that is potentially associated with two covariate vectors, x and z. The first, x, is straightforward to obtain and we have a large sample $\mathcal{B}$ of data on (y, x). The second, z, is more expensive or difficult and we have only a relatively small sample $\mathcal{L}$ of data on (y, x, z). Typically x might be demographic characteristics, treatments, phenotypes etc, whereas z might be genetic or omic information. For instance McTeer et al. [12] have an application where y is a measure of liver function, x includes age, gender, BMI and pre-existing health conditions, and z is genomic sequence data. We assume that (y, x, z) are independently drawn from a common population. Letting g denote group membership ($\mathcal{B}$ or $\mathcal{L}$), we require $f(g \mid x, z) = f(g \mid x)$, which means the decision whether or not to measure z depends only upon observed confounders x. We also require $f(y \mid x, z, g) = f(y \mid x, z)$, so that the response y can depend on x and z but not on the decision to measure z.

We are interested in $f(y \mid x, z)$, which can be estimated directly from $\mathcal{L}$, albeit unreliably when the number of observations in $\mathcal{L}$ is small. Our proposal is to add strength to estimation by making use of reliable information on $f(y \mid x)$ obtained from the large sample $\mathcal{B}$. Space restrictions mean that only an outline of the ideas, methods and results will be given here.

We start with models for $f(y \mid x, z)$ and $f(y \mid x)$, referring to the latter as the "marginal", meaning marginalised over z. We write

$$E[y \mid x, z] = \theta(x, z), \qquad E[y \mid x] = \theta(x)$$

and suppress notation on other parameters. Care needs to be taken that models for $\theta(x, z)$ and $\theta(x)$ are compatible. For example if y is binary then we cannot have logistic models with linear predictors for both $f(y \mid x, z)$ and $f(y \mid x)$ except in trivial special cases. A fully nonparametric approach might be adopted for $\theta(x)$ given that we have assumed a large amount of data is available but for $\theta(x, z)$ a flexible parametric model is likely to be preferred. Our choice is

$$\theta(x, z) = \text{expit}(D\beta)$$

where D is a design matrix made up of p B-splines in x and z. Following Eilers and Marx [13] we choose a large number of equidistant knots but then penalise roughness in the coefficients of adjacent B-splines. Hence our first estimation method, using $\mathcal{L}$ only, is to find β that maximises

$$\begin{aligned} R_1(\beta) &= \ell(\beta; y, D) + \lambda_1 \sum_{j=1}^{p} \left(\Delta^{(2)} \beta_j\right)^2 \\ &= \ell(\beta; y, D) + \lambda_1 \beta^T P^T P \beta \quad \text{say.} \end{aligned} \tag{1}$$

Here $\ell(\beta; y, D)$ is a log-likelihood or other reward function, λ_1 is a smoothing parameter, $\Delta^{(2)}\beta_j = \beta_j - 2\beta_{j-1} + \beta_{j-2}$ is a second difference measure of roughness and P is a matrix of coefficients needed to form second differences in vector/matrix form.

Now let $\hat{\theta}_{\mathcal{B}}(x)$ be an estimator of $\theta(x)$ obtained from $\mathcal{B}$. We can estimate the same thing from $\mathcal{L}$ at any x_0 using

$$\hat{\theta}_{\mathcal{L}}(x) = \sum_{i \in \mathcal{L}} k\left(\frac{x_i - x_0}{\sigma_k}\right) \hat{\theta}_{\mathcal{L}}(x_i, z_i) \Big/ \sum_{i \in \mathcal{L}} k\left(\frac{x_i - x_0}{\sigma_k}\right),$$

where $k(.)$ is a kernel function and σ_k is a smoothing parameter. For our second estimation method we propose adding an additional penalty term to (1) to encourage estimates for which $\hat{\theta}_{\mathcal{L}}(x)$ is close to $\hat{\theta}_{\mathcal{B}}(x)$. Specifically, we choose β to maximise the doubly penalised reward

$$R_2(\beta) = R_1(\beta) + \lambda_2 \left(\hat{\theta}_{\mathcal{L}}(x_{test}) - \hat{\theta}_{\mathcal{B}}(x_{test})\right)^T \left(\hat{\theta}_{\mathcal{L}}(x_{test}) - \hat{\theta}_{\mathcal{B}}(x_{test})\right), \quad (2)$$

where x_{test} is a set of user-selected values and λ_2 is a second smoothing parameter. Perperoglou and Eilers [14] have a different form of double penalty technique but much of their discussion of computational aspects applies to (2).

To close we give a brief summary of a simple simulation experiment. We initially took $n = 400$ observations (x, y) on a regular grid over $(0,1)^2$. Response y was Gaussian with mean function $\theta(x, z)$ shown in Fig. 3. Half of the observations were selected to form $\mathcal{L}$, with the remainder held back to determine prediction error. We used the true marginal mean $\theta(x)$ in the second penalty term, assuming that $\mathcal{B}$ is sufficiently large for estimation error to be negligible.

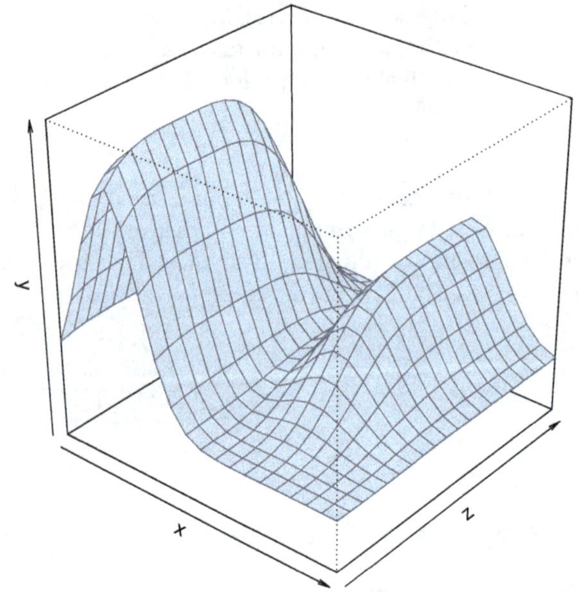

Fig. 3. Simulation $E[y \mid x, z] = \theta(x, z)$.

Figure 4 shows the true marginal mean $\theta(x)$ together with, for a typical dataset, the corresponding estimates using unsmoothed B-splines, the single smoothing method (1) and the double smoothing method (2). For the latter we have added a simultaneous confidence band [15] modified by the Copas and Eguchi double-the-variance rule [16] to bring robustness to local model misspecification. Details are omitted.

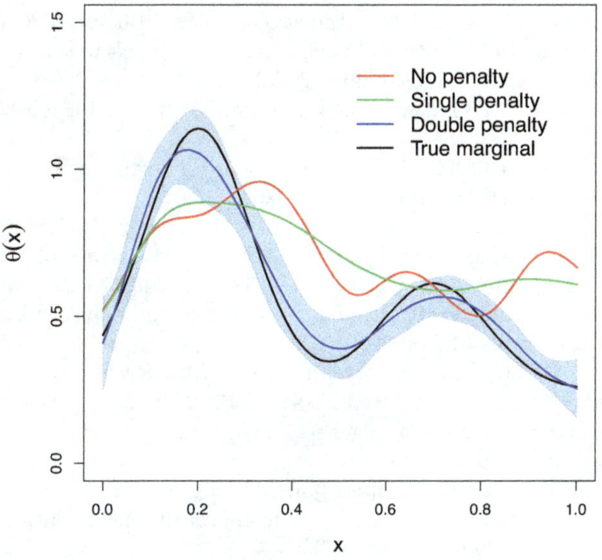

Fig. 4. Illustration of marginal estimates

Table 2 summarises the performance of the single and double smoothing methods, using mean square prediction error for the holdout sample. Results are based on 200 replicates, in 192 of which the double penalty method outperformed the single penalty technique. The new method seems to work well.

Table 2. Mean square prediction error (×100) for single and double smoothing methods

		Mean	Std. dev.	Min.	Max.
Single penalty	MSPE_1	9.4	2.8	4.2	19.6
Double penalty	MSPE_2	7.3	2.0	4.1	17.1

Acknowledgements. Thanks to Matt McTeer for discussion and collaboration on some of the material in Sect. 4.

References

1. Wu, C. F. J.: Statistics = Data Science? University of Michigan inaugural lecture (1997). https://www2.isye.gatech.edu/~jeffwu/presentations/.pdf
2. Cleveland, W.S.: Data science: an action plan for extending the technical areas of the field of statistics. Int. Stat. Rev. **69**, 21–26 (2001)
3. Donoho, D.: 50 years of data science. J. Comput. Graph. Stat. **26**, 745–766 (2017)

4. Breiman, L.: Statistical modeling: the two cultures. Stat. Sci. **16**, 199–231 (2001)
5. DHSC, Department of Health and Social Care: Handbook to the NHS Constitution for England, 1 October 2023 update (2023)
6. Boyle, A., Mason, S.: What has the 4-hour access standard achieved? Br. J. Hosp. Med. **11**, 620–622 (2014)
7. Department of Health: The NHS Plan: a plan for investment, a plan for reform. National Archives UK, reference dh_4002960 (2000)
8. Mason, S., Weber, E.J., Coster, J., Freeman, J., Locker, T.: Time patients spend in the emergency department: England's 4-hour rule - a case of hitting the target but missing the point? Ann. Emerg. Med. **59**, 341–349 (2012)
9. Schemper, M., Henderson, R.: Predictive accuracy and explained variation in Cox regression. Biometrics **56**, 249–255 (2000)
10. Harrell, F.E., Califf, R.M., Pryor, D.B., Lee, K.L., Rosati, R.A.: Evaluating the yield of medical tests. J. Am. Med. Assoc. **247**, 2543–2546 (1982)
11. Nagelkerke, N.J.D.: A note on a general definition of the coefficient of determination. Biometrika **78**, 691–692 (1991)
12. McTeer, M., Henderson R., Anstee, Q.M., Missier, P.: Handling overlapping asymmetric data sets: a twice penalized P-spline approach. Mathematics **12**, 777 (2024). https://doi.org/10.3390/math12050777
13. Eilers, P.H.C., Marx, B.D.: Flexible smoothing with B-splines and penalties. Stat. Sci. **11**, 89–121 (1996)
14. Perperoglou, A., Eilers, P.H.C.: Penalized regression with individual deviance effects. Comput. Stat. **25**, 341–361 (2010)
15. Crainiceanu, C.M., Staicu, A.-M., Ray, S., Punjabi, N.: Bootstrap based inference on the difference in the means of two correlated processes. Stat. Med. **31**, 3223–3240 (2011)
16. Copas, J.B., Eguchi, S.: Local model uncertainty and incomplete-data bias (with Discussion). J. Roy. Stat. Soc. B **67**, 459–513 (2005)

Semi-Markov Multistate Model with Interval-Censored Transition Times

Xavier Piulachs[1(✉)], Klaus Langohr[2], and Guadalupe Gómez[2]

[1] Polytechnic University of Catalonia, Campus Terrassa, 08222 Terrassa, Spain
xavier.piulachs@upc.edu
[2] Polytechnic University of Catalonia, Campus Nord, 08034 Barcelona, Spain

Abstract. A Cox-based multistate model is proposed for analyzing a multicohort event history process with interval-censored transition times. The cohort is included as a stratum variable when modeling each transition hazard, while testing the compliance with the Markov property conditional on the prognostic covariates. Whenever the Markovian assumption does not hold for a given transition, the time of entry into the current state is incorporated in the modeling procedure, yielding a semi-Markov process. To deal with interval censoring, an easy-to-implement procedure is based on performing a multiple imputation of the unknown transition times within the specified intervals. The corresponding artificially completed datasets are separately fitted using the proposed multistate model, each providing inference on the target population quantity. Finally, the overall collected information is properly combined. The described methodology is applied to a three-wave dataset of COVID-19-hospitalized adults.

Keywords: semi-Markov multistate model · interval-censored data · multiple imputation · COVID-19

1 Introduction

Within the scope of multicohort biomedical studies, interest may lie in modeling the elapsed time until the occurrence of intermediate events, for which multistate models provide a powerful tool (e.g., [1]). The transition hazards can be properly estimated under independent right censoring conditional on the covariates. We assume a stratum-cohort Cox model, addressing potential departures from the Markovian assumption by considering the time of entry into the current state. This yields a semi-Markov multistate process. There may be situations, however, where the intermediate transition times are only known to have occurred within a specified interval, resulting in interval-censored data. A common practice is to impute a single value for each unobserved transition time, but this practice leads to biased estimates and too small standard errors. This work explores alternative approaches such as multiple imputation techniques, which offer an appealing solution for correcting the lack of uncertainty when using a single

J. Einbeck et al. (Eds.): IWSM 2024, CONTRIB.STAT., pp. 255–262, 2024.
https://doi.org/10.1007/978-3-031-65723-8_39

datum. Once multiple imputation is performed, we obtain a set of time-to-event datasets, each of which is fitted using a multistate model via standard inference procedures. The population quantity of interest is finally obtained by properly combining the results of these multiple analyses.

2 Methodology

2.1 General Framework

Consider a finite set of mutually exclusive states $\mathcal{R} = \{1, \ldots, R\}$, along with the stochastic process that indicates the state occupied by the ith subject at a particular time point $t \geq 0$, $\{Y_i(t), t \geq 0\}$, $i = 1, \ldots, n$. Consider also a heterogeneous population involving $G > 1$ cohorts of subjects. The ith subject's cohort, $g = 1, \ldots, G$, is controlled by $G - 1$ indicators, $\{c_{gi},\ g \geq 2\}$, so $c_{gi} = 1$ if the subject is actually in cohort $g \in \{2, \ldots, G\}$, and $c_{gi} = 0$ otherwise. For the particular case $c_{2i} = \ldots = c_{Gi} = 0$, the subject is part of the first cohort, $g = 1$. The method of accounting for cohort information enables us to consider potential inter-cohort heterogeneity within the target population. This ultimately leads to infer cohort-specific medical conclusions.

The multistate structure can be fully described by the transition hazard between consecutive states $\{\ell, m\} \in \mathcal{R}, \ell \neq m$, defined as the ith subject's instantaneous cause-specific hazard per time unit of time, going from the state ℓ to the state m. Formally,

$$h_i^{\ell m}\{t \mid \mathbf{x}_i, \mathcal{H}_i(t), c_{gi} = 1\} = \lim_{dt \to 0} \frac{\Pr\{Y_i(t + \mathrm{d}t) = m \mid Y_i(t) = \ell;\ \mathbf{x}_i, \mathcal{H}_i(t), c_{gi} = 1\}}{\mathrm{d}t}, \tag{1}$$

where the above hazard-based measure is conditioned on: the current time t, a p-dimensional vector of baseline prognostic covariates (possibly different for each transition), $\mathbf{x}_i = (x_{1i}, \ldots, x_{pi})^\top$, and the historical information up to immediately before time t, $\mathcal{H}_i(t) = \{Y_i(u),\ 0 \leq u \leq t\}$. As another key element within the multistate modeling framework, one can define the transition probability between any pair of states, even if they are not subsequent. This is postulated as the ith subject's probability of being in state m at time t conditional on occupying the state ℓ at time s, with $s < t$, along with the subject's characteristics $\mathbf{x}_i$ and $\mathcal{H}_i(s)$:

$$P_i^{\ell m}(t \mid s, \mathbf{x}_i, \mathcal{H}_i(s), c_{gi} = 1) = \Pr\{Y_i(t) = m \mid Y_i(s) = \ell,\ \mathbf{x}_i, \mathcal{H}_i(s), c_{gi} = 1\}, \quad s < t. \tag{2}$$

Typically, the underlying multistate process is assumed to be Markovian conditional on the transition-specific covariates, so the effect of $\mathcal{H}_i(t)$ disappears, and the parameter estimation procedure is greatly simplified. However, this is not necessarily true and must be checked for each transition.

Throughout, the whole multistate process is modeled by separately fitting a Cox model for each transition hazard. Under this framework, a subject's past history can easily be considered in the $\ell \to m$ transition by including time $t_{\ell i}$ at which the current state ℓ is reached. Estimates for regression coefficients are found by maximizing the Cox partial log-likelihood function for the transition at hand, while the Breslow estimator [2] provides a nonparametric estimate for the corresponding cumulative baseline hazard function.

2.2 Semi-Markov Multistate Modeling Approach

The cohort is included as a stratum variable within each transition, thus providing flexibility to estimate transition-specific underlying risks according to the different cohorts. Additionally, the time of entry into the current state is incorporated as a fixed covariate to accommodate semi-Markov processes. This yields the following stratum-cohort Cox regression model whenever a given subject i is in the cohort g:

$$\begin{aligned} &h_i^{\ell m}(t \mid \mathbf{x}_i, t_{\ell i}, c_{gi} = 1) \\ &\qquad = h_{0g}^{\ell m}(t) \exp\left\{(\boldsymbol{\beta}^{\ell m})^\top \mathbf{x}_i + \gamma^{\ell m} t_{\ell i} + \eta_{g \times x_q}^{\ell m} x_{qi}\right\}. \end{aligned} \tag{3}$$

Here, $h_{0g}^{\ell m}(t)$ is the baseline hazard function specific to the gth cohort, $\mathbf{x}_i = (x_{1i}, \ldots, x_{pi})^\top$ is a vector of baseline covariates, $\boldsymbol{\beta}^{\ell m} = (\beta_{x_1}^{\ell m}, \ldots, \beta_{x_p}^{\ell m})^\top$ is a vector of p unknown regression coefficients corresponding to $\mathbf{x}_i$, and $\gamma^{\ell m}$ is an unknown coefficient related to $t_{\ell i}$; whenever the Markovian rule holds, $\gamma^{\ell m} = 0$. Furthermore, the interaction between the gth cohort and a particular covariate x_q, $q \in \{1, \ldots, p\}$, can be included through the term $\eta_{g \times x_q}^{\ell m}$; note that the case $g = 1$ entails $\eta_{g \times x_q}^{\ell m} = 0$. Following [3], we test the Markov property conditional on the covariates when modeling a particular $\ell \to m$ Cox-based transition hazard. This procedure involves a global test score, computed in a summarized manner from a family of local log-rank tests whose p-values are obtained via subsampling techniques. When the null hypothesis is rejected, a subject's past history can be easily considered by including the time of entry $t_{\ell i}$. A significant non-zero estimate for $\gamma^{\ell m}$ is then directly obtained.

Assuming x_q as a continuous covariate, we might be interested in assessing whether or not a common effect for x_q exists across the G cohorts. That is, our interest would focus on testing the hypothesis $\mathrm{H}_0\colon \eta_{g \times x_q}^{\ell m} = 0$ for $g = 1, \ldots, G$, which can be effectively conducted using a likelihood ratio test. A rejection of H_0 would suggest an interaction effect between the gth cohort and x_q, and the hazard ratio $\mathrm{HR}_{x_q|g}^{\ell m} = \exp\left\{\left(\beta_{x_q}^{\ell m} + \eta_{g \times x_q}^{\ell m}\right)\Delta\right\}$ would allow us to quantify differences between cohorts with respect to the effect of a Δ-unit increase in x_q.

2.3 Interval-Censored Transition Times from Intermediate States

Consider an intermediate state S through which $j = 1, \ldots, n_j \leq n$ subjects pass from state L to state U, with true transition times T_{Lj}^* and T_{Uj}^*, respectively. Additionally, suppose there are n_{obs} observed times, which include both known and right-censored times, and n_{ic} interval-censored times, so $n_j = n_{obs} + n_{ic}$; thus, the subject index j may be rewritten as $j = \{1, \ldots, n_{obs}\} \cup \{1, \ldots, n_{ic}\}$ for notational clarity. We denote by T_j^* a possibly right- and interval-censored, nonnegative random variable which provides the transition time into state S for the n_j subjects under consideration. Our primary focus is on the n_{ic} subjects providing interval-censored transition times, for which $T_j^* \in (T_{Lj}^*, T_{Uj}^*)$ with $0 \leq T_{Lj}^* < T_j^* < T_{Uj}^* < \infty$, where intervals (T_{Lj}^*, T_{Uj}^*) may randomly overlap. The Cox partial likelihood function cannot be employed under interval censoring, so alternative methods for estimating (3) are required. A possible solution is based on multiply imputing these unknown times within the specified intervals and applying a procedure $D \geq 2$ times. The process as a whole consists of the following three computational steps.

Step 1
The true transition times into the S state are assumed to have an underlying Weibull distribution [4]. That is, $T_j^* \sim \mathrm{We}\{\lambda(\mathbf{x}_j), \kappa\}$, where $\lambda(\mathbf{x}_j) > 0$ is the shape parameter conditional on the covariates, and $\kappa > 0$ is the constant scale parameter. This Weibull distribution gives rise to the log-linear regression

$$\log T_j^* = \gamma_0 + \boldsymbol{\gamma}^\top \mathbf{x}_j + \sigma\, \varepsilon_j, \tag{4}$$

where now γ_0 and σ are the location and scale parameters for the $L \to S \to U$ path, respectively, while ε_j denotes the independent stochastic errors which follow a standard Gumbel distribution, $\varepsilon_j \sim \mathrm{G}(0, 1)$. Importantly, there is a direct correspondence between (3) and (4) when the baseline hazard function of the former is Weibull distributed. Maximum likelihood estimates for $\{\gamma_0, \boldsymbol{\gamma}, \sigma\}$ can be derived from the available data using the R package `survival`, which allows us to obtain the Weibull parameters via the transformations $\lambda(\mathbf{x}_j) = \exp[-\{\gamma_0 + \boldsymbol{\gamma}^\top \mathbf{x}_j\} / \sigma]$, and $\kappa = 1/\sigma$.

Step 2
The D imputed values for each interval-censored transition time are obtained by independently drawing from the predictive Weibull distribution, confined to (T_{Lj}^*, T_{Uj}^*). This results in D datasets with either known or right-censored data. The dth artificially completed dataset, $d = 1, \ldots, D$, is then fitted using a multistate model, providing D parameter estimates on the population quantity θ to be estimated and accompanying standard errors; i.e., $\{\hat{\theta}_1, \ldots, \hat{\theta}_D\}$ and $\{\widehat{\mathrm{SE}}(\hat{\theta}_1), \ldots, \widehat{\mathrm{SE}}(\hat{\theta}_D)\}$. The R package `mstate` [5] is used to fit the transition hazards as proposed in (3). For further details on parameter estimation, the reader is referred to [6].

Step 3
The multiple sets of estimates for θ, $\{(\hat{\theta}_d, \widehat{\mathrm{SE}}(\hat{\theta}_d)),\ d = 1, \ldots, D\}$, are properly pooled to obtain a repeated-imputation inference [7]. Specifically, the average estimate for θ is

$$\hat{\theta}_{av} = \frac{1}{D} \sum_{d=1}^{D} \hat{\theta}_d, \tag{5}$$

while the combined variability is

$$\widehat{\mathrm{SE}}_{av}(\hat{\theta}) = \left\{ \frac{1}{D} \sum_{d=1}^{D} \widehat{\mathrm{SE}}^{2}(\hat{\theta}_d) + \frac{(D+1)}{D} \frac{1}{(D-1)} \sum_{d=1}^{D} (\hat{\theta}_d - \hat{\theta}_{av})^2 \right\}^{1/2}. \quad (6)$$

Interestingly, (6) has two components to assess the true uncertainty. The first component estimates the within-imputation variability as usual, while the second one accounts for the between-imputation variability, introducing the correction $(D+1)/D$ for small values of D. However, assuming a sufficiently large D, this correction becomes negligible, allowing us to construct confidence intervals for parameter θ as $\mathrm{IC}_{1-\alpha}(\theta) = \{\hat{\theta}_{av} - z_\alpha \widehat{\mathrm{SE}}_{av}(\hat{\theta}), \hat{\theta}_{av} + z_\alpha \widehat{\mathrm{SE}}_{av}(\hat{\theta})\}$, with z_α denoting the (1 - α) quantile of the standard normal distribution.

3 Three-Wave COVID-19 Data

The real data comprise $n = 3290$ COVID-19-hospitalized adults (without a ceiling of care), admitted to the hospital during the first three pandemic waves in the Barcelona metropolitan area. As a particular feature of our data, none of the individuals were lost to follow-up after hospital admission; they were all monitored until either hospital discharge or death. Figure 1 shows the unidirectional multistate model of subject flow in COVID-19 hospitalizations across the three waves, including the number of individuals in each wave. Upon hospital admission (state 0), subjects are assigned to No Severe Pneumonia, NSP (state 1) or Severe Pneumonia, SP (state 2); thus, all subjects are in one of these two states at $t = 0$. They can then pass through Recovery (state 3), Noninvasive Mechanical Ventilation, NIMV (state 4), or Invasive Mechanical Ventilation, IMV (state 5). Finally, subjects move to Discharge (state 6) or Death (state 7).

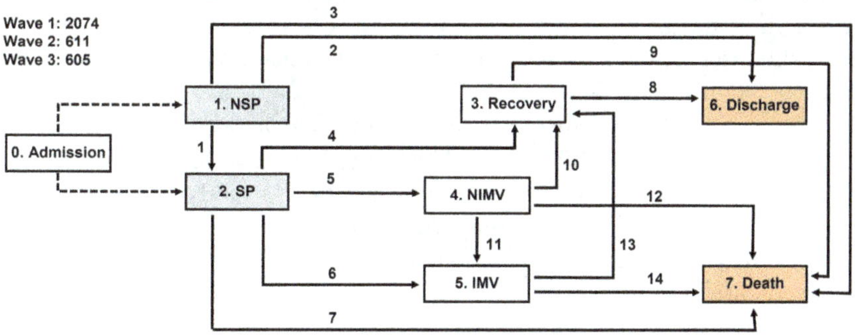

Fig. 1. The in-hospital course of COVID-19 is divided into seven states: 1. No severe pneumonia (NSP), 2. Severe pneumonia (SP), 3. Recovery, 4. Noninvasive mechanical ventilation (NIMV), 5. Invasive mechanical ventilation (IMV), 6. Discharge, and 7. Death. The model has 14 possible transitions (solid arrows) between a pair of states.

The prognostic covariates potentially included at a given transition are sex, age, and the percentage of inspired oxygen (21% at room air), along with the time of entry into the SP state for the non-Markovian transitions, i.e., SP $\rightarrow$ NIMV and SP $\rightarrow$ IMV. Moreover, since interaction terms between wave and any covariate are allowed, the quantitative prognostic covariates are centered around their means. An appealing aspect of the multistate modeling framework relies on using the hazard transition estimates to produce tailored predictions for the event history process. For example, let us consider a fictitious subject, say k, from our target population but not included in the COVID-19 dataset, known to occupy the ℓ = SP state at time $s = 0$. Our population parameter of interest is the subject-specific conditional probability of occupying at time $t > 0$ a future state m, either Discharge or Death, conditional on: the prognostic features, the time of entry into SP set to zero, and the wave, $g = 1, 2, 3$:

$$\begin{aligned}\theta(t) &\equiv P_k^{\ell m}(t \mid s = 0,\, \mathbf{x}_k,\, t_{\ell k} = 0,\, c_{gk} = 1) \\ &= \Pr\{Y_k(t) = m \mid Y_k(s = 0) = \ell,\, \mathbf{x}_k,\, t_{\ell k} = 0,\, c_{gk} = 1\}, \quad t > 0. \qquad (7)\end{aligned}$$

For illustration, we examine the evolution of two hypothetical profiles within each wave: a low-risk and a high-risk 50-year-old male, each with markedly different health forecasts. Nevertheless, some of the transition times to the S = Recovery state are interval censored, which poses a major challenge for modeling our COVID-19 data. Among subjects transitioning to the Recovery state at any time, interval censoring may be encountered in those who follow two specific paths within their global trajectories: $n_{ic1} = 9$ of the $n_{j1} = 409$ who arrive from L_1 = SP and $n_{ic2} = 150$ of the $n_{j2} = 263$ who arrive from L_2 = NIMV, with all ultimately transitioning to U = Discharge after S = Recovery. We assume a Weibull distribution for the event times within each path, $T_{j1}^* \sim \text{We}\,\{\lambda_1(\mathbf{x}_{j1}),\, \kappa_1\}$ and $T_{j2}^* \sim \text{We}\,\{\lambda_2(\mathbf{x}_{j2}),\, \kappa_2\}$, postulate the corresponding log-linear regression models, and obtain estimates for the Weibull parameters. Subsequently, we impute $D = 25$ values to replace each interval-censored observation, resulting in 25 completed datasets. The multistate model postulated in (3) is then individually fitted to each dataset. This model serves as the basis for estimating the transition hazards for low- and high-risk profiles within each wave, computing (7) at prespecified time points. Particularly, we obtain $\{\hat{\theta}_d(t = 10), \ldots, \hat{\theta}_d(t = 50)\}$ and $\{\widehat{\text{SE}}(\hat{\theta}_d(t = 10)), \ldots, \widehat{\text{SE}}(\hat{\theta}_d(t = 50))\}$, $d = 1, \ldots, 25$, for each profile and wave. These estimates are then properly averaged to derive $\{\hat{\theta}_{av}(t = 10), \ldots, \hat{\theta}_{av}(t = 50)\}$ and $\{\widehat{\text{SE}}(\hat{\theta}_{av}(t = 10)), \ldots, \widehat{\text{SE}}(\hat{\theta}_{av}(t = 50))\}$, allowing us to reconstruct the evolution of the conditional prediction probabilities in each case (Fig. 2).

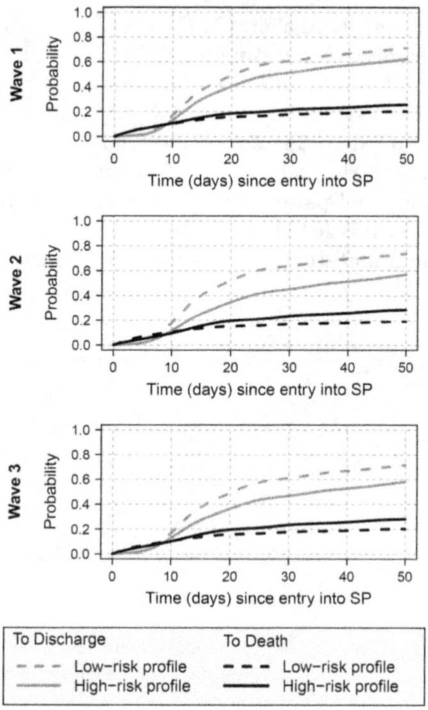

Fig. 2. Prediction probabilities for low-risk and high-risk profiles in each wave, obtained from multiply imputing the transition probabilities at $t \in \{10, 20, 30, 40, 50\}$.

4 Conclusions

The current work involves a preliminary approach to multiple imputation methods within the scope of a Cox-based multistate modeling framework. However, certain aspects would deserve further investigation. It would be advisable to analyze the performance of the method across different numbers of imputations, as well as its dependence on the specification of a particular parametric model for interval-censored transition times. Additionally, the introduction of subject-specific random effects could be considered to capture unobserved features.

References

1. Cook, R.J., Lawless, J.F.: Multistate Models for the Analysis of Life History Data. Chapman & Hall/CRC, Boca Raton (2018)
2. Breslow, N.E.: Contribution to the Discussion of the paper by D. R. Cox. J. Roy. Stat. Soc. Ser. B **34**, 216–217 (1972)
3. Titman, A.C., Putter, H.: General tests of the Markov property in multi-state models. Biostatistics **23**, 380–396 (2022)

4. Alarcón-Soto, Y., Langohr, K., Fehér, C., García, F., Gómez, G.: Multiple imputation approach for interval-censored time to HIV RNA viral rebound within a mixed effects Cox model. Biom. J. **61**, 299–318 (2019)
5. Putter, H., Fiocco, M., Geskus, R.B.: Tutorial in biostatistics: competing risks and multi-state models. Stat. Med. **26**, 2389–2430 (2007)
6. de Wreede, L.C., Fiocco, M., Putter, H.: The mstate package for estimation and prediction in non- and semi-parametric multi-state and competing risks models. Comp. Meth. Prog. Bio. **99**, 261–274 (2010)
7. Rubin, D.B.: Multiple Imputation for Nonresponse in Surveys. John Wiley & Sons, Hoboken (2004)

A Distance-Based Statistic for Goodness-of-Fit Assessment

Darshana Jayakumari[1(✉)], Jochen Einbeck[2], John Hinde[3], and Rafael A. Moral[1]

[1] Maynooth University, Maynooth, Ireland
darshana.jayakumari.2021@mumail.ie
[2] Durham University, Durham, UK
[3] University of Galway, Galway, Ireland

Abstract. The modelling of count data in real world scenarios often requires models that address over-dispersion. Within the generalized linear modeling framework, various over-dispersion models are available as extensions of the basic Poisson model. Graphical assessment of goodness-of-fit commonly involves half-normal plots, for which a simulated envelope can be added to aid interpretation. The simulated envelope is such that, under a well-fitted model, the majority of points should fall within its bounds. Nonetheless, closely related models tend to produce very similar graphs. Here, we propose an objective statistic based on half-normal plots with a simulated envelope to aid goodness-of-fit assessment.

Keywords: Count data · Half-normal plot · Model selection

1 Introduction

In ecological studies it is very prevalent to find count data of many types. For example, counts of animals (abundance) can be used to study habitat preference; fertility (number of eggs of a pest insect) can be used to investigate the effectiveness of an organic insecticide; number of fish captured at different ages can be used to study the migratory patterns of fish stock [4]. The basic model that can mathematically capture the varying patterns in count data is the Poisson model. But in real world scenarios the inability of the Poisson model to handle over -dispersion (or under -dispersion) makes it unsuitable for many cases. Many one-parameter extensions of the Poisson model have been proposed in the literature which can handle over- or under-dispersion. These include the negative binomial (with a linear or quadratic variance function, hereafter referred to as NB-lin and NB-quad, respectively) [2], the quasi-Poisson, Conway-Maxwell Poisson, generalized Poisson, among other models. Another common feature of count datasets is an inflated number of zeros when compared to the frequency of zeros expected by a Poisson model. This can be accommodated by zero-inflated (ZI) extensions of the Poisson, such as the ZI Poisson (ZIP) and ZI negative binomial (ZINB) [7].

J. Einbeck et al. (Eds.): IWSM 2024, CONTRIB.STAT., pp. 263–268, 2024.
https://doi.org/10.1007/978-3-031-65723-8_40

One important discerning feature of the many proposed extensions to the Poisson model, is the resulting variance function, which may accommodate over- or under-dispersion in different ways. After fitting a model, the next step is to employ a relevant diagnostic test to assess model fit, typically involving a model diagnostic, such as residuals of different types. Graphical methods give a comprehensive overview of the pattern of residuals and an insight into the variability in the data [3]. The half-normal plot is a class of residual plots that plots the absolute value of the model statistics against the expected order statistics of a half-normal distribution [5]. The expected order statistics of the half normal distribution can be approximated as:

$$\Phi^{-1}\left(\frac{i+n-\frac{1}{8}}{2n+\frac{1}{2}}\right) \tag{1}$$

where $\Phi^{-1}(\cdot)$ is the inverse of the Gaussian cumulative distribution function, i is the $i-$th order statistic, $1 \leq i \leq n$, and n is the sample size. The application of half normal plots to use as a model selection method commenced with the usage of guardrails and later it was recommended to use simulated envelopes as a better technique [1].

The simulated envelope is constructed by (i) simulating 99 or more response variables using the same distribution, design matrix, and fitted coefficients; (ii) re-fitting the same model to each simulated sample; (iii) calculating the same type of residuals, in absolute value and in order; and (iv) computing desired percentiles for each order statistics (usually 2.5% and 97.5%). The median is also computed, and shown as a dashed line in the plot.

Although they are a useful tool to identify whether the observed data is a plausible realisation of a fitted model, they may bring forth the error of subjective bias when similar model fits are being compared. In this work, we developed a statistic to be used as a complement for half-normal plots with a simulated envelope to mitigate this inefficiency. The method is expected to clearly distinguish between similar models and also be able to compare true and quasi-likelihood based models, for which widely accepted information criteria (such as AIC or BIC) cannot be calculated.

2 Material and Methods

2.1 Proposed Distance Metric

We developed a metric based on distances of the residual points from the median of the envelope $\mathcal{E}_i = \{x \in \mathcal{R} | x \in (l_i, u_i)\}$, where u_i and l_i are the upper and lower bounds. The metric is given by:

$$d = \sum_{i=1}^{n} d_i = \sum_{i=1}^{n} |r_i - m_i|^p$$

where r_i is the $i-$th ordered residual, m_i is the the median of the envelope corresponding to the $i-$th ordered residual, n is the sample size and p is the distance norm considered (i.e. $p = 1$ corresponds to the L_1 norm, and $p = 2$ to squared Euclidean distance).

2.2 Simulation Studies and Application to Real Data

We carried out an extensive simulation study where 1000 simulated samples were generated from the Poisson model and a number of Poisson extensions, namely the NB-lin, NB-quad, ZIP, and ZINB. This was done for three sample sizes (20, 50, and 100) and the distance statistic was computed using the two distance norms. We also present two case studies as applications of the proposed distance metric. The first dataset considered was obtained from the R package `mvabund` [6], and included the abundance of hunting spiders from the species *Alopecosa accentuata* that were caught in 100 pitfall traps (1m radius) over a period of 60 weeks as the response variable, and the soil dry mass as a covariate of interest. The covariate was $\log(x + 1)$ transformed prior to model fitting. We fitted Poisson, quasi-Poisson, NB-lin, NB-quad, ZIP, and ZINB models. The half normal plots corresponding to the fitted models were constructed 100 times and the median estimate of the distance metric was used to compare the model fits.

The second dataset explores the effect of six sugars at five different doses on the induction of somatic embryos from callus cultures in a tissue culture experiment [5]. The experiment was doing using the orange variety named Caipira. The whole experimental setup consisted of a randomised block design with five blocks and six sugars (maltose, glucose, galactose, lactose, sucrose and glycerol) at five dose levels. The following linear predictor was used in modelling:

$$\log(\mu_{ijk}) = \beta_0 + b_j + \beta_{1k} d_i + \beta_{2k} d_i^2,$$

where β_0 denotes the intercept, b_j is the effect of the j−th block, $j = 1, \ldots, 5$, d_i is the i−th dose, $i = 1, \ldots, 5$ and β_{1k} and β_{2k} are the linear and quadratic dose effects for the k−th sugar, $k = 1, \ldots, 6$.

We fitted the same models as used in first example. The half normal plots corresponding to the fitted models and the distance metric were computed to compare the model fits.

3 Results and Discussion

3.1 Simulation Studies

We explore one scenario from the simulation study when the parent model is the negative binomial model with a linear variance function (NB-lin) and the dispersion parameter value is equal to 7, which could be considered as strong over-dispersion. A well-fitted model is expected to have a minimum value for the distance metric and in this case the results showed that the NB-lin and quasi-Poisson models gave the minimum value for all the sample sizes considered. The similar performance of the quasi-Poisson model is expected as both models have a linear variance function. Another result which takes into account the number of times the distance metric has been computed be minimum in a single simulation run shows that L_1 norm realises the parent model and squared Euclidean distance model shows a mixture of the Quasi Poisson and NB-lin for all the sample sizes. After comparing the distance metric with the BIC, where available, the distance metric has shown to perform in line with the BIC values, or sometimes better in small samples.

3.2 Case Studies

For the spider dataset the calculated distance metric for the two distance norms for the various fitted models, and the associated BIC values for comparison, are presented in Table 1.

Table 1. Median distance metric obtained from 100 half-normal plots generated for six different models fitted to the spider data, with two values of p, and associated BIC values

Model	$p = 1$	$p = 2$	BIC
Poisson	34.66	91.62	246.18
Quasi-Poisson	2.69	0.69	–
NB-lin	2.19	0.34	141.83
NB-quad	2.97	1.14	148.82
ZIP	13.22	14.26	194.09
ZINB	1.29	0.46	147.11

The potential subjective bias in selecting the best model motivates the need to have an additional quantitative metric and in this case the squared Euclidean distance norm of the distance metric prefers NB-lin and is in line with the BIC values. The L_1 norm of the distance metric prefers ZINB and this is expected as the estimate of zero-inflation parameter is 2.75×10^{-5} which is equivalent to zero, or no zero-inflation present.

For the orange tissue culture dataset the calculated distance metric for the two distance norms for the various fitted models, and the associated BIC values, are presented in Table 2. The half normal plots corresponding to the fitted models shown in Fig. 1 that there is a subjective bias in finding the best model among the considered models. As a next step we calculated the proposed distance metric associated with the fitted models. The distance metric values are given in Table 2. It is clearly evident that NB-lin is the better performing model as it has a linear variance function, and this is in line with BIC values. A closely related model to the NB-lin would be the Quasi-Poisson. The distance metric gives a clear comparison between the models that have full likelihood and quasi-likelihood as opposed to the BIC.

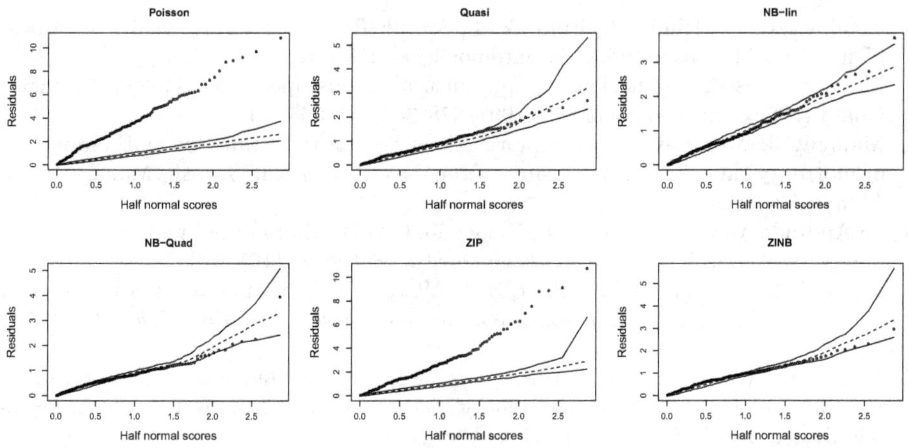

Fig. 1. Half-normal plots with a simulated envelope for fitted models for orange data

Table 2. Distance metric computed from half-normal plots generated for six different models fitted to the orange data, with varying values of p, and associated BIC values

Model	$p = 1$	$p = 2$	BIC
Poisson	346.67	1207.65	3053.53
Quasi-Poisson	14.63	2.16	–
NB-lin	6.88	0.58	1382.47
NB-quad	8.88	1.54	1397.53
ZIP	228.23	646.6	2728.29
ZINB	11.05	1.68	1438.8

4 Future Directions

The future directions of this work will include expanding the simulation framework to explore mis-specified link functions and covariates. Other possibilities would be to extend the approach to mixed models and to explore the use of different forms of residuals and other diagnostics, such as Cook's distances.

Acknowledgments. Special Thanks for the financial support of Science Foundation Ireland under Grant number 18/CRT/6049 for funding this project.

References

1. Atkinson, A.C.: Plots, Transformations and Regression; An Introduction to Graphical Methods of Diagnostic Regression Analysis, p. 282. Clarendon Press, Oxford (1985)
2. Hilbe, J.M.: Modeling Count Data. Cambridge University Press, Cambridge (2014)

3. Jayakumari, D., Hinde, J., Einbeck, J., Moral, R.A.: Tools for assessing goodness of fit of GLMs: case studies in entomology. In: Moral, A.R., Godoy, W.A. (eds.) Modelling Insect Populations in Agricultural Landscapes, pp. 211–235. Springer, Cham (2023). https://doi.org/10.1007/978-3-031-43098-5_11
4. Mainguy, J., Moral, R.D.A.: An improved method for the estimation and comparison of mortality rates in fish from catch-curve data. North Am. J. Fish. Manag. **41**(5), 1436–1453 (2021)
5. de Andrade Moral, R., Hinde, J., Demétrio, C.G.B.: Half-normal plots and overdispersed models in R: the hnp package. J. Stat. Softw. **81**(10) (2017)
6. Wang, Y.I., Naumann, U., Wright, S.T., Warton, D.I.: mvabund–an R package for model-based analysis of multivariate abundance data. Meth. Ecol. Evol. **3**(3), 471–474 (2012)
7. Yau, K.K., Wang, K., Lee, A.H.: Zero-inflated negative binomial mixed regression modeling of over-dispersed count data with extra zeros. Biometr. J. J. Math. Methods Biosci. **45**(4), 437–452 (2003)

Author Index

J. Einbeck et al. (Eds.): IWSM 2024, CONTRIB.STAT., pp. 269–270, 2024.
https://doi.org/10.1007/978-3-031-65723-8

Printed in the USA
CPSIA information can be obtained
at www.ICGtesting.com
CBHW051523280724
12322CB00003B/82

9 783031 657221